T0259999

"An exciting innovative new addition to the occupational therapy sensory integration literature. Theoretically sound practical case-based application to intervention. A must for the practicing pediatric occupational therapist."

— **Sharon A. Cermak, EdD, OTR/L, FAOTA**, *professor of Occupational Science and Occupational Therapy, University of Southern California*

"This book will appeal to pediatric therapists seeking to enhance their clinical reasoning for the treatment of children with complex sensory conditions including neuromotor that restrict participation and diminish quality of life. The reader is taken on a journey that begins with an inviting overview of the holistic and integrated intent of the book and proceeds to a clearly articulated model of clinical reasoning. Throughout the journey, the model is applied to a broad spectrum of sensorimotor diagnoses establishing the importance of using a holistic and integrated approach to treatment planning and intervention. The journey culminates with a presentation of community-based programs designed to enhance participation and improve quality of life for children who navigate these multifaceted sensory and neuromotor challenges daily."

— **Gay L. Girolami, PT, PhD, c/NDT**, *clinical professor, Department of Physical Therapy, University of Illinois in Chicago (UIC)*

"I love that this book describes clear pathways for providing meaningful, evidence-based practice, without over-simplifying the complexity and importance of clinical reasoning in occupational therapy. As a clinical director, it is a useful resource for mentoring employees who are newly entering practice or changing their area of practice."

— **Cheryl L. Ecker, MA, OTR/L, BCP, SWC**, *clinical director, Therapy in Action; co-author,* Sensory Processing Measure, Sensory Processing Measure-Preschool, and Sensory Processing Measure-2, SPM-2 Quick Tips Infant-Toddler (User Guide)

"For ten years I have been waiting for this new book – exactly since the moment I learned that its predecessor wouldn't be updated. I loved the book about combining SI with NDT that helped me as a young clinician develop my skills in combining SI with strategies from other approaches. The new book still maintains the focus on combining approaches and practical relevance. It is a treasure chest drawing on the expertise of a plethora of master clinicians and scholars, mainly from the field of Occupational Therapy. Its richness addresses the fact that we see much more complex cases in our clinics today. A single approach usually cannot fulfill these children's and families' needs. I highly recommend this book to the OT and other health professionals who have specialized in one method and are interested in educating themselves about other approaches. This book provides clinicians with guidance on how to combine approaches with inspiration for providing the best individualized interventions we can. As I have learned from my friend and mentor, Erna, and her mantra for therapists, 'Be clear in your head and eclectic with your hands,' which is a principle reflected in this book about combining intervention approaches. It allows us to provide the best therapy for each individual child."

— **Elisabeth Soechting, MA, OTR,** *owner of SpielStudio and SI-SeminarInstitut; president of Austrian SI Organization GSIÖ e.V.*

"Absolutely recommended. This is a clear and concise textbook that responds to what, why, and when to apply a combination of approaches used by occupational therapists and other health professionals in childhood. Based on evidence and clinical reasoning this work guides you to achieve the best intervention results."

— **Sara Jorquera, PhD, TO**, *director Centro de Atención Temprana y Desarrollo Infantil AYTONA, Madrid, Spain*

"This book meets the needs of students and professionals updating knowledge for evidence based clinical practice in Sensory Integration and other intervention models used with children with different pathologies. This book describes the importance of context and how to facilitate the creation of transformative environments so that sensations are integrated at different levels, from intrinsic motivation to the therapist's behaviors while facilitating active participation in occupations. Children teach us a different world; this book teaches us to improve that world."

— **Marcos Chiang, TO,** *máster en Integración de Personas con Discapacidad, director, Crecimiento y Desarrollo, adjunct professor Universidad Autónoma de Chile y Universidad Santo Tomás*

An Evidence-Based Guide to Combining Interventions with Sensory Integration in Pediatric Practice

This book offers practical ideas on the combination of sensory integration theory principles with other evidence-based approaches in the evaluation and treatment of multifaceted issues in children with disabilities.

Using the ICF Model, a Clinical Reasoning Model, and featuring numerous case studies, the opening chapters focus on the evidence for combining intervention approaches for diagnoses most often encountered in clinical practice. The latter half of the book covers the delivery of services using blended intervention approaches in different settings, such as the school, the hospital, and in nature. Featured are existing community programs illustrating the combination of approaches in practice. Appendices include reproducible resources, a guide to assessments, and approaches.

The text will guide occupational therapists and other health professionals working with children and adolescents across a variety of settings in using clinical reasoning skills in a systematic manner that will lead to better interventions.

Erna Imperatore Blanche, PhD, OTR/L, FAOTA, faculty in the Division of Occupational Science and Occupational Therapy at the University of Southern California and co-director, Therapy West, Inc. She is an international expert in sensory integration theory and interventions.

Clare Giuffrida, PhD, OTR/L, FAOTA, adjunct faculty, Rush University, is recognized internationally for her scholarship and research linking sensory processing with motor learning.

Mary Hallway, BS, OTR/L, SWC, C/NDT, advanced NDTA-OT instructor, is an internationally recognized educator, consultant, and clinician with expertise in neurodevelopmental treatment and sensory processing/integration.

Bryant Edwards, OTD, MA, OTR/L, BCP, MPH, is Director of Clinical Services – Rehabilitation and Professional Specialties at Children's Hospital Los Angeles. He is an expert in applying principles of sensory integration theory in hospital and community settings.

Lisa A. Test, OTD, OTR/L, FAOTA, is Coordinating Therapist for OT and PT Program, Los Angeles Unified School District with expertise in applying principles of sensory integration theory in different school contexts and community settings.

An Evidence-Based Guide to Combining Interventions with Sensory Integration in Pediatric Practice

Edited by Erna Imperatore Blanche, Clare Giuffrida, Mary Hallway, Bryant Edwards, and Lisa A. Test

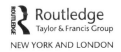

NEW YORK AND LONDON

First published 2022
by Routledge
605 Third Avenue, New York, NY 10158

and by Routledge
2 Park Square, Milton Park, Abingdon, Oxon, OX14 4RN

Routledge is an imprint of the Taylor & Francis Group, an informa business

Library of Congress Cataloging-in-Publication Data
Names: Blanche, Erna I., editor.
Title: An evidence-based guide to combining interventions with sensory integration in pediatric practice / Erna Imperatore Blanche, Clare Giuffrida, Mary Hallway, Lisa A. Test, Bryant Edwards.
Description: New York : Routledge, 2021. | Includes bibliographical references and index.
Identifiers: LCCN 2021017561 (print) | LCCN 2021017562 (ebook) | ISBN 9780367506902 (hardback) | ISBN 9780367506889 (paperback) | ISBN 9781003050810 (ebook)
Subjects: LCSH: Movement disorders in children—Treatment. | Sensorimotor integration.
Classification: LCC RJ496.M68 E95 2021 (print) | LCC RJ496.M68 (ebook) | DDC 618.92/83—dc23
LC record available at https://lccn.loc.gov/2021017561
LC ebook record available at https://lccn.loc.gov/2021017562

ISBN: 978-0-367-50690-2 (hbk)
ISBN: 978-0-367-50688-9 (pbk)
ISBN: 978-1-003-05081-0 (ebk)

DOI: 10.4324/9781003050810

Typeset in NewBaskerville
by Apex CoVantage, LLC

This book is dedicated to our teachers: the children and their families, our colleagues and mentors who have guided us, and our students who have consistently challenged us in our practice. Finally, we dedicate and give profound thanks to our families, friends, and colleagues who have supported us through the process.

Contents

Contributors

M. Angelica Barraza, BS, OTR/L, C/NDT, Co-founder and Director of Clinical Services, Kidnectivity, Chicago, Illinois

Kim Barthel, BMR, OTR, Advanced NDTA-OT Instructor; President, Relationship Matters Consultancy Inc., Victoria, British Columbia, Canada

Erna Imperatore Blanche, PhD, OTR/L, FAOTA, Clinical Professor of Occupational Therapy, Chan Division of Occupational Science and Occupational Therapy, University of Southern California; Director of Research and Program Development, Therapy West, Inc., Los Angeles, California

Stefanie C. Bodison, OTD, OTR/L, Assistant Professor of Research, joint appointment in the Keck School of Medicine, Pediatrics and Chan Division of Occupational Science and Occupational Therapy, University of Southern California, Los Angeles, California

Leah Dunleavy, MA, BCBA, OTR/L, OTD, Clinic Director, Eyas Landing, Chicago, Illinois

Bryant Edwards, OTD, MA, OTR/L, BCP, MPH, Director, Clinical Services – Rehabilitation and Professional Specialties, Children's Hospital Los Angeles, Los Angeles, California

Joanne Flanagan, ScD, OTR/L, Associate Professor, Dr. Pallavi Patel College of Health Care Sciences, Department of Occupational Therapy Tampa, Nova Southeastern University (NSU), Florida

Clare Giuffrida, PhD, MS, OTR/L, C/NDT, FAOTA, Adjunct Clinical Assistant Professor, Department of Physical Medicine and Rehabilitation, Rush College of Medicine, Rush University Chicago, Illinois; Early Intervention Specialist, Occupational Therapist, Chicago, Illinois

Alexa Greif, OTD, MS, OTR/L, Head of Program Development, Blue Bird Day, LLC, Chicago, Illinois

Kimberly Grenawitzke, OTD, OTR/L, SCFES, IBCLC, CNT, Occupational Therapist II, Lucile Packard Children's Hospital at Stanford Children's Health, Palo Alto, California

Janet S. Gunter, OTD, OTR/L, Director of Clinical Services, Therapy West, Inc., Clinical Assistant Professor of Occupational Therapy, Chan Division of Occupational Science and Occupational Therapy, University of Southern California, Los Angeles, California

Mary Hallway, BS, OTR/L, SWC, C/NDT, Advanced NDTA-OT Instructor, President, The Hallway Group, Inc., Newport Beach, California

Erin Harvey, OTD, OTR/L, Clinic Director—North Center, Blue Bird Day, LLC, Chicago, Illinois

Sarah Hirschman, MOT, OTR/L, Clinic Director—West Loop, Blue Bird Day, LLC, Chicago, Illinois

Karrie L. Kingsley, OTD, OTR/L, Associate Professor, University of Southern California, Los Angeles, California

Laura Kula OTD, MS, OTR/L, Occupational Therapist, Shirley Ryan Ability Lab, Glenview, Illinois, Occupational Therapist, Round Tree School District #116, Chicago, Illinois

Eirini V. Liapi, PT, MSc, c/PhD, Lecturer of Occupational and Physical Therapy Department, Metropolitan College of Thessaloniki in Collaboration Queen Margaret University, Thessaloniki, Greece

Sophia Magaña, OTD, OTR/L, Clinical Supervisor, Coordinator of Early Intervention Group Programs, Therapy West, Inc, Los Angeles, California; supervisor, rehabilitation services, Stanford Children's Health, Palo Alto, California

Laura Mraz, OTD, OTR/L, Executive Director, Blue Bird Day, LLC; Occupational Therapist, Blue Bird Day & Eyas Landing, Chicago, Illinois

Bonnie Nakasuji, OTD, OTR/L, FAOTA, Co-founder and Director of Administration, Fieldwork Coordinator, Therapy West Inc, Los Angeles, California

Michele Parkins, MS, OTR, STAR Institute Faculty, Founder and Director, Great Kids Place Rockaway, New Jersey

Gustavo Reinoso, PhD, OTR/L, Associate Professor, Nova Southeastern University, Tampa, Florida

Lisa R. Reyes, MSCS, MS, OTR/L, Occupational Therapy Consultant, Chicago, Illinois

Anna Sampsonidis M.A., OTR, Program Leader, Occupational Therapy Department, Metropolitan College of Thessaloniki in Collaboration

Queen Margaret University; director of practice, Syn-Ergasia, Therapeutic Intervention Ltd.; director, The Hellenic Scientific Association for Sensory Integration, Thessaloniki, Greece

Sarah A. Schoen, PhD, OTR, Director of Research; STAR Institute for Sensory Processing, Centennial, Colorado

Takako Shiratori, PhD, DPT, PT, Physical Therapist, The Polyclinic, Seattle, Washington

Virginia Spielman, PhD, MSOT, Executive Director, STAR Institute for Sensory Processing, Centennial, Colorado

Shelby Surfas, OTD, OTR/L, Associate Professor of Clinical Occupational Therapy, Program Area Lead and Director of Occupational Therapy, USC University Center for Excellence in Developmental Disabilities, Children's Hospital Los Angeles, Los Angeles, California

Joan Surfus, OTD, OTR/L, SWC, Adjunct Assistant Clinical Professor of Occupational Therapy, Chan Division of Occupational Science and Occupational Therapy, University of Southern California, Los Angeles, CA, Clinical Coordinator of Occupational Therapy, Pediatric Therapy Network, Torrance, California

Lisa A. Test, OTD, OTR/L, FAOTA, Coordinating Therapist Occupational Therapy and Physical Therapy Program, Los Angeles Unified School District, Los Angeles, California

Artwork

Gary Roland Hill
Los Angeles, California

Reviewers

Teresa May-Benson ScD, OTR/L, FAOTA, President, TMB Educational Services, Philadelphia, Pennsylvania

Elizabeth Carley, OTD, OTR/L, Program Coordinator and Mental Health Consultant Northwest Center Kids IMPACT, Seattle, Washington

Thomas Decker, OTD, OTR/L, Associate Professor, Department of Occupational Therapy Nova Southeastern University, Tampa, Florida

Cara Gelfand, MEd, Early Childhood Special Education, Los Angeles Unified School District, Los Angeles, California

Janet S. Gunter, OTD, OTR/L, Director of Clinical Services, Therapy West, Inc., Clinical Assistant Professor of Occupational Therapy, Chan Division of Occupational Science and Occupational Therapy, University of Southern California, Los Angeles, California

Denise Hogrefe, MA, OTR/L, Clinical Advising Therapist, Los Angeles Unified School District, Los Angeles, California

Elise Holloway MPH, OTR/L, SWC, IBCLC, NTMTC, Occupational Therapy Clinical Specialist, Maternal-Child Services, Huntington Hospital, Pasadena, California; occupational therapy consultant Early Start Program, Eastern Los Angeles Regional Center, Alhambra, California

Dominique Blanche Kiefer, OTD, OTR/L, Director of Administration Therapy West, Inc., Los Angeles, California, Occupational Therapist, Lake Highland Preparatory School, Orlando, Florida

James Koontz, EdD, Coordinator, Moderate Severe and LRE Programs, Los Angeles Unified School District, Los Angeles, California

Amy Lynch, PhD, TBRI® Educator, SCFES, OTR/L, Associate Professor, Program in Occupational Therapy, Department of Health and Rehabilitation Sciences, Temple University, Philadelphia, Pennsylvania

Kary Rappaport, OTR/L, MS, SCFES, IBCLC, Co-owner, Feeders & Growers, Portland, Oregon

Gustavo Reinoso, PhD, OTR/L, Associate Professor, Nova Southeastern University, Tampa, Florida

Aneeta Sagar, MA, OTR/L, Director, Kinder Center, Los Angeles, California

Nora Chun-Uba MS, OTR/L, Assistant Director Rehabilitation Services, UCSF Medical Center/ Benioff Children's Hospital, San Francisco, California

Preface

This book began with a passion for sensory integration theory and its application to treatment as taught by A. J. Ayres. Therefore, authors and editors were recruited to augment a variety of clinical expertise in the application of theoretical content. By knowing Dr. Ayres and learning from her example, we understood that sensory integration was not the only way to address the problems we encountered in practice. The need to provide interventions that most closely align with the needs of children and families and the complexity of clinical practice requires a combination of clinical approaches and attention to research. Sensory integration is a fundamental approach to meeting the needs of many children, but the needs of many children are beyond the scope of only using a sensory integration approach.

Dr. Ayres understood the importance of a child's engagement with others and with environmental challenges that she called "just the right challenge." The principles of her approach are central to the themes developed throughout this book. Sensory integration principles remain at the center of what we do and how we consider the child's mental and physical health in the environment. By blending treatment approaches, we move from a singular approach to a methodology that considers other interventions that together provide the best fit for fostering children's self-determination.

Beyond a doubt, practice has changed immeasurably during the last 30 years. There is a need to be faster, more systematic in data gathering, and more efficacious in measuring interventions' outcomes. Answering those needs requires the clinician to be creative in blending intervention approaches in a systematic manner guided by current evidence.

We offer a model to systematize both the data gathering process and the hypotheses derived from them. What follows are examples of different populations, their challenges, and the evidence for best practices throughout the evaluation and treatment process. The book includes exemplars of several contexts where sensory integration treatment is combined with other approaches. It ends with an overview of community programs that blend interventions to be more impactful in their deliveries. The authors of these chapters are professionals who have rich experiences, crossing boundaries between education, research, and practice. This book is our testimony to the openness of Dr. Ayres' thinking and to her implementation of the science and art of therapy.

Part 1

Foundations for Clinical Reasoning

1 The Pieces of the Whole

Erna Imperatore Blanche and Clare Giuffrida

Sarah, a newly hired occupational therapist working in a community setting, receives a referral for Luke, a 2-year-old boy who is developmentally delayed and shows signs of autism. Luke lives with his mother and 14-year-old sister in subsidized housing. His mother works the early shift at a local grocery store and leaves the house before the children are up so that in the early afternoon she can come home, prepare a meal for her children, and go to a second part time job at a local restaurant. The mother relies on her daughter to put Luke to bed, and to get him up in the morning to take him to his daycare before she goes to school. The daycare staff referred Luke to a state agency because he is delayed in his motor skills, is clumsy, and does not interact well with the other children. Sarah does not quite know where to start. She questions whether Luke has signs of autism spectrum disorder (ASD) and/or a coordination problem or is just tired and hungry. She wonders whether, because the family is stressed, Luke does not receive sufficient care and support at home.

Facing multifaceted cases, such as the foregoing example, is a common dilemma encountered by health care workers in the present health care environment. With increasing complexity of service delivery, several aspects need to be considered: the needs of the child and family, the socioeconomic status affecting available funding for intervention, and the research evidence available to support the use of the specific interventions chosen to ameliorate the child's problems. Furthermore, when assessing the child and the family needs, the practitioner must consider the relationships among the diagnosis, the functional limitations, and the child's participation in home, school, and community.

This book is written for pediatric clinicians with intermediate levels of experience treating clients where there are multiple factors to consider. The primary focus is on the application of the Reasoning in Action Model (RAM, Chapter 2) to a variety of diagnoses. The model incorporates the challenges of service delivery, family and child goals, and participation issues. The book also focuses on the sensory integration approach, one of the most fundamental interventions in pediatrics, and its combination with other approaches using evidence-based clinical practice and applicable research findings. Informing each chapter is

DOI: 10.4324/9781003050810-2

terminology associated with the International Classification of Function, Disability and Health: Children and Youth version (ICF-CY), an inclusive international framework useful in characterizing pediatric health conditions across many dimensions and in various contexts. The ICF-CY is used to classify the function and health of the developing child, and to describe the impact of context on some of the most common pediatric health conditions (World Health Organization, 2007) as presented herein and as seen by therapists.

The choices of relevant intervention models depend upon how and to what degree the child's health condition has impacted functioning at home, in school, and in the community. For example, a practitioner cannot choose to utilize sensory integration as traditionally described when addressing the needs of a child with cerebral palsy. Alternatively, a practitioner cannot focus solely on sensory processing when intervening with a child with ASD. In the case of a child with cerebral palsy, the child's fine and gross motor difficulties require the inclusion of neuromotor approaches. Possible intervention strategies could include sensory strategies developed within a sensory integration approach and positioning strategies developed within a biomechanical approach. In the case of a child with ASD, it is likely the clinician will also need to include behavioral strategies thus incorporating a behavioral approach within the intervention plan. These strategies need to optimize participation of the child in the family's daily living context; therefore, the positioning devices, and behavioral and sensory strategies, respectively, need to be practical for parent/guardian implementation. Furthermore,

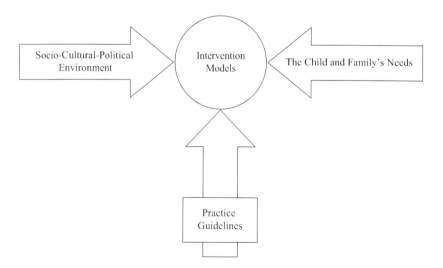

Figure 1.1 Multiple Influences on Daily Clinical Practice

practitioners' intervention schedule will be dictated by the health care delivery or educational system in which they practice. For example, to promote self-determination, the school practitioner would collaborate with the student and the educational team to ensure that appropriate supports are embedded throughout the school routine, including recess and lunch time. A practitioner in an outpatient facility might provide direct intervention to a child once or twice a week, while supplementing it with a therapeutic program for the family to incorporate at home. In summary, the complexity of current practice requires threading together multiple pieces to provide the most comprehensive interventions using the most relevant and available options (See Figure 1.1).

The Pieces of the Whole

Sensory integration treatment (SIT) is one of the most utilized evidence-based approaches in pediatric practice (Monez et al., 2019) and the most commonly researched individualized (and singular) intervention. However, current literature supports the use of multiple frames of reference in daily treatment planning, either theoretically (Reynolds et al., 2017), through research that combines sensory integration with other approaches (Blanche et al., 2016; Schoen et al., 2018), or through the combination of multiple approaches in the conceptualization of randomized intervention studies with a variety of populations (Prizant et al., 2003; Rogers et al., 2012). Combining different approaches with sensory integration principles also requires consideration of the socioeconomic environment dictating practice, the family's needs, and the best available evidence.

Socioeconomic Environment and Funding

We navigate a range of different political systems and an ever-changing global environment, as highlighted by the occurrence of the unprecedented, international pandemic, COVID-19 in 2020. The pandemic drastically impacted health care and the global economy. Such pivotal events influence everyday life, which dictate and dominate not only health care delivery models, but the ability of people in various socioeconomic brackets to readily access them. In the case of COVID-19, many settings transitioned from traditional health care, where therapists provided direct face-to-face services, to telehealth when it was possible and appropriate.

Other and more traditional shifts prompting changes in health care have included ongoing changes in funding priorities and an ongoing need for research evidence to guide clinical practice. However, the overarching issue has been specific to several international initiatives highlighted by the World Health Organization's (WHO) introduction of the ICF (2001) and the ICF-CY (2007), two international frameworks designed to guide health care practice and research for adults and children while accounting for all aspects of function across various contexts.

International Trends

In the last 30 years of health care, two major models of disablement emerged to guide clinical practice: the medical model and the social model. For many years the medical model, the primary model for health care, focused on pathology and examining the causes of impairments leading to disability. The medical model of disablement reflects a treatment approach focused on the body (i.e., muscle shortening) impairment level, and clinical intervention (muscle elongation and stretching) focused on improving dysfunction. However, a competing model, the social model of disablement, views disability as a composite of factors and conditions, many of which are caused by society and act as barriers to the individual's participation in society.

Clinically, the medical model impacts the selection of interventions that are focused on the impairment level, along with the lessening of impairments and concomitant functional limitations. On the other hand, the social model prioritizes the need for social interventions to enable all persons to participate in society regardless of their disabilities. While the medical and social models both highlight different aspects of the ability-disability continuum, neither fully captures a person's capabilities and, their health and participation in society. However, the ICF and the ICF-CY (WHO's approach for measuring health and disability), does capture both for adults and children. Endorsed by WHO in 2001, the ICF provides a comprehensive, internationally accepted framework to describe health related functioning across different conditions. In 2007, a child and youth version of the ICF (i.e., ICF-CY) was developed to capture functional abilities and disabilities in developing individuals by building on the descriptions of the ICF categories (WHO, 2007). With its functional emphasis, the ICF-CY provides a common language, useful across disciplines, as well as national boundaries to advance services, policy and research on behalf of children and youth (WHO, 2013).

The ICF-CY (2007) version, similar to the ICF (2001) framework, consists of two sections: part one contains elements of "functioning and disability," and part two includes "contextual factors." Each section impacts the health condition/disorder and interacts with the other. Functioning is described as a complex interacting system that takes into account the fundamental components of the framework, descriptive of the child's health condition, including body structure and functions, activities/ participation and context, and the personal and environmental factors specific to the child's health condition (Darsaklis et al., 2013). The ICF-CY is based upon an interactive biopsychosocial model of functioning that focuses on functioning beyond the medical or biological by taking into account other influences such as the environment and an array of contextual factors (Adolfsson et al., 2018) (Figure 1.2 shows a schematic representation of the two-part ICF-CY model with accompanying definition of terms) See Table 1.1.

Part one of the ICF-CY focuses on issues that are more directly related to a child's health condition. It is divided into two components: (1) body functions and structures, and (2) activity and participation. However, sometimes activity and participation are separated in this model to further the discussion of the impact of specific health conditions on measurable child-specific outcomes. In the ICF-CY framework, these three components (body functions and structure; activity; and participation) are neutral or positive terms that underscore the components of health while also reducing the stigma that use of negative terms can have on framing the impact of a disability (WHO, 2007, 2014).

Part two of the ICF-CY framework is comprised of two contextual factors: environmental and personal. According to WHO (2007), environmental factors refer to the physical, social and attitudinal environments in which an individual conducts his/her life. Personal factors refer to

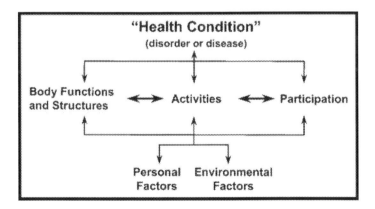

Figure 1.2 ICF-CY Model

Source: Copyright 2001 by the World Health Organization (WHO), reprinted with permission.

Table 1.1 Terms and Definitions of Health and Disability in ICF-CY (2007)

TERM	DEFINITION
In the context of health:	
Functioning	An umbrella term for body functions, body structures, activities, and participation. It denotes the positive aspects of the interaction between an individual (with a health condition) and that individual's contextual factors (environmental and personal factors).
Disability	An umbrella term for impairments, activity limitations and participation restrictions. It denotes the negative aspects of the interaction between an individual (with a health condition) and that individual's contextual factors (environmental and personal factors).
Body functions	The physiological functions of body systems (including psychological functions).
Body structures	Anatomical parts of the body such as organs, limbs, and their components.
Impairments	Problems in body function and structure such as significant deviation or loss.
Activity	The execution of a task or action by an individual.
Participation	Involvement in a life situation.
Activity limitations	Difficulties an individual may have in executing activities.
Participation restrictions	Problems an individual may experience in involvement in life situations.
Environmental factors	The physical, social, and attitudinal environment in which people live and conduct their lives. These are either barriers to or facilitators.

other attributes of the individual apart from those directly related to health conditions, such as gender, age, social background, individual psychological assets, experience, etc. Although these two contextual factors are not related to a child's health condition directly, they may influence the child's perception of his/her health condition (e.g., acceptance of disability or past experience), and may have an effect on the outcomes of his/her health condition and quality of life (e.g., age, habit, or others' support). The ICF-CY model helps us to describe the multi-dimensional circumstances of real-life experience, rather than focusing on the functional limitations and restrictions associated with having a disability (Ueda & Okawa, 2003). Moreover, research associated with this framework has generated an increasing number of outcome measures assessing the different factors that define the child's functioning and participation across domains (see Assessments Table in Appendix).

The ICF-CY is not only congruent with the fundamental assumption of pediatric therapy, but is also aligned with the recent shifts in the rehabilitation literature that view disability not as a disease, but rather as a condition characterized by limitations in function and performance as well as adaptation to environmental demands. It provides a framework for describing an individual's level of function and health beyond pathology, while guiding practitioners to select interventions that enable the person to participate fully in life. The ICF-CY framework can also guide the practitioner's selection of outcome measures designed to assess the impact of blended interventions on the child's functioning at many levels, and in different contexts. Using the ICF-CY framework, the clinician can begin an assessment by gaining an understanding of the child's participation in everyday activities. Once the child's participatory needs are highlighted, the clinician continues to define the child's activity limitations and underlying body structures and/or functional factors that are limiting the child's participation. Throughout this text chapter, authors will use terms from the ICF-CY framework as they discuss clinical practice and reasoning, evidence-based research, and health care outcomes associated with a clinician's delivery of health care at the individual and population level.

Sarah, informed by the ICF-CY model with its emphasis on functioning and the need to know more about Luke's activities and participation in daycare and at home, interviews the day care staff about Luke's routines as well as his participation in day care and activities during the day. Sarah also visits the family's home in order to uncover possible contextual supports for, and barriers to, Luke's participation in and performance of activities at home and in day care. The day care staff is concerned that Luke is often irritable, sleepy, and hungry, and wonder if the child receives opportunities for engagement in cognitive and physical activities. Sarah notices that the physical context in the day care center is clean and organized, toys are neatly stacked on low shelves allowing the children to freely choose and reach for them. When Sarah visits the home, she notices that there are few developmentally appropriate toys available for Luke to choose, dishes are in the sink, and the physical space for a family of three is limited. The mother, who holds two jobs in order to support her family, discusses her concerns about the child's irritability. Most of the time that she spends with Luke is on weekends when she only goes to one of her jobs and has more time to interact with him.

In order to further identify Luke's functional abilities, limitations, and impairments, Sarah administers to Luke a standardized developmental assessment, the Bayley-4. She also gives both the mother and day care staff a sensory processing questionnaire, Toddler Sensory Profile 2, to fill out about sensory-based emotional and motor behaviors demonstrated by Luke at home or in the day care center. Sarah has the mother and the staff at daycare discuss Luke from their perspectives and from within the context in which they see him function and participate. Also, by having Luke's mother and the day care staff complete different outcome measures specific to Luke's functioning, each contributes their view of Luke and how he acts in different contexts and with different people. As Sarah puts together a comprehensive picture of Luke at home and in day care, she develops a hypothesis over time about Luke and his functioning in these contexts. She will further develop this profile as she puts the various pieces of information together about Luke's functional performance and participation in everyday activities.

Evidence-Based Clinical Practice

Along with the introduction of the ICF-CY model framing different health conditions, another impactful and recent trend in medicine, health care and other arenas is the adoption of evidence-based clinical practice. The classic description of evidence-based practice highlights three basic elements: finding and using the best scientific evidence available to assess and intervene, respecting and working with the values and preferences of the client, and using the practitioner's expertise developed through ongoing clinical practice, education, and reflection (Sackett, 1997). For the practitioner in pediatrics, this means selecting the best intervention approach according to the evidence supporting the intervention's effectiveness and efficacy. However, research evidence in support of interventions used in pediatrics is limited. Thus, the practitioner is required to integrate practice guidelines developed by experts, and research that may not yet meet the criteria for scientific rigor as defined by the gold standard of evidence-based practice, the randomized controlled trial (Hariton & Locascio, 2018). Furthermore, it means that the practitioner needs to collect outcomes to support future use of different paradigms, or combinations of paradigms, to support future use of the different interventions in pediatrics. In the following chapters, we present several different approaches to assessing and intervening in pediatric practice. In each area where supporting evidence is available for the intervention, pertinent evidence is compared and contrasted in context. The evidence is provided not only so that the reader becomes more familiar with the principles of the different approaches, but so that the reader becomes more critically aware of the current state of research supporting practice as well as the application of this research to everyday practice.

Sarah reviews the results of the evaluation, and on the developmental assessment, Luke is functioning more than one standard deviation (SD) below the mean in the cognitive, motor and language areas. Additionally, on the sensory processing caregivers' reports, the scores suggest poor regulation of behavior, with responses fluctuating between hyper and hypo responsiveness to visual, auditory, movement, and proprioceptive input. Integrating different forms of ongoing clinical reasoning, Sarah continues to review the literature and realizes that children from lower socioeconomic environments tend to exhibit lower scores in developmental assessments, and that they catch up quickly when early intervention is provided. However, Sarah is concerned that Luke's scores on the parent sensory questionnaire reveal poor regulation and significant sensory processing problems.

Arranging the Pieces Through Clinical Reasoning

Clinical reasoning, the hallmark of an advanced clinician, is defined as the therapist's thought process, seldom documented, but pivotal when making decisions about client care (Schell & Schell, 2017). It is based on critical thinking, an intellectually disciplined process that is unique to the individual and entails a mode of thinking that is self-guided, self-disciplined and attempts to reason at the highest level of quality in a fair-minded way. Throughout the practice process, the practitioner uses multiple forms of clinical reasoning. These forms include: scientific, based on the literature and existing research; narrative, focusing on the therapist's everyday storytelling about the patient's problems (Mattingly & Fleming, 1994); pragmatic, which requires fitting the current realities of service delivery into treatment planning – for example, the socioeconomic environment at a given time; ethical, focusing on ethical dilemmas; interactive, focusing on communication between service providers and others; and conditional reasoning, which is considered to be a blending of all other forms of reasoning that enables the clinician to project client outcomes and eventualities across multiple areas (Mattingly & Fleming, 1994; Schell & Schell, 2017).

From the beginning of the therapeutic encounter, the therapist engages in various forms of critical thinking that evolve in conjunction with the various challenges and demands faced by the client, as well as the environment in which the therapist works. These could be the school system, the hospital setting, private practice, home care, or the community.

After evaluating Luke both at home and in daycare, and speaking with his mother and teachers, Sarah discusses her results with the family and the referral team. This results in a request for funding from the state agency to provide individual intervention twice per week, once in the home and once in the childcare agency. In consultation with the mother and daycare workers, Sarah collaboratively sets goals to increase Luke's developmentally appropriate participation in home and day care everyday activities. The outcome measures she chooses to use to monitor progress are the same developmental assessments used in the evaluation. The results from standardized assessments are used in conjunction with behavioral observations and measurable, functional goals already established with Luke's mother. The method of delivery includes individualized intervention at home and at daycare. The intervention approaches utilized include sensory integration, Developmental Individualized Relationship (DIR), and a developmental cognitive learning approach addressing executive functions, all of which include ongoing parent and staff education and training. All these interventions utilize play as the context for the intervention; therefore, Sarah feels that the interventions are compatible with each other. Lastly, the contexts chosen are the home and daycare settings; in order to provide the necessary intervention services, Sarah has to schedule home visits on Saturday mornings, the day the mother is not working.

In summary, Sarah utilizes different forms of clinical reasoning in her evaluation and choice of intervention methods. Her evaluation is informed by current best assessment practices, the choice of funding and setting is informed by pragmatic reasoning, and the choice of interventions by scientific reasoning. She is also aware of her own narrative about the child and the mother's life situation. She uses an interactive reasoning method to deliver a playful interaction with the child, but also an empathic and supportive interaction with the mother.

After 6 months, Sarah re-evaluates Luke with the same developmental assessment, the Bayley-4, utilized in the prior evaluation. Luke is functioning at age level in gross- and fine-motor development. Additionally, he has made gains in receptive language and adaptive areas, but he is still more than 1 SD behind his age. Sarah decides to refer the child to a speech-language pathologist, requesting a diagnostic evaluation to rule out ASD, and she continues with her intervention plan to address adaptive skills, with a re-evaluation in 6 months. Sarah is pleased with the progress and discusses this with Luke's mother, his sister, and the daycare staff, reinforcing the importance of their contribution to his progress.

This case illustrates how the present health environment requires the incorporation of a variety of skills and multiple intervention approaches. Sarah's choice of using an approach informed by sensory integration theory combined with a DIR approach, and a developmental approach focusing on executive functions, requires her to understand the underlying premises of all approaches. She uses sensory integration to address the irritability that the child presented towards sensory stimuli, a DIR approach to address the social-interactive issues, and a developmental approach focusing on executive functions to address goal-oriented behaviors. To measure progress across many dimensions, Sarah uses outcome measures associated with the different levels of the ICF-CY model. Using the ICF-CY framework, she identifies some of Luke's impairments at the body structure and body functions level, such as limited regulatory skills, and inadequate sensory responsiveness, and she examines how his body structural and functional impairments were affecting his engagement and participation in developmentally appropriate activities across contexts. She also considers to what degree his overall functioning and health has been impacted by different factors in the contexts of both the home and daycare environments.

In addition to introducing a data informed clinical reasoning model, RAM, this book also focuses on the interaction between treatment approaches, but primarily the interaction between sensory integration treatment and other approaches. There is a focus on specific populations of children with disorders (ASD, developmental coordination disorder, cerebral palsy) frequently seen in pediatric clinical practice. We also focus on different settings in which children are seen for intervention where combined approaches are used; and we highlight programs that use structured methods of combining those approaches. The success of treatment, and ultimately the best outcomes for each child such as Luke, depends on the following: including the needs of children and their families into the decision-making process; being current on the empirical research supporting choices made in the intervention process; incorporating evidence-based practice (EBP) into ongoing treatments; and using sound clinical reasoning to optimize best practice for each child and their family.

References

Adolfsson, M., Sjoman, M., & Bjorck-Akesson, E. (2018). ICF-CY as a framework for understanding child engagement in preschool. *Frontiers in Education*, *3*(36), 1–12. doi:10.3389/feduc.2018.00036

Blanche, E., Chang, M., Gutiérrez, J., & Gunter, J. (2016). Effectiveness of a sensory-enriched early intervention group program for children with developmental disabilities. *American Journal of Occupational Therapy*, *70*(5), 1–8. doi:10.5014/ajot.2016.018481

Darsaklis, V., Snider, L., Majnemer, A., & Mazar, B. (2013). Assessments used to diagnose developmental coordination disorder: Do their underlying constructs match the diagnostic criteria. *Physical and Occupational Therapy in Pediatrics*, *33*(2), 186–198. doi:10.3109/01942638.2012.739268

Hariton, E., & Locascio, J. J. (2018). Randomized controlled trials – The gold standard for effectiveness research. *BJOG: An International Journal of Obstetrics and Gynecology*, *125*(13), 1716. doi.org/10.1111/1471–0528.15199

Mattingly, C., & Fleming, M. H. (1994). *Clinical reasoning: Forms of inquiry in a therapeutic practice* (p. 37). FA Davis.

Monez, B. U., Houghton, R., Law, K., & Loss, G. (2019). Treatment patterns in children with autism in the United States. *Autism Research*, *12*(3), 517–526. doi:10.1002/aur.2070

Prizant, B. M., Wetherby, A. M., Rubin, E., & Laurent, A. C. (2003). The SCERTS model: A transactional, family-centered approach to enhancing communication and socioemotional abilities of children with autism spectrum disorder. *Infants & Young Children*, *16*(4), 296–316.

Reynolds, S., Glennon, T. J., Ausderau, K., Bendixen, R. M., Kuhaneck, H. M., Pfeiffer, B., Watling, R., Wilkinson, K., & Bodison, S. C. (2017). The issue is – Using a multifaceted approach to working with children who have differences in sensory processing and integration. *American Journal of Occupational Therapy*. doi:10.1016/j.jaac.2012.08.003

Rogers, S. J., Estes, A., Lord, C., Vismara, L., Winter, J., Fitzpatrick, A., Guo, M., & Dawson, G. (2012). Effects of a brief Early Start Denver Model (ESDM) – based parent intervention on toddlers at risk for autism spectrum disorders: A randomized controlled trial. *Journal of the American Academy of Child & Adolescent Psychiatry*, 51(10), 1052–1065. doi:10.1016/j.jaac.2012.08.003

Sackett, D. L. (1997, February). Evidence-based medicine. In *Seminars in perinatology* (Vol. 21, No. 1, pp. 3–5). WB Saunders. https://doi.org/10.1016/S0146-0005(97)80013-4

Schell, B. A. B., & Schell, J. W. (2017). *Clinical and professional reasoning in occupational therapy* (2nd ed.). Lippincott Williams & Wilkins.

Schoen, S. A., Miller, L. J., & Flanagan, J. (2018). A retrospective pre-post treatment study of occupational therapy intervention for children with sensory processing challenges. *The Open Journal of Occupational Therapy*, 6(1), 4. https://doi.org/10.15453/2168-6408.1367

Ueda, S., & Okawa, Y. (2003). The subjective dimensions of functioning and disability: What is it and what is it for? *Disability and Rehabilitation*, 25(11–12), 596–601. doi:10.1080/0963828031000137108

World Health Organization. (2001). *International classification of functioning, disability and health (ICF)*. World Health Organization. https://app.who.int

World Health Organization. (2007). *International classification of functioning, disability and health for children and youth (ICF-CY)*. World Health Organization. https://app.who.int

World Health Organization. (2013). *How to use the ICF: A practical manual for using the international classification of functioning, disability and health (ICF). Exposure draft for comment*. World Health Organization. https://app.who.int

World Health Organization. (2014). *International classification of functioning, disability and health (ICF)*. https://app.who.int

2 Reasoning in Action Model (RAM)

A Data-Based Model of Clinical Reasoning

Erna Imperatore Blanche

Years ago, I visited a newly established clinic. While passing by an ongoing session, I observed a therapist treating a boy who appeared to enjoy being on a swing. She stopped the swing and asked the child a question. He did not acknowledge the therapist's presence or respond to the question, and the therapist continued swinging him.

I remember that experience and compared it with Jean Ayres' treatment in which she posed a challenge and expected the child to respond successfully with what we call an *adaptive response*. After the child responded to the challenge, Ayres reinforced the response by providing feedback, either verbally or by increasing the sensory experience the child sought and needed (in some cases it was vestibular input). With those children, I thought Ayres combined sensory integration treatment (SIT) with a behavioral approach. On other opportunities, she suggested using SIT with neurodevelopmental treatment (NDT), specifically to address the issues presented by a child with cerebral palsy (CP). I learned from her that sometimes it was essential to combine intervention approaches with SIT.

As time goes by, I have realized that successful clinicians often choose more than one intervention approach to be most effective. However, when intervention approaches are combined, the clinician needs to understand the basic principles of each and why certain combinations should be utilized to solve a clinical problem. Recent intervention studies support the use of a combination of intervention practices. For example, Schoen et al. (2018) combined sensory integration (SI) with other behavioral and parent interventions to produce measurable changes in children with developmental disorders (see chapter 14). Combining and blending intervention approaches also happens in daily clinical practice. A review of 2677 treatment notes from 171 clients diagnosed with autism spectrum disorder (ASD) in a clinical setting, revealed that clinicians commonly use multiple approaches in practice. In that review, in more than 90 percent of the notes, clinicians reported using SIT in conjunction with other intervention approaches (Ellis, 2016; unpublished master's thesis).

DOI: 10.4324/9781003050810-3

In this book we focus on the interaction between theoretical perspectives, primarily the interaction between SIT and other approaches. We emphasize that the success of an intervention depends on the use of the best evidence; that is, incorporating the needs of children and their families, sound clinical reasoning, and empirical research supporting the choices made in the intervention process (Sackett et al., 1996; Sackett, 1997). Utilizing multiple approaches requires the intervener to understand the basic science and disciplines supporting the development of the relevant intervention, the main principles of the intervention utilized, the areas addressed by the intervention approach, and the research behind it. Appendix B provides a summary of the most often utilized intervention approaches in pediatrics.

Reasoning in Action Model (RAM): A Clinical Reasoning Model of Analysis

In this chapter we present a model of analysis, the Reasoning in Action Model (RAM), used to evaluate and plan interventions for children with a variety of disorders. Other writers have described similar models as either theory-driven, data-driven intervention models, or clinical reasoning frameworks (Ashburner et al., 2014; Blanche, 2006, 2010; Faller

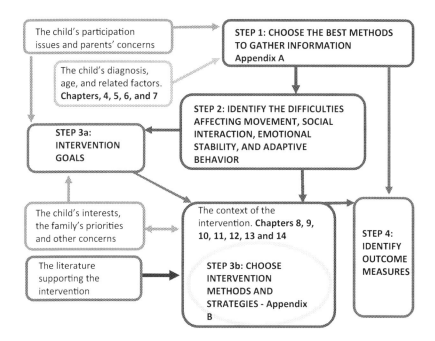

Figure 2.1 Data-Based Reasoning in Action Model (RAM)

et al., 2016; Schaaf & Blanche, 2012; Schaaf, 2015). The model is based on current literature and best practice (Sniderman et al., 2013), and encompasses four steps intended to assist clinical reasoning:

1. Gathering information
2. Identifying difficulties and barriers affecting participation and functional performance
3. Choosing the best evidence to support intervention strategies
4. Identifying outcome measures

Each step builds on the previous one and requires careful analysis of the child's needs and strengths to guide the information gathering process and the selection of interventions strategies (Blanche, 2006, 2010).

Step 1: Gathering Information

Step one in the model entails considering the child's participation issues when selecting the most relevant assessment tools to be used in evaluating the child's performance. The initial information received is typically the intake form, which serves as the first point of departure in the process.

Reason for Referral or Participation Issues

A complete referral history should include a diagnosis (if one exists), the parents' and teachers' concerns with clear, specific examples of decreased participation, and reduced functional performance. For example, being unable to button or having problems entering the school cafeteria are examples of functional performance and participation issues; tactile defensiveness is not. The evaluator needs to assess the importance that the family places on the participation issues, how they relate to the child's diagnosis, and the methods used to measure progress with regard to participation. The next section describes this process.

Methods Available to Gather Information

A comprehensive evaluation includes information gathered through a comprehensive standardized assessment data collection process; surveys and questionnaires completed by the parents and the referral source; skilled observations including clinical structured and unstructured observations, and ecological observations made in a naturalistic setting. The child's diagnosis and age often dictate the assessment tools utilized. As an example, for a toddler with ASD, the assessments might include a developmental assessment such as the Bayley Scales of Infant Toddler Development Fourth edition (Bayley-4) (Bayley, 2019), a sensory processing parent survey such as the Toddler Sensory Profile 2 (Dunn & Daniels, 2002; Dunn, 2014), and unstructured observations of the child's interactions with tasks and people in the environment (Blanche, 2002/2010). The assessment tools utilized for an older child with motor difficulties may include a Bruininks-Oseretsky Test of Motor Proficiency Second edition (BOT-2) (Bruininks & Bruininks, 2005) or the Movement Assessment Battery for Children (MABC) (Henderson et al., 2007), and observations of postural control and muscle tone.

Surveys and questionnaires completed by the parents or community members inform the assessor about the child's performance in daily activities. Most of these questionnaires focus on specific areas of performance, such as sensory processing, motor development, behavioral adaptations, and emotional regulation. For example, the Sensory Profile 2 (Dunn, 1999, 2014) focuses on sensory processing specifically concerning registration and modulation of sensory input; it is utilized for children with Attention Deficit Hyperactivity Disorder (ADHD), ASD, and mild motor difficulties. On the other hand, the Developmental Coordination Disorder Questionnaire (DCDQ) (Wilson, 2010) focuses on motor performance, and the Pediatric Evaluation of Disability Inventory-Computer Adapted Test (PEDI-CAT) focuses on functional performance in daily activities, mobility, social/cognition and responsibility, and has a section specific to children with autism (Coster et al., 2016; Dumas et al., 2012). (For a list with descriptions of the most often utilized assessment tools, surveys, and questionnaires in practice, please refer to the assessment table in Appendix A).

Clinicians use observations in naturalistic situations (described as ecological observations) as well as in a clinical environment (described as clinical observations) to assess the child's sensory preferences and avoidances, play styles, functional limitations, and the strategies utilized while interacting with the environment. Ecological, clinically structured, and unstructured observations provide essential qualitative data accompanying any evaluation; sometimes, they are the only means of gathering information (Ayres, 1984; Blanche, 2002/2010). Moment-to-moment observations are flexible and can provide information on the child's abilities and compensations in specific contexts. The therapist can then use in-the-moment clinical judgment to alter the type and order of the data collection (Dunn, 1981).

Standardized, normed referenced, and criterion-referenced evaluation tools focus on specific skills as they relate to functional performance. Standardized evaluations include developmental assessments; evaluations of body functions focusing on motor performance, sensory processing, behavioral, cognitive, and social skills; evaluations of functional performance and participation; and evaluations of quality of life and sense of well-being. Standardized tools provide an objective measure of the child's behavior in comparison to peers of the same age; they are useful when identifying a child's issues and measuring the progress of an intervention.

Step 2: Identifying Difficulties Affecting Participation and Functional Performance: Social Interactions, Emotional Stability, Motor Performance, Play and Adaptive Behavior

This step in the process relies heavily on the clinician's reasoning and clinical judgment described in Chapter 1. This step encompasses four phases that help organize the analysis of the information collected. Each of these phases answers a question in the reasoning process. These are:

- First Phase – Identifying troublesome issues: What are the child's observable behaviors that appear problematic, what are the activity limitation and participation issues, and what is the data obtained from Step 1?
- Second Phase – Generating Hypotheses: How are the observations related to behavior regulation, cognitive skills, motor control, and sensory processing?
- Third Phase – Weighing the Number of Data Points Supporting a Hypothesis and Offering a Conclusion: What are the main difficulties presented by the child and how they relate to cognition, executive functions, motor performance, behavior regulation, and sensory processing problems?
- Fourth Phase – Relating the identified issues to participation: How does the conclusion derived from the data relate to the reason for the referral?

The hypothesis generation form in Table 2.1 helps organize the information.

First Phase: Listing the Data Obtained Through Parent Interviews, Observable Behaviors, and Testing

Blanche (2002/2010) previously described this first method of data analysis as entailing the listing of behaviors observed and other data in one column and relating these to specific difficulties in the next column. What is essential for the success of this step is for the clinician to ensure that the behaviors listed are objective observations of behaviors in context, and not interpretations of behaviors.

The case depicted in Box 2.1 provides an example of this method of reasoning.

Table 2.1 includes the therapist's ecological observations and the data obtained through standardized testing and structured observations. The

Box 2.1　Luke's Case Study

Luke is a 6-year-old boy referred to occupational therapy by his teacher because he does not attend during class, fights with others, and exhibits decreased academic performance. During the therapist's observation in the classroom, Luke became fidgety during circle time and pushed children sitting next to him. During free play, Luke ran around aimlessly or moved from one activity to the other without finishing any of them. However, when the therapist asked him to copy the construction of a block structure, he was able to do it. The therapist's hypothesis initially was that Luke's difficulties with attention were probably due to arousal issues, since he was able to attend when motor abilities were required in a controlled sensory environment. In order to clarify her hypothesis, the therapist chose to assess the child by administering a parent sensory questionnaire (SPM), tactile subtests from the Sensory Integration and Praxis Test (SIPT), the Post-Rotary Nystagmus (PRN) Test, and structured clinical observations.

Once in the specialized clinical setting, Luke's behavior became disorganized during free play. He ran and threw himself onto a large ball without regard to his safety. When the therapist provided choices, Luke preferred the platform swing to swirl around, and crash on the pillows. During the administration of structured observations, Luke had difficulty maintaining his balance on one foot with eyes closed, exhibited decreased extensor tone, and was unable to catch a ball, skip, or imitate sequential finger touching, alternating forearm movements, or jumping jacks.

Table 2.1 Hypothesis Generation Form

First Phase: Data (Issues in participation, observations, other available information)	Second Phase: Hypotheses Generation/ Interpretations
Reason for referral: *Does not attend in class*	Decreased attention linked to increased or decreased arousal Decreased attention linked to executive functions
Reason for referral: Fidgety, runs around	Decreased attention Seeks movement linked to hyporesponsiveness to vestibular input
Sensory questionnaire and interview	Hyporesponsiveness to vestibular input Hyperresponsiveness to touch.

(Continued)

First Phase: Data (Issues in participation, observations, other available information)	Second Phase: Hypotheses Generation/Interpretations
Observations in the classroom: *Seems lost during transitions*	Decreased attention Decreased ideation Decreased organizational skills
Observation in the classroom: Punches others *during circle time*	Antisocial behaviors Hyperresponsivity to tactile input Seeks proprioceptive input
Observation in the specialized setting (clinic): Enjoys swinging and turning, poor safety awareness	Hyporesponsiveness to vestibular input Decreased attention
Observation in the specialized setting: Avoids shaving cream	Hyperresponsiveness to tactile input
Observation in specialized setting: Moves away when the therapist guides him by touching his shoulder	Hyperresponsiveness to tactile input
Observation in a specialized setting: Decreased antigravity extension	Decreased postural control Hyporesponsiveness to vestibular input
Observation in the specialized setting: Falling and crashing	Decreased postural control Seeks proprioceptive input
Observation in the specialized setting: Tremor during fine motor tasks	Tremor due to neuromotor control
Structured observations in specialized setting: Difficulties with Jumping jacks and skipping	Decreased bilateral motor coordination Decreased sequencing abilities Decreased motor planning
Structured observations in specialized setting: Difficulties with sequential finger touching and alternating forearm movements (Diadochokinesis)	Decreased sequencing abilities Decreased motor planning
Structured observations in specialized setting: Difficulties with slow ramp movements	Decreased perception of proprioceptive feedback
Standardized testing: Low scores in the movement ABC ball play and postural control items	Decreased ability to anticipate movements Decreased postural control
Standardized testing: low scores in bilateral motor coordination test (BMC) and Post-rotary Nystagmus Test (PRN)	Decreased bilateral motor coordination Hyporesponsiveness to vestibular input
Observations during administration of tactile discrimination tests: Becomes fidgety and appears to avoid touch.	Hyperresponsiveness to tactile input

Therapist's initial hypothesis: Increased responsivity to tactile input, decreased responsivity to vestibular and proprioceptive input affecting bilateral motor coordination and sequencing. Child may exhibit attention and organizational issues linked to executive functioning.

left column describes the observations and the right column, the possible interpretations, which are discussed further in phase two. The therapist's initial hypothesis is shown at the bottom of Table 2.1.

Second Phase of Analysis: Organizing Observations and Generating Hypotheses

When providing interpretations, it is helpful to identify at least two interpretations or hypotheses for each behavior. For example, the behavior of "punches others during circle time" can relate to at least two hypotheses: antisocial behavior and hyperresponsiveness to tactile. Also, the behavior of "*falling and crashing*" can have two hypotheses: seeking proprioceptive input and having difficulties with postural control. Once the clinician identifies at least 10 problematic behaviors and their hypotheses, the clinician, guided by existing evidence, links the behaviors to either sensory processing or other explanations. For example, if the child is presenting difficulties in postural control and the clinician has ruled out a neuromotor impairment, the postural issues may relate to vestibular processing if other indicators of inadequate responsivity to vestibular input are present. Alternatively, if the child exhibits aggression when encountering large groups of people and the clinician has ruled out antisocial behaviors, the behavior may be related to an increase in the child's level of arousal due to tactile processing difficulties. In this phase, the clinician explores the question of how the difficulties presented by the child link to behavior regulation, motor control, cognition, or sensory processing, and considers how these observations relate to each other.

Attention and behavioral organization may be affected by executive functions, arousal regulation, and sensory processing, among other reasons. Motor control difficulties may relate to sensory processing or other systems influencing motor control such as muscle tone abnormalities, strength, skeletal problems, and fatigue. Considering other potential impairments helps the therapist decide which intervention approaches to utilize, and whether using SI as a frame of reference should be the primary or secondary choice. Thus, the question to ask when organizing information at this phase of analysis is: How *are the presenting difficulties related to other areas of functional performance, sensory processing, or other impairments?* Table 2.2 shows how the data can be organized to derive a conclusion.

Third Phase: Counting Data Points and Culminating in a Conclusion

In this phase, the clinician weighs the number of data points supporting a specific hypothesis by counting the number of behaviors backing each

Table 2.2 Hypotheses Generation Form With Conclusion

First Phase: Data (Issues in participation, observations, other available information)	*Second Phase: Hypotheses Generation/ Interpretations*	*Third Phase: Counting Data Points and Conclusion*
Reason for referral: *Does not attend in class*	Decreased attention (possibly linked to increased or decreased arousal or to executive functions) ◇	
Reason for referral: Fidgety, runs around	Decreased attention ◇ / Seeks movement linked to hypo responsiveness to vestibular input #	◇ Overall decreased attention (4)
Sensory questionnaire and interview	Hyporesponsiveness to vestibular input # / Hyperresponsiveness to tactile input ≡ / Decreased attention ◇ / Decreased ideation ∧ / Decreased organizational skills ∞ / Antisocial behaviors %	# Hyporesponsiveness to vestibular input (6)
Observations in the classroom: *Seems lost during transitions*		∧ Decreased ideation (1) / ∞ Decreased organizational skills (1)
Observation in the classroom: Punches others *during circle time*	Hyperresponsivity to tactile input ≡ ○ / Seeks proprioceptive input ○	≡ Hyperresponsiveness to tactile input (6)
Observation in the specialized setting: Enjoys swinging and turning, poor safety awareness	Hyporesponsiveness to vestibular input # / Decreased attention ◇	
Observation in the specialized setting: Avoids shaving cream	Hyperresponsiveness to tactile input ≡	
Observation in specialized setting: Moves away when the therapist guides him by touching his shoulder	Hyperresponsiveness to tactile ≡	
Observation in a specialized setting: Decreased antigravity extension	Decreased postural control ↔ / Hyporesponsiveness to vestibular input #	←Decreased postural control (3)
Observation in the specialized setting: Falling and crashing	Decreased postural control ↔ / Seeks proprioceptive input ○	○Seeks proprioceptive input (2) and decreased proprioceptive feedback (1)

(Continued)

Table 2.2 (Continued)

First Phase: Data (Issues in participation, observations, other available information)	Second Phase: Hypotheses Generation/ Interpretations	Third Phase: Counting Data Points and Conclusion
Observation in the specialized setting; Tremor during fine motor tasks	Tremor due to neuromotor control	TOTAL proprioception (3)
Structured observations in specialized setting; Difficulties with Jumping Jacks and skipping	Decreased bilateral motor coordination ‖	‖ Decreased bilateral motor coordination (3)
Structured observations in specialized setting; Uneven, dysrhythmic movement in sequential finger touching	Decreased sequencing abilities T̄ Decreased motor planning P Decreased sequencing abilities T̄	T̄ Decreased sequencing (3) P Decreased motor planning (2)
Structured observations in specialized setting; Difficulties with sequential finger touching and Alternating Forearm Movements (Diadochokinesis)	Decreased sequencing abilities T̄ Decreased motor planning P	
Structured observations in specialized setting; Difficulties with Slow Ramp Movements	Decreased perception of proprioceptive feedback ○	
Parent completed sensory questionnaire: Identified increased responses to tactile input and decreased responses to vestibular input.	Hyperresponsiveness to tactile input ≡ Hyporesponsiveness to vestibular input #	
Standardized testing; Low scores in the Movement ABC ball play and postural control items	Decreased ability to anticipate movements Decreased postural control ↪	
Standardized testing; low scores in bilateral motor coordination test (BMC) and Post-rotary Nystagmus Test (PRN)	Decreased bilateral motor coordination ‖ Hyporesponsiveness to vestibular input #	
Observations during administration of tactile discrimination tests; becomes fidgety and appears to avoid touch.	Hyperresponsiveness to tactile input ≡	

hypothesis (see the number in parentheses after each interpretation). The hypothesis supported by the most data points is weighed against those with fewer points. The clinician should also identify additional hypotheses supported by the data that needs to be explored further. In Luke's example presented in Table 2.2, a summary of data points follows:

- Hyporesponsiveness to vestibular input = 6
- Functions related to proprioceptive processing =3
- Hyperresponsiveness to touch = 6

Functions related to vestibular/proprioceptive processing:

- Decreased postural control=3
- Bilateral motor coordination and sequencing=3

Now the therapist feels more confident about the conclusions presented in Box 2.2.

Part of this phase also requires further examination of the data collected. The therapist needs to answer the following questions: *What other information do I need to take into consideration to answer the reason for referral?*

Fourth Phase: Relating the identified difficulties to the reason for referral, or participation

In this phase, the examiner needs to tie the culminating conclusion to the reason for referral, or the participation issues. In this case, the therapist reports that:

- The attention difficulties observed in the classroom are probably due to modulation of the level of arousal linked to hyperresponsiveness

---

Box 2.2 The Therapist Feels Confident of the Following Conclusions

The child is hyporesponsive to vestibular input which may impact attention, postural control, and bilateral motor coordination.

The child presents proprioceptive processing difficulties that may also impact postural control and sequencing.

The child presents with hyperresponsiveness to tactile input that may relate to social difficulties and decreased attention.

Ideation and attention as part of executive functions need to be further assessed.

to tactile input as supported by published research (Dunn & Bennett, 2002; Pfeiffer et al., 2015).

- Decreased attention and excessive movements interfering with classroom participation can also be related to hyporesponsiveness to vestibular input.
- Decreased postural control, decreased bilateral motor coordination, and decreased sequencing abilities may be related to vestibular/proprioceptive processing.
- The impact of executive functions on attention and ideation need to be further explored.
- Tremor during fine motor tasks may be related to motor control issues not related to sensory processing.

The goals and outcome measures include skills affecting participation as they relate to the intervention method utilized. This step is discussed in the next section.

Steps 3a and 3b: Choosing the Best Evidence to Support Intervention Strategies: Intervention Goals and Intervention Planning

Step 3 encompasses two aspects: (a) choosing the intervention goals based on the reason for referral and the issues identified during the evaluation process, which will be discussed later in this chapter, and (b) identifying the intervention methods to be utilized, the context in which the intervention will be delivered, and, once in the treatment session, the process of blending interventions and its relationship to the overall goals. Incorporating multiple frames of reference into the intervention process requires understanding both the basic tenets of each, and how these can be combined with other treatment approaches. Because this book is about blending approaches with sensory integration theory, the basic elements of SI intervention will be covered and how other approaches can complement it.

SI Intervention: Basic Elements of SI Intervention

Ayres (1972, 1979, 1984) identified the following elements as central to Sensory Integration Treatment (SIT): the sensory experience, the adaptive response, the sensory enriched physical environment, the context of play, and the therapeutic alliance. If all five components are present, the intervener is committed to using an SI approach. When using a classic or traditional SI intervention, the specialized sensory-rich environment is also required. Figures 2.2 and 2.3 illustrate the relationship between these elements. In Figure 2.2, the sensory experience is central and embedded in the adaptive response. Adaptive responses (AR) are embedded in a context of play through the therapeutic alliance, co-created between the

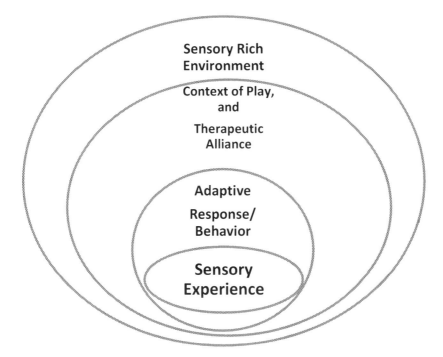

Figure 2.2 The Basic Elements of SIT

child and the intervener. When an intervener combines SIT with other approaches, attention to these elements is essential.

However, there are components not included in SIT that need to be addressed. In Table 2.3, the column on the right suggests areas that can be further explored to complement a pure SI based intervention. This table does not exclude SI theory from attending to these areas.

Sensory Experiences

The first and most central component in SI Intervention is the use of sensory experiences based on an understanding of the sensory difficulties presented by the child. When considering sensory experiences, the therapist needs to determine which equipment to make available for the child to choose from based on the following factors:

- the child's sensory processing difficulties
- the impact of the sensory processing difficulties on performance
- the impact of sensory input on the child's level of arousal
- the place where the intervention occurs

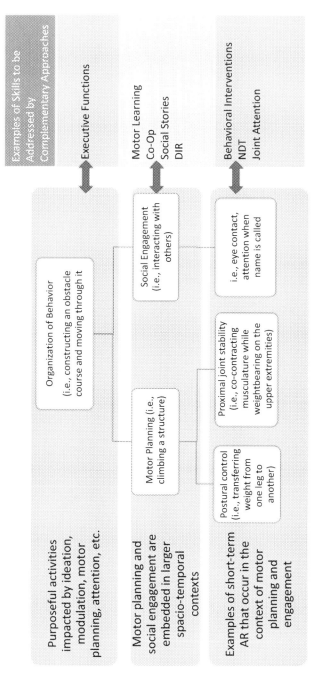

Figure 2.3 Nesting Adaptive Responses/Behaviors

Table 2.3 The Relationship Between Principles of SIT and Areas Not Addressed in Traditional SIT

SI PRINCIPLES	USED IN TRADITIONAL SI INTERVENTION	SUGGESTIONS FOR FURTHER ELABORATION
THE SENSORY SYSTEMS	Tactile Vestibular Proprioceptive	What about other senses? Visual Auditory Olfactory Interoceptive
ADAPTIVE RESPONSE/ CHALLENGE	Adaptive responses utilize sensory experiences Focus on motor and behavior	Motor: what about cognition, posture, and movement quality? Behavior: what about ideation and executive functions?
CONTEXT OF PLAY/ CHILD CENTERED	Intrinsic motivation Enjoyable Spontaneous	What about an in-depth understanding of child-centered interventions and the incorporation of all elements of play?
THERAPEUTIC ALLIANCE	A partnership: Child-directed, therapist modified	Exploring the most successful ways to develop the therapeutic alliance?
ENRICHED PHYSICAL ENVIRONMENT	Sensory rich gym type environments	Is that enough? What about interventions in the community?

For example, in a clinical setting, if the child is hyporesponsive to vestibular input, the intervener hangs swings for the child to choose from; but if the child exhibits tactile discrimination difficulties, the intervener makes tactile media available for the child. This is easier said than done, as children may not choose what is presented to them but may select something that the therapist doesn't consider to be the best choice for that child. In that case, the intervener needs to ensure that the activity has a purpose, and that sensory experiences are part of it. In a video of Jean Ayres and the child named Ray, he chose to climb on a swing in the shape of a horse even when the swing was unstable, and even though the child presented signs of gravitational insecurity. Once the child was on the swing, he immediately chose to come down, but Dr. Ayres made sure that the child stayed on the swing for a few minutes by stabilizing the swing; thus, increasing the amount of input he received while making sure that he maintained an upright position. In that situation, she was aware of the sensory experience (being off the ground and moving) embedded in the adaptive response, which required the child to integrate the sensory information (control his anxiety while being off the ground and maintaining postural stability).

When blending approaches, the intervener needs to consider the following points:

- How is the sensory experience utilized in other approaches?

For example, in neurodevelopmental treatment (NDT) based on the work of Bobaths (1967), the sensory experience is part of the facilitation techniques utilized. The intervention does not necessarily address sensory processing difficulties, but when facilitating movement, it is essential to understand the type and intensity of the sensory input and how it needs to be altered.

- Will a sensory experience increase the feedback of an undesired behavior or motor response?

In the example provided at the beginning of this chapter in which the therapist moved the swing even after the child did not respond to her request, the intervener did not understand that from a behavior analysis frame of reference, if a request for a response is made, then it is imperative to wait and help the child produce the response; otherwise the lack of response is reinforced with the sensory input provided.

Adaptive Responses and Adaptive Behaviors

The second component of the intervention is the AR or responses to the challenges tailored by the therapist to address the child's participation difficulties. The challenges are subtle and at a level that the child can perform, also referred to as the "just right challenge." The AR is the most challenging element to elicit in the intervention process, as it must be related to the child's participation difficulties and the treatment goals. Ayres (1984, unpublished notes) described adaptive "responses" as lower-level actions to counteract the challenges presented by the therapist or the environment. These "responses" could also be automatic. She added that adaptive "behaviors" were actions initiated by the individual to solve problems in the environment, but not necessarily as a "response" to environmental demand. As examples, she described postural reactions as responses, and initiating the construction of an obstacle course as adaptive behavior. Adaptive behaviors are more complex interactions with the environment. At present, the term "adaptive responses" is used in both cases; however, it is essential to distinguish between lower and higher-level interactions, as the therapist needs to target AR or the "just-right-challenge" during interventions. This refers to the level in which the child is challenged but not overburdened. The combination of "challenge and success" (Ayres, 1972, p. 259) provides a sense of fulfillment that is an important part of the therapeutic process, while also contributing to strengthening the therapeutic alliance.

When challenging the child to produce an AR, the therapist needs to answer the following questions:

- *What are the functional and participation issues presented by the child, and what are the family's concerns represented in the goals?*

The treatment goals reflecting the participation issues and family's concerns issues are the end products of the intervention, while the challenges posed to the child to produce AR during the intervention session relate to impairments hindering participation. For example, if a child is referred to intervention because of handwriting problems, but the evaluation results point to motor planning issues and postural control issues, the AR will center around gross and fine motor planning and postural control. The intervention approaches utilized should include SIT, an understanding of motor learning theories, and NDT principles. The challenges and the AR posed in each intervention approach are different (see Figure 4). Similarly, if the child is referred because of stereotyped behaviors, the goal may target the reduction of these behaviors in community settings (principles related to the behavioral approach), and the AR should target purposeful interactions while integrating the sensory experiences the child may seek and need.

- *What are underlying challenges to the performance/participation issues that need to be posed to the child during the therapeutic session? And How can the complexity of the AR be increased?*

During the intervention, the therapist may present challenges at different levels and target adaptive responses and behaviors that vary in complexity (see Figure 2.3). For example, a child navigating through an obstacle course might need to climb on equipment. At the lowest level (see Figure 2.3), the therapist may present short-term challenges requiring, for example, momentary proximal joint stability while leaning on hands to get out the equipment; or joint attention if the therapist points to a place where the child needs to go; and postural control if the therapist facilitates weight shifts while the child is mounting the equipment. At the next level, the child may be challenged by having to complete motor planned actions to mount and dismount equipment. Furthermore, at the highest level, the child can be challenged by the need to have a purpose and carry it to completion (i.e., getting to the other end of the obstacle course). Doing that requires: filtering external distractions, modulating sensory information, ideation, keeping the purpose in short term and working memory, and organizing the actions through multiple steps to get to the endpoint. In sensory integration, we refer to these actions as organization of behavior (OR). In the general literature, they are described as actions that require executive functioning.

The complexity of the AR also relates to the spatial and temporal context in which they occur; that is, AR that last seconds and occur in a confined physical environment (i.e., playing in a bin filled with balls) are often less complex than an AR that requires the person to move through a larger physical space and maintain the purpose of the action in mind for a prolonged period of time (i.e., moving through an obstacle course with several pieces of equipment) (Blanche & Parham, 2001). It is also important to note that when combining approaches, the different levels of the AR can be addressed by separate intervention approaches. For example, the term "organization of behavior" (OR) utilized in SIT is an executive function (EF) that requires understanding the influences on goal-oriented behavior; sensory processing influences on OR; and social-emotional influences on goal-oriented behaviors. Thus, addressing OR requires a combination of interventions.

Context of Play

The third component is the context of the intervention, a playful situation that requires the inclusion of the characteristics of play (intrinsic motivation, spontaneous, pleasurable, active). The context of play requires a physical environment that motivates children to direct their actions towards exploration, mastery, and play, and is often labeled as actions that are "*child directed.*" The experience of play requires a child to consider the activity as self-selected, self-directed, spontaneous or in the moment, pleasurable, active, including aspects of novelty, sometimes considered exciting, and, most importantly, for an activity to be considered play the pleasure is derived from doing it (Blanche & Knox, 2008). Thus, in a session, the more a clinician includes these characteristics into the activity, the more it is perceived as playful for the child. Chapter 13 focuses on the context of play and the therapeutic alliance and offers recommendations for creating it in the therapeutic process.

The Therapeutic Alliance/Use of Self

The fourth element is the one that makes the session possible: the therapeutic alliance requires the therapist to read the child's cues, respond to them and find the suitable challenge (Bundy & Hacker, 2020). The therapeutic alliance is a common theme in the literature (Taylor, 2008). It requires careful consideration of the therapist's preferred style of interaction and the intervention approach to be utilized. In most intervention approaches, the intervener needs to respond to the child's signals; responding may require changing one's preferred interaction styles. For example, while using some rehabilitation intervention approaches, the therapist is required to use an instructive style; whereas, in relationship-based approaches, the therapist may need to use a collaborative or supportive style. Thus, the frame of reference utilized influences the interaction style required. While the context of sensory integration intervention requires a therapist to cooperate with the child's choices, the context of other approaches requires a therapist to be more structured and directive. Chapter 13 will explore these principles in more detail. Based on the conclusions of Luke's therapist based on the assessment, intervention was informed by SIT as the primary approach, blended with other approaches as presented in Box 2.3.

Box 2.3

In preparation for the first session, the therapist sets up a few pieces of suspended equipment, the ball pit, and some brushes, and climbing equipment. Upon entering the room, Luke immediately climbed on the platform swing and attempted to move it with his feet. The therapist corrected the position by asking him to sit cross-legged on the swing and pump it with his upper extremities. In this way, the therapist encouraged Luke to use bilateral motor coordination and sequencing. The therapist shook the swing in play so Luke would fall on the pillows and she would then have the opportunity to provide deep pressure as part of the treatment to address tactile hyperresponsiveness.

The therapist then offered Luke the opportunity to play bumper cars on the tire swings with another child. When they agreed, she asked them to count before bumping. By doing this, the therapist planned to work on Luke's ability to maintain attention, anticipate an action, organize his behavior, take turns, socialize with another child in play, and increase the amount of proprioception, vestibular and tactile input he received. Both children were enthusiastic about the game, but Luke's arousal increased, and he started kicking the other child in an attempt to bump. The therapist corrected this behavior once; when Luke continued kicking, the therapist stopped the activity, using a behavioral approach to stop the maladaptive behavior of kicking or punching others.

In a subsequent session, Luke informed the therapist that he had just read a comic book about spider man where the character climbs a building and crosses over a bridge to save a child. The clinician used this opportunity to have Luke figure out how he could replicate the story in the comic book. In this way, she targeted executive functions of visualization, ideation, and organization.

Components of Successful Interventions

In order to create the most effective intervention, the clinician needs to consider evidence from published research literature supporting the choice of intervention, the clinician's clinical reasoning (Steps 1 and 2), the client's (and family's) expectations (Sackett et al., 1996), and the context of the intervention. The outcomes of these steps are clear treatment objectives and contextual treatment choices.

Use the Literature

Different types of literature serve as evidence supporting the choices of intervention. The evidence includes descriptive studies focusing on sensory processing issues presented by different diagnoses; effectiveness studies using individualized sensory integration treatment as defined by Ayres; and effectiveness studies focusing on specific sensory experiences that can be used as part of any intervention. Descriptive studies have provided rich information on the presence of sensory processing issues associated with a variety of diagnoses, including ASD, attention deficit disorder, developmental coordination disorder (DCD), cerebral palsy (CP), learning disabilities, and other developmental disorders. In Luke's case, the therapist used information provided by descriptive studies on the presence of tactile deficits in children with attention difficulties (Dunn & Bennett, 2002). More specific information about research on sensory processing issues in specific diagnoses is provided in the chapters describing ASD, DCD, and CP.

Effectiveness studies include studies using sensory strategies to address modulation issues, enriched environment studies, and large randomized studies using traditional one-to-one classic sensory integration intervention (SIT). SIT refers to a one-to-one intervention in a specialized setting utilizing Ayres description of SIT. In some cases, it is referred to as Ayres Sensory Integration ®. Sensory strategies refer to the use of specific contextual choices that may alter the child's behavior in the moment (see Chapter 3).

The effectiveness of SIT was originally studied by Ayres (1968; Ayres & Mailloux, 1981) and later studied by others (Miller et al., 2007; Pfeiffer et al., 2011; Schaaf et al., 2014) Although effectiveness studies focusing on the delivery of individualized sensory integration interventions have become more scientifically sound during the last 10 years (Miller et al., 2007; Pfeiffer et al., 2011; Schaaf et al., 2014), current trends towards interventions delivered in natural environments may require the use of manualized intervention programs that include multiple frames of references across multiple environments. SIT is presently considered to be an evidence-based intervention for children with ASD (Schoen et al., 2019; Steinbrenner et al., 2020) and the outcome measures utilized to support its use include a variety of standardized measures.

The Family's Expectations and Motivations

The family's interests and expectations are important when choosing the goals to be addressed. An initial interview and continuous communication with the parents are pivotal, both when addressing the family's needs and when assuring their participation during the intervention process. It is important to include assessments that tap into the parents' views of the children's progress. Measurements such as the Vineland Adaptive Behavior Scales (Sparrow et al., 2005) and the PEDI-CAT (Dumas et al., 2012) are based on parent reports, and have been used successfully to collect information about the child's progress.

The Context of the Intervention

The context of the intervention includes the physical environment where the intervention will be provided, the time of the day, and other variables such as the funding sources, the child's and the parents' schedule, the access to specialized equipment, and other factors. The context of the intervention influences the choice of delivery of the intervention (as well as moderating the goals); that is, if the child requires individualized SIT, environmental modifications, or the use of sensory strategies, or if other intervention approaches are combined with SIT.

Establishing Clear and Measurable Treatment Objectives

When establishing treatment objectives, it is essential for them to be related to functional performance and determined with the parents. Objectives need to be clearly stated so they can be used to measure progress. They need to include the behavior that needs to be changed, the setting and task in which it will be assessed, and the conditions that will be considered. Some of the outcome measures described in the following can be used to measure progress.

Step 4: Identify Outcome Measures

Every intervention needs to establish measurable treatment objectives that are related to difficulties in participation, and to the skills addressed during the intervention. There are several types of outcome measures; those most often utilized are pre- and post-treatment standardized assessments. Goal Attainment Scaling (GAS) has become a popular alternative to standardized measures utilized to measure the results of sensory integration treatment (Mailloux et al., 2007; Miller et al., 2007; Pfeiffer et al., 2011; Schaaf et al., 2014). Other forms of collecting ongoing information during treatment include single-subject designs (SSD) (Ottenbacher, 2016), the utilization of coding treatment videos, and using highly structured treatment notes (Collins & Dworkin, 2011; Thompson & Blanche, 2015).

Conclusion

Blending sensory integration intervention principles with other approaches such as NDT, Motor Learning or ABA requires careful analysis of the child's functional and participation problems, the results of the evaluation, the context of the intervention, and the goals to be attained. In this chapter we have presented a model of analysis (RAM) that can help therapist organize the assessment information and plan intervention.

References

Ashburner, J. K., Rodger, S. A., Ziviani, J. M., & Hinder, E. A. (2014). Optimizing participation of children with autism spectrum disorder experiencing sensory challenges: A clinical reasoning framework. *The Canadian Journal of Occupational Therapy, 81*(1), 29–38.

Ayres, A. J. (1968). Learning disabilities and the vestibular system. *Journal of Learning Disabilities, 11*(1), 30–41.

Ayres, A. J. (1972). *Sensory integration and learning disorders.* Western Psychological Services.

Ayres, A. J. (1979). *Sensory integration and the child.* Western Psychological Services.

Ayres, A. J. (1984). *The adaptive response.* Unpublished document.

Ayres, A. J., & Mailloux, Z. (1981). Influence of sensory integration procedures on language development. *American Journal of Occupational Therapy, 35,* 383–390.

Bayley, N., & Aylward, G. P. (2019). *Bayley scales of infant and toddler development* (4th ed.). Pearson.

Blanche, E. I. (2002/2010). *Observations based on sensory integration theory.* Pediatric Therapy Network.

Blanche, E. I. (2006). Clinical reasoning in action: Designing intervention. In R. Schaaf & S. Smith-Roley (Eds.), *Sensory integration: Clinical reasoning for diverse populations* (pp. 91–106). Therapy Skill Builders.

Blanche, E. I., & Knox, S. H. (2008). Learning to play: Promoting skills and quality of life in individuals with cerebral palsy. *Clinics in Developmental Medicine, 178*(1), 357–370.

Blanche, E. I., & Parham, L. D. (2001). Praxis and the organization of behavior in time and space. In S. Smith-Roley, E. Blanche, & R. Schaaf (Eds.), *Understanding the nature of sensory integration with diverse populations* (pp. 183–201). Therapy Skill Builders.

Bobaths, B. (1967). The very early treatment of cerebral palsy. *Developmental Medicine & Child Neurology, 9*(4), 373–390.

Bruininks, R. H., & Bruininks, D. B. (2005). *Bruininks – Oseretsky test of motor proficiency* (2nd ed.). Pearson Assessment.

Bundy, A. C., & Hacker, C. (2020). The art of therapy. In A. C. Bundy & S. J. Lane (Eds.), *Sensory integration theory and practice* (3rd ed.). F.A. Davis.

Collins, A., & Dworkin, R. J. (2011). Pilot study of the effectiveness of weighted vests. *American Journal of Occupational Therapy, 65*(6), 688–694.

Coster, W. J., Kramer, J. M., Tian, F., Dooley, M., Liljenquist, K., Kao, Y. C., & Ni, P. (2016). Evaluating the appropriateness of a new computer-administered measure of adaptive function for children and youth with autism spectrum disorders. *Autism, 20*(1), 14–25.

Dumas, H. M., Fragala-Pinkham, M. A., Haley, S. M., Ni, P., Coster, W., Kramer, J. M., Kao, Y-C., Moed, R., & Ludlow, L. H. (2012). Computer adaptive test performance in children with and without disabilities: Prospective field study of the PEDI-CAT. *Disability and Rehabilitation, 34*(5), 393–401.

Dunn, W. (1981). *A guide to testing clinical observations in kindergartners.* American Occupational Therapy Association.

Dunn, W. (1999). *The sensory profile manual.* The Psychological Corporation.

Dunn, W. (2014). *The sensory profile2 manual.* The Psychological Corporation.

Dunn, W., & Bennett, D. (2002). Patterns of sensory processing in children with attention deficit hyperactivity disorder. *OTJR: Occupation, Participation and Health, 22*(1), 4–15.

Dunn, W., & Daniels, D. B. (2002). Initial development of the infant/toddler sensory profile. *Journal of Early Intervention, 25*(1), 27–41.

Ellis, K. (2016). *Data mining: Gathering data a pediatric occupational therapy practice.* A Thesis Presented to the Faculty of the Graduate School at the University of Southern California in partial fulfillment of the requires for the degree of Master of Arts (Occupational Therapy).

Faller, P., Hunt, J., van Hooydonk, E., Mailloux, Z., & Schaaf, R. (2016). Application of data-driven decision making using ayres sensory integration® with a child with autism. *American Journal of Occupational Therapy, 70*(1).

Henderson, S. E., Sugden, D. A., & Barnett, A. (2007). *Movement assessment battery for children* (Movement ABC-2) (2nd ed.). Pearson/Psych-Corp.

Mailloux, Z., May-Benson, T. A., Summers, C. A., Miller, L. J., Brett-Green, B., Burke, J. P., Cohn, E. S., Koomar, J. A., Parham, L. D., Smith Roley, S., Schaaf, R. C., & Schoen, S. A. (2007). Goal attainment scaling as a measure of meaningful outcomes for children with sensory integration disorders. *American Journal of Occupational Therapy, 61*(2), 254–259.

Miller, L. J., Coll, J. R., & Schoen, S. A. (2007). A randomized controlled pilot study of the effectiveness of occupational therapy for children with sensory modulation disorder. *American Journal of Occupational Therapy, 61*(2), 228–238.

Ottenbacher, K. J. (2016). Republication of "when is a picture worth a thousand p values? A comparison of visual and quantitative methods to analyze single subject data". *The Journal of Special Education, 50*(3), 133–140.

Pfeiffer, B. A., Daly, B. P., Nicholls, E. G., & Gullo, D. F. (2015). Assessing sensory processing problems in children with and without attention deficit hyperactivity disorder. *Physical & Occupational Therapy in Pediatrics, 35*(1), 1–12.

Pfeiffer, B. A., Koenig, K., Kinnealey, M., Sheppard, M., & Henderson, L. (2011). Effectiveness of sensory integration interventions in children with autism spectrum disorders: A pilot study. *American Journal of Occupational Therapy, 65*(1), 76–85.

Sackett, D. L. (1997, February). Evidence-based medicine. In *Seminars in perinatology* (Vol. 21, No. 1, pp. 3–5). WB Saunders.

Sackett, D. L., Rosenberg, W. M. C., Gray, J. A. M., Haynes, R. B., & Richardson, W. S. (1996). Evidence based medicine. *BMJ: British Medical Journal, 313*(7050), 170–171.

Schaaf, R. C. (2015). The issue is – Creating evidence for practice using data-driven decision making. *American Journal of Occupational Therapy, 69*, 6902360010. http://dx.doi.org/10.5014/ajot.2015.010561

Schaaf, R. C., Benevides, T., Mailloux, Z., Faller, P., Hunt, J., Van Hooydonk, E., & Kelly, D. (2014). An intervention for sensory difficulties in children with autism: A randomized trial. *Journal of Autism and Developmental Disorders, 44*(7), 1493–1506

Schaaf, R. C., & Blanche, E. I. (2012). Emerging as leaders in autism research and practice: Using the data-driven intervention process. *American Journal of Occupational Therapy, 66*(5), 503–505. doi:10.5014/ajot.2012.006114.

Schoen, S. A., Lane, S. J., Mailloux, Z., May-Benson, T., Parham, L. D., Smith Roley, S., & Schaaf, R. C. (2019). A systematic review of Ayres sensory integration intervention for children with autism. *Autism Research, 12*(1), 6–19.

Schoen, S. A., Miller, L. J., & Flanagan, J. (2018). A Retrospective pre-post treatment study of occupational therapy intervention for children with sensory processing challenges. *The Open Journal of Occupational Therapy, 6*(1), Article 4. https://doi.org/10.15453/2168-6408.1367

Sniderman, A. D., LaChapelle, K. J., Rachon, N. A., & Furberg, C. D. (2013). The necessity for clinical reasoning in the era of evidence-based medicine. *Mayo Clinic Proceedings, 88*(10), 1108–1114.

Sparrow, S. S., Cicchetti, D. V., & Balla, D. A. (2005). *Vineland adaptive behavior scales* (2nd ed.). Pearson.

Steinbrenner, J. R., Hume, K., Odom, S. L., Morin, K. L., Nowell, S. W., Tomaszewski, B., Szendrey, S., McIntyre, N. S., Yucesoy-Ozkan, S., & Savage, M. N. (2020). *Evidence-based practices for children, youth, and young adults with autism.* The University of North Carolina at Chapel Hill, Frank Porter Graham Child Development Institute, National Clearinghouse on Autism Evidence and Practice Review Team.

Taylor, R. R. (2008). *The intentional relationship: Outpatient therapy and use of self.* FA Davis.

Thompson, B., & Blanche, E. I. (2015). The effects of vestibular activity during sensory integration intervention on spontaneous affect and communication within the therapy session. *Sensory Integration Special Interest Quarterly, 38*(2), 1–4.

Wilson, B. N., & Crawford, S. G. (2010). *Developmental coordination disorder questionnaire 2007.* Alberta Health Services & Alberta Children's Hospital Foundation.

3 Sensory Processing

A Conceptual Model

Erna Imperatore Blanche and
Stefanie C. Bodison

Sensory integration theory derives knowledge from different disciplines which likely contributes to confusion surrounding the terminology utilized by occupational therapy clinicians, educators, and researchers (Blanche et al., 2019; Bodison et al., 2019). Furthermore, clinicians combine interventions in different ways creating a puzzle of terms that are sometimes ill defined. In this short chapter, we define concepts and present a conceptual model that attempts to organize terms utilized in the literature, including sensory integration therapy (SIT), Sensory Integration, sensory-based therapies, sensory processing interventions, sensory diets, and Ayres Sensory Integration ® (ASI™), among others. The indiscriminate use of these terms fosters confusion as the casual reader assumes all these terms describe the same thing. One of the most important terms to be clarified is the difference between sensory integration theory and sensory integration treatments/interventions and the difference between sensory processing and sensory integration. Table 3.1 offers a summary of these terms and the conceptual model on Figure 3.1 organizes the concepts.

The model is divided in three areas: the issue being addressed, the theories/frames of reference and intervention models utilized to address the issue, and examples of interventions derived from the theoretical models and frameworks. In this model, we see that the issue or area of concern is sensory processing. See Table 3.1 for a definition of sensory processing. All the interventions described in the model address sensory processing in different sensory systems and in different ways. The next level represents frames of reference, theories or models that are used to address sensory processing challenges. The lower level represents specific examples of interventions based on models of intervention. The arrows indicate the proposed historical connection between terms. The arrow between perceptual motor approaches and sensory integration theory illustrates the influence of one over the development of the other. The arrow from sensory integration theory to sensory processing suggests an influence of sensory integration theory, as the first theory

DOI: 10.4324/9781003050810-4

Table 3.1 Summary of Terms

TERM	BRIEF DESCRIPTION
Sensory Processing	"Overarching construct to summarize various neuronal interactions in the brain associated with incoming sensory signals from the environment or body and the subsequent responses resulting from that input" (Ayres, 1979/2005; Baranek et al., 2006; Dunn, 2001; Miller et al., 2009; Parham et al., 2007; Schauder & Bennetto, 2016; Bodison et al., 2019, p. 5).
	The term "sensory processing" is used to describe peripheral and central nervous system processes in all sensory systems (Ahn et al., 2004). Sensory Processing Disorders have been classified by different authors, including Miller et al. (2007), Baranek et al. (2006), and Dunn (2001, 2014).
Sensory Integration Theory	A theory originally developed by A. Jean Ayres, PhD that continues to evolve. Its focus is on responsiveness and unimodal or multimodal integration of sensations in three main systems (tactile, proprioceptive, and vestibular) and their contributions to behavior organization, emotion regulation, and motor performance.
	Ayres included a model of development (Ayres, 1972, 1979/2005) focusing on the impact of the vestibular, proprioceptive and tactile systems on participation (end products), a description of dysfunctions in discrimination and modulation of arousal (Ayres, 1972, 1979/2005; Bundy et al., 2002; Bundy & Lane, 2020), and evaluation and intervention guidelines. In order to differentiate sensory integration theory from sensory integration treatment (SIT), a definition of SIT is provided in the next row.
Sensory Integration Treatment (SIT)	An intervention based on the theory of sensory integration defined as "interventions that target a person's ability to integrate sensory information [either in unimodal or multimodal domains] (visual, auditory, tactile, proprioceptive, and vestibular) from their body and environment in order to respond using organized and adaptive behavior" (Steinbrenner et al., 2020, page 29); also referred to as Ayres Sensory Integration® Intervention
Environmental Modifications/ Strategies	Environmental supports (i.e., changes in lighting, sensory rooms) and sensory strategies (i.e., weighted blankets, weighted vests) alter sensory input to address arousal/ emotion regulation and stress reduction in specific environments (Bodison, 2018).
Perceptual-Motor Approaches	Evaluation tools and intervention approaches focusing on altering sensory-motor skills through the performance of fine and gross motor activities. Repetition of activities is encouraged for learning and it can be delivered in small groups.

(*Continued*)

TERM	BRIEF DESCRIPTION
Cognitive/ Behavioral Approaches Focusing on Self-Regulation	Training programs focusing on increasing individuals' awareness of their level of arousal and responses to sensory events and involves teaching cognitive strategies to change behavioral responses. These programs target self-regulation and may or may not be based on the individual evaluation of sensory processing issues.
Other Sensory-Based Interventions	Auditory training Massage Other

to systematically focus on sensory processing disorders, influencing the interdisciplinary interest in sensory processing as an area of study.

In this model, the theory and intervention originally developed by Ayres can be systematically delivered through SIT or ASI™, interventions focusing primarily on improving vestibular, proprioceptive, and/or tactile functions. SIT and ASI™ are differentiated from other practices in research through the use of specific fidelity scales (Parham et al., 2007). SIT can be delivered in combination with other intervention approaches in clinical practice (Blanche et al., 1995).

Environmental adaptations can be differentiated from sensory strategies in that environmental adaptations are applied distally to the physical environment, while sensory strategies are applied to individuals. Environmental adaptations include altering lighting or sound such as in Snozelen and sensory rooms to impact anxiety. Environmental adaptations are often used in mental health settings (Seckman et al., 2017). Sensory strategies include the use of equipment such as weighted vests (Bodison, 2018; Lin et al., 2014), adapted seating (Metz et al., 2020; Schilling & Schwartz, 2004), or other forms of directly altering the person's active interaction with the sensory experience. In this model, these modifications are represented as different from SIT although they can be embedded in SIT. For example, using vestibular input to increase vocalizations, eye contact and general arousal (Kantner et al., 1982; Ray et al., 1988; Magrun et al., 1981) can be used as part of an active interaction during SIT (Thompson & Blanche, 2015) or as a modification of the specific seating material in the classroom (Schilling & Schwartz, 2004; Rollo et al., 2019). Studies focusing on tactile input in the form of passive massage have supported its use in regulating arousal and increasing attention (Bodison, 2018; Edelson et al., 1999; Field, 1998). These studies have contributed to our understanding of the effects of deep pressure during the intervention process but are not considered part of SIT. The main difference between strategies

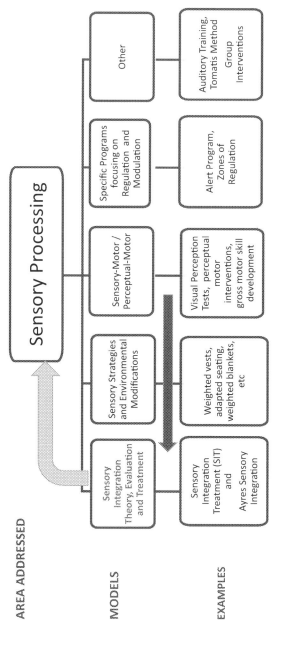

Figure 3.1 Conceptual Model Sensory Processing

Source: Blanche and Bodison, 2020

utilized as part of SIT and environmental adaptations/strategies is that while the first one is embedded within an active challenge during a child-directed therapeutic session, the latter is prescribed by a clinician/teacher and applied in isolation to enhance performance in a very specific environment.

More recently, Cermak and colleagues have demonstrated that the use of sensory strategies in the form of a weighted blanket and adaptations to the dental environments in the form of lighting and sound, has a significant effect on children with ASD during teeth cleaning (Cermak et al., 2015). These studies contribute to our understanding of the effects of modifying the sensory experiences in the environment on arousal, stress, and general performance.

Perceptual motor approaches (PMA) are often more prescriptive than SIT and are commonly used to address specific sensory motor difficulties that can be delivered either individually or in small groups. These approaches include visual perception tasks, fine motor/hand manipulation activities, visual-motor tasks, and gross motor tasks such as those initially developed by Frostig, Kephard, Getman, and Barsch (Parush & Hahn-Markowitz, 1997). Ayres' initial work included elements of perceptual motor approaches.

Cognitive behavioral approaches are also often utilized in conjunction with SIT. These approaches utilize specific training programs to gage one's own sensory responses and arousal level and actively change them. Examples include the Alert Program (How Does Your Engine Run) (Williams & Schellenberger, 1996); Zones of Regulation (Kuypers, 2011), Sense-Ability Program (Moore, 2005), Curriculum for Self-Regulation (Moore, 2015), and wellness programs that include sensory strategies (Gardner et al., 2012). Many of these programs are found in pediatric settings; however, some of these programs are also used in adult mental health practice.

Lastly, there are other approaches that also relate to sensory processing such as auditory training programs, specific forms of massage, and activity programs such as yoga and aqua therapy. These approaches acknowledge the impact of sensory experiences on performance.

In summary, this conceptual model offers an organization of concepts related to sensory processing and sensory integration. As a working model, it clarifies terminology and the relationship between diverse intervention models.

References

Ahn, R. R., Miller, L. J., Milberger, S., & McIntosh, D. N. (2004). Prevalence of parents' perceptions of sensory processing disorders among kindergarten children. *American Journal of Occupational Therapy*, 58(3), 287–293.

Ayres, A. J. (1972). *Sensory integration and learning disorders*. Western Psychological Services.

Ayres, A. J. (1979/2005). *Sensory integration and the child* (25th anniversary ed.). Western Psychological Service.

Baranek, G. T., David, F. J., Poe, M. D., Stone, W. L., & Watson, L. R. (2006). Sensory experiences questionnaire: Discriminating sensory features in young children with autism, developmental delays, and typical development. *Journal of Child Psychology and Psychiatry and Allied Disciplines, 47*, 591–601.

Blanche, E. I., Bodison, S. C., Stein Duker, L. I., & Cermak, S. (2019). An examination of sensory-related terminology across disciplines: Part two. *SIS Quarterly Practice Connections, 4*(3), 5–7.

Blanche, E. I., Botticelli, T. M., & Hallway, M. K. (1995). *Combining neuro-developmental treatment and sensory integration principles – An approach to pediatric therapy.* Therapy Skill Builders.

Bodison, S. C. (2018). A comprehensive framework to embed sensory interventions within occupational therapy practice. *SIS Quarterly Practice Connections, 3*(2), 14–16.

Bodison, S. C., Stein Duker, L. I., Cermak, S. A., & Blanche, E. I. (2019). An examination of sensory-related terminology across disciplines: Part one. *SIS Quarterly Practice Connections, 4*(2), 5–7.

Bundy, A. C., & Lane, S. J. (Eds.). (2020). *Sensory integration: Theory and practice* (3rd ed.). F. A. Davis Company.

Bundy, A. C., Lane, S. J., & Murray, E. (2002). *Sensory integration – theory and practice* (2nd ed.). F. A. Davis Company.

Cermak, S. A., Duker, L. I. S., Williams, M. E., Dawson, M. E., Lane, C. J., & Polido, J. C. (2015). Sensory adapted dental environments to enhance oral care for children with autism spectrum disorders: A randomized controlled pilot study. *Journal of Autism and Developmental Disorders, 45*(9), 2876–2888.

Dunn, W. (2001). The sensations of everyday life: Empirical, theoretical, and pragmatic considerations. *American Journal of Occupational Therapy, 55*(6), 608–620. https://doi.org/10.5014/ajot.55.6.608

Dunn, W. (2014). *Sensory profile™ 2 user's manual.* Pearson.

Edelson, S. M., Edelson, M. G., Kerr, D. C., & Grandin, T. (1999). Behavioral and physiological effects of deep pressure on children with autism: A pilot study evaluating the efficacy of Grandin's hug machine. *American Journal of Occupational Therapy, 53*(2), 145–152.

Field, T. M. (1998). Massage therapy effects. *American Psychologist, 53*(12), 1270.

Gardner, J., Dong-Olson, V., Castronovo, A., Hess, M., & Lawless, K. (2012). Using wellness recovery action plan and sensory-based intervention: A case example. *Occupational Therapy in Health Care, 26*(2–3), 163–173.

Kantner, R., Kantner, B., & Clark, D. (1982). Vestibular stimulation effect on language development in mentally retarded children. *American Journal of Occupational Therapy, 36*, 36–41.

Kuypers, L. (2011). *The zones of regulation.* Think Social Publishing.

Lin, H. Y., Lee, P., Chang, W. D., & Hong, F. Y. (2014). Effects of weighted vests on attention, impulse control, and on-task behavior in children with attention deficit hyperactivity disorder. *American Journal of Occupational Therapy, 68*(2), 149–158.

Magrun, W. M., Ottenbacher, K., McCue, S., & Keefe, R. (1981). Effects of vestibular stimulation on spontaneous use of verbal language in developmentally delayed children. *American Journal of Occupational Therapy, 35*, 101–104.

Metz, A. E., DeMarco, M., Khalsa, A., Kreuz, N., Stock, R., & Westfall, A. (2020). The effects of ball chair seating during an instructional period in first grade classrooms. *Journal of Occupational Therapy, Schools, & Early Intervention*, 1–15.

Miller, L. J., Anzalone, M. E., Lane, S. J., Cermak, S. A., & Osten, E. T. (2007). Concept evolution in sensory integration: A proposed nosology for diagnosis. *American Journal of Occupational Therapy*, 61(2), 135–140.

Miller, L. J., Nielsen, D. M., Schoen, S. A., & Brett-Green, B. A. (2009). Perspectives on sensory processing disorder: A call for translational research. *Frontiers in Integrative Neuroscience*, 3, Article 22.

Moore, K. (2005). *The sensory connection handbook & manual*. Therapro.

Moore, K. (2015). *The sensory connection program: Curriculum for self-regulation*. Therapro.

Parham, L. D., Ecker, C., Miller Kuhaneck, H., Henry, D. A., & Glennon, T. J. (2007). *Sensory processing measure manual*. Western Psychological Services.

Parush, S., & Hahn-Markowitz, J. (1997). A comparison of two settings for group treatment in promoting perceptual-motor function of learning disabled children. *Physical & Occupational Therapy in Pediatrics*, 17(1), 45–57.

Ray, T., King, L., & Grandin, T. (1988). The effectiveness of self-initiated vestibular stimulation in producing speech sounds in an autistic child. *Occupational Therapy Journal of Research*, 8, 187–190.

Rollo, S., Crutchlow, L., Nagpal, T. S., Sui, W., & Prapavessis, H. (2019). The effects of classroom-based dynamic seating interventions on academic outcomes in youth: A systematic review. *Learning Environments Research*, 22(2), 153–171.

Seckman, A., Paun, O., Heipp, B., Stee, M., Keels-Lowe, V., Beel, F., & Delaney, K. R. (2017). Evaluation of the use of a sensory room on an adolescent inpatient unit and its impact on restraint and seclusion prevention. *Journal of Child and Adolescent Psychiatric Nursing*, 30(2), 90–97.

Schauder, K. B., & Bennetto, L. (2016). Toward an interdisciplinary understanding of sensory dysfunction in autism spectrum disorder: An integration of the neural and symptom literatures. *Frontiers in Neuroscience*, 10, Article 268.

Schilling, D. L., & Schwartz, I. S. (2004). Alternative seating for young children with autism spectrum disorder: Effects on classroom behavior. *Journal of Autism and Developmental Disorders*, 34, 423–432.

Steinbrenner, J. R., Hume, K., Odom, S. L., Morin, K. L., Nowell, S. W., Tomaszewski, B., Szendrey, S., McIntyre, N. S., Yucesoy-Ozkan, S., & Savage, M. N. (2020). *Evidence-based practices for children, youth, and young adults with autism.* The University of North Carolina at Chapel Hill, Frank Porter Graham Child Development Institute, National Clearinghouse on Autism Evidence and Practice Review Team.

Thompson, B., & Blanche, E. I. (2015). The effects of vestibular activity during sensory integration intervention on spontaneous affect and communication within the therapy session. *Sensory Integration Special Interest Quarterly*, 38(2), 1–4.

Williams, M., & Schellenberger, S. (1996). *How does your engine run? A leader's guide to the alert program for self-regulation*. Therapy Works.

Part 2

Pediatric Populations

4 Combining Approaches

Autism Spectrum Disorders

Joanne Flanagan, Gustavo Reinoso, and Erna Imperatore Blanche

Autism spectrum disorder (ASD) is a complex neurodevelopmental disability appearing during the first three years of life as a result of a neurological disorder that affects development in social interaction and communication (Autism Society of America, 2012). The reported number of cases during the last 20 years has increased, with a recent estimate of one in 54 children (Maenner et al., 2020). ASD is highly heritable (Hallmayer et al., 2011), with a recurrence risk of 18.7 percent in the same family (Ozonoff et al., 2011). Families of children with ASD report more significant health care needs and have greater financial, employment, and time burdens compared with families with children with other diagnoses (Kogan et al., 2018). The multifaceted issues presented by this population, make the work of health professionals increasingly more complex, and may be best addressed by family-centered approaches. The objectives of this chapter are:

- To briefly review the core features of ASD and how they relate to sensory processing challenges seen in children with ASD
- To describe early indicators of autism and strengths and challenges across the lifespan
- To present the RAM clinical reasoning model for the evaluation and intervention process of children with ASD
- Discuss evidence-based approaches for the treatment of children with ASD
- To exemplify the utilization of blending different treatment approaches for optimal outcomes

The new criteria for the DSM-V (American Psychiatric Association [APA], 2013) describes two symptoms for the diagnosis of ASD: social communication and interaction deficits and restricted and repetitive behaviors and interests (RRB). In addition, hyper- or hyporesponsiveness to sensory input is now one of four sub-criteria under the restrictive/repetitive behavior domain. Currently several diagnostic tools are

DOI: 10.4324/9781003050810-6

utilized in research and clinical practice. See Table 4.1 for selected diagnostic instruments.

Children with ASD present impairments across many areas leading to challenges in participation in daily tasks (Bölte et al., 2019; Watling et al., 2005). The sensory processing issues that may be linked to these impairments and participation issues include hyper and hypo responsiveness to tactile, auditory, vestibular, olfactory, proprioceptive, and visual input affecting emotion regulation, attention, language, social communication, and motor performance (Ausderau et al., 2016; Baranek et al., 2006; Foss-Feig et al., 2012; Schoen et al., 2009; Tomchek et al., 2015). Understanding the link between sensory processing and the presence of functional and participation issues related to ASD is an ongoing dilemma affecting the choice of interventions used in clinical practice. Table 4.2 provides evidence of the relationship between sensory processing and core ASD symptoms.

In the developmental course, impairments challenge the child's performance in different ways. Children under 12 months often present with motor delays that may be the most salient impairments in participation early on. Decreased postural control and abnormal movement patters are often some of the earliest signs of disruption in the development

Table 4.1 Selected Instruments Commonly Used to Diagnose Individuals With ASD or Assess ASD Symptoms

Instrument, Author(s) & Publisher	*Type of instrument*
Autism Diagnostic Observation Schedule-2 (ADOS-2). (Lord et al., 2012)	Performance diagnostic test, considered a gold standard in children from 12 mo. to adulthood
Autism Diagnostic Interview-Revised (ADI-R). (Le Couteur et al., 2003)	Interview for caregivers of children and adults (mental ages from about 18 months and above)
Social Responsiveness Scale (SRS-2). (Constantino & Gruber, 2012)	Rating scale of social behaviors completed by caregivers or teachers for children from 4 to 18 years of age
Childhood Autism Rating Scale, Second Edition (CARS-2). (Schopler et al., 2010)	Clinician's rating scales and one form for caregivers for children 2 years and up
Gilliam Autism Rating Scale – Second Edition (GARS-3). (Gilliam, 2014)	A rating scale used with parents, teachers and clinicians for ages 3 to 22 years
The Modified Checklist for Autism in Toddlers, Revised with Follow-Up (M-CHAT-R/F) (Robins et al., 2009)	Free caregiver questionnaire for children ages 16–30 months
Screening Tool for Autism in Toddlers and Young Children (STAT™) (Stone et al., 2000)	A play-based screening instrument for children 2–3 years of age

Table 4.2 Sensory Processing Difficulties Related to Core Symptoms of ASD

CORE SYMPTOMS OF ASD	RELATIONSHIP TO SENSORY PROCESSING
Social Communication and Interaction Domain • Deficits in social-emotional reciprocity • Deficits in nonverbal communicative behaviors • Deficits in developing, maintaining, and understanding relationships)	Sensory dysregulation impacts social functioning (Thye et al., 2018) Tactile sensitivity is associated with attention difficulties, including inattentive and hyperactive symptoms (Ashburner et al., 2008) Tactile, olfactory, and auditory hypo responsiveness and total scores in the Short Sensory Profile (SSP) – related to decreased communication (Baker et al., 2008; Tomchek et al., 2015) Sensory seeking related to decreased socialization (Baranek et al., 2018; Tomchek et al., 2015) Hyper responsiveness related to decreased socialization (Liss et al., 2006)
Repetitive and Restrictive Behaviors Domain • Repetitive speech or motor movements or use of objects • Insistence on sameness • Restricted interests • Hyper- or hypo-responsiveness to sensory input) (APA, 2013).	Maladaptive behaviors related to patterns of sensory processing (Baker et al., 2008; Lane et al., 2010) Hyper response to touch relates to rigid and inflexible behaviors, repetitive verbalizations, visual stereotypes, abnormally focused attention (Baranek et al., 1996; Foss-Feig et al., 2012) Somatosensory discrimination related to motor deficits (Zetler et al., 2019)

of the nervous system and suggest a later diagnosis of ASD (Estes et al., 2015; Flanagan et al., 2012; Nickel et al., 2013).

As the child grows, the impairments impacting participation change. School-age children with ASD often present impairments in social skills, executive functions, emotion regulation, and praxis that play an important role in establishing relationships and feelings of competence; difficulties in these areas have been linked to decreased participation in physical, and social leisure activities (Hilton et al., 2008; Maddox et al., 2018; Orsmond & Kuo, 2011; Potvin et al., 2013).

In adolescence and adulthood, mental health issues become the most salient impairments affecting participation. Individuals with ASD are at higher risk for depression, anxiety, and other psychosocial issues (Strang et al., 2012; White et al., 2018). These challenges have been linked to social isolation and poor academic and job performance (see Table 4.3

Table 4.3 ASD Features According to ICF (based on Bölte et al., 2019)

	Body Structures and Functions	Activity	Participation
Under 36 months	Decreased muscle tone Atypical motor and postural development Sensory processing anomalies including decreased tolerance of touch or auditory input Repetitive behaviors, Poor digestive functions Delayed speech Hyper- or hypo-responsiveness	Feeding difficulties Delays in social interactive play (i.e., pointing, orientation to name, anticipation) Decreased copying and imitation skills used in language and simple ADLs.	Decreased participation in play Delayed acquisition of IADL such self-feeding, dressing,
36 months to adolescence	Hyper and hypo responsiveness to sensory experiences become more evident Impairments in executive functions and emotional regulation results in decreased drive/motivation, decreased attention, memory, basic and higher cognitive functions necessary for organized behavior Decreased perceptual-motor functions affect praxis.	Decreased social skills and language development. Maladaptive behaviors become more salient. Copying and imitations skills are delayed Difficulty learning to write and read. Difficulty handling stress	Ability to develop and understand relationships Decreased engagement in diverse physical, organized sports, and social leisure activities Decreased ability to participate in IADL (toileting, dressing, preparing a meal, using transportation Decreased classroom and community participation
Adolescence and adulthood	Anxiety Depression Difficulties with emotion regulation, slow processing, and executive functions.	Depression and other psychosocial issues Behavioral issues interpersonal interactions?	Increased isolation Decreased participation in leisure activities Social communication Difficulty getting and maintaining a job. Poor academic performance

for examples of autism specific impairments and associated activity and participation restrictions according to the ICF-CY).

Impairments, activity limitations, and decreased participation highlight the need for a comprehensive assessment of functional deficits followed by a combination of intervention approaches focusing on primary neurophysiologic disorders and secondary behavioral anomalies and how these deficits affect participation (Perrot-Beaugerie et al., 1990).

Step 1: Gathering Information on the Child's Functional Problems and Diagnostic Considerations

Functional and participation difficulties tied to the reason for consulting an occupational therapist may include maladaptive behaviors, emotional dysregulation, decreased attention, poor social skills, decreased ideational abilities, and decreased imitation and motor planning skills. One of the goals during the evaluation is to assess if the child's functional issues relate to sensory processing, as the choice of intervention approaches will partially depend on these factors.

A comprehensive evaluation includes information obtained from the caregiver and the referral source; skilled clinical observations preferably in a naturalistic setting; and standardized testing data if possible. The assessment tools administered are often determined by the child's age and ability to follow directions. Commonly used assessments with this population are:

- Ages and Stages Questionnaire (ASQ-3™, ASQ:SE-2™)
- Bayley IV
- MSEL
- PDMS-2
- MABC-2
- BOT-2
- Vineland Adaptive Behavior Scales – Third Edition (VABS-3)
- Pediatric Evaluation of Disability Inventory-Computer Adaptive Test for Autism Spectrum Disorders

Refer to the assessment table in Appendix A for more information.

Children may present with a variety of sensory processing disorders, requiring assessment of the child's responses to sensory input with a variety of methods including non-structured and structured observations, parent questionnaires and, when possible, standardized measures of sensory processing. The sensory evaluation tools chosen to assess the child need to focus on all sensory systems and discern between hypo and hyper responsiveness to specific sensory inputs as affecting arousal regulation, social interaction, and adaptive behaviors.

Step 2: Identify Difficulties Affecting Movement, Social Interactions, Emotional Stability, and Adaptive Behavior

This step relies heavily on the clinicians' reasoning and clinical judgment to complete the four phases that help organize the analysis of the information collected during Step 1. The following case (Box 4.1) provides an example of this method of reasoning, organizing information gathered from Step 1 and then encompassing the four phases of Step 2.

First Phase: Listing Observable Problematic Behaviors

In the left-hand column, Jenny's clinician organizes the information by listing objective observations of behaviors obtained through standardized parent questionnaires, background information, parent interview of the occupational history, and clinical observations (See Table 4.1).

Second Phase: Organizing Observations and Generating Hypotheses

Next, Jenny's clinician identifies at least two hypotheses for each problematic behavior. For example, the behavior of "*waving hands*" can have the hypotheses of seeking proprioceptive input for modulation (which could be compared to scores on the COP-R), or "poor regulation of behaviors," and the behavior of "*temper tantrums*" may be related to sensory modulation or decreased motor planning. The following list includes the therapist's observations on the left column and the possible interpretations on the right column (see Table 4.4). The therapist uses existing evidence to link the behaviors to sensory processing or to other areas of development. Weighing in other potential issues will help her decide which intervention approaches to utilize and if using SI as a frame of reference should be the primary or secondary choice.

Third Phase: Counting Data Points and Culminating in a Conclusion

Jenny's occupational therapist weighs the number of data points supporting a specific hypothesis by counting the number of behaviors backing each hypothesis (see number in parentheses after each interpretation in bottom of Table 4.4). In Jenny's case, motor planning difficulties are supported by seven behaviors, postural control is supported by four behaviors, proprioceptive issues are supported by five behaviors, hyper responsiveness to touch is supported by five behaviors, and decreased attention is supported by five behaviors. In addition, there are a number of behaviors linked to the diagnosis of ASD which may be related to signs of sensory-motor issues. The standardized data supporting the

Box 4.1   Jenny's Case Study

Jenny is a 5-year-old girl diagnosed with ASD, who was referred to occupational therapy because of temper tantrums, tendency to falls and crashes, emotional outbursts, and aggressive behaviors. She attended an Applied Behavioral Analysis (ABA) based preschool program where the focus was on expressive language development. During the evaluation in the pre-school setting, the therapist realized that Jenny became frustrated during challenging motor tasks. Her vocalizations became high-pitched screaming sounds which got louder as she became frustrated. When asked to copy a construction with blocks during the administration of standardized testing, Jenny did not try to imitate building a four-block train but stacked blocks. The clinician was unable to complete standardized performance-based assessment. In the classroom, Jenny held her hands over her ears when peers were loud and made high-pitched vocalizations when touched. Stereotypical behaviors were also observed such as flicking and waving her fingers in front of her face.

The therapist observed Jenny in a sensory gym and noticed Jenny's poor proximal joint alignment and a tendency to support herself on available surfaces. Jenny also tended to walk on her toes and elevate her shoulders. During motor activities, she had difficulty balancing and performing motor activities, such as jumping and hopping, climbing over objects, and catching a ball. Jenny's therapist also completed the Comprehensive Observations of Proprioceptive Processing (COP-R).

From administering the SSP, COP-R and parent interview, the therapist found that Jenny was a picky eater and did not like soft, lumpy slimy foods. She also did not like to wear socks, have her hair washed or cut, and screamed when her mother put lotion on her body. She had less of a response to bumping into things or falling than children her own age. She did not appear to hear what was said to her and also did not tend to notice others leaving or entering a room. She also had difficulty donning and doffing clothing.

During fine motor activities, Jenny made high-pitched sounds when presented with finger paint. Additionally, she was not observed to use appropriate pressure with objects, such as balls and crayons, and imitated lines but was unable to copy simple shapes. The following list includes the therapist's observations, the left column describes the observations and the right column the possible interpretations. The therapist's hypothesis focused on Jenny's difficulties in relating to objects and people, motor planning possibly related to sensory responsiveness and discrimination difficulties and decreased proprioceptive processing.

Table 4.4 Reasoning in Action Model: Jenny

First Phase: Data (Issues in participation, observations, other available information)	Second Phase: Hypotheses Generation/ Interpretations
Reason for referral: *wave hands and flicks fingers in front of face*	Poor regulation Seeking proprioception/hypo-responsive to proprioception Stress
Parent interview: temper tantrums when teeth are brushed *or during grooming tasks*	Hyper responsiveness to touch Decreased attention
Parent interview: *history of toe walking, which was also observed in the clinic*	Idiopathic toe walking control Proprioceptive seeking Hyper responsiveness to touch
Parent interview: *does not like lotion on her body*	Hyper responsiveness to touch
Parent interview*: does not assist in donning and doffing clothing*	Decreased motor planning Decreased attention
Parent interview and observation: *emotional outburst without apparent reason*	Task is challenging – decreased motor planning Change in the environment (novelty) Unrelated stress Hyper-responsiveness to sensory input Physical ailment
Parent interview: *bumping into things or falling does not appear to bother the child*	Hyporesponsiveness to proprioception/ somatosensation, seeking input Decreased attention Decreased postural control Decreased motor planning
Parent interview: *does not respond to name, does not appear to hear what is said to her*	Hyporesponsiveness to auditory input Decreased level of arousal
Parent interview: *does not tend to notice others leaving or entering a room*	Hyporesponsiveness to visual input Decreased level of arousal Decreased attention
Observation in the classroom: *sat in chair briefly, but often wandered around classroom*	Poor postural control affecting the ability to sit still Decreased attention Poor regulation
Observation in the classroom: *when tapped lightly on the back, child makes a high-pitched screaming sound*	Hyperresponsive to touch
Observation in the classroom: *inadequate joint alignment when holding a pencil and immature grasp*	Decreased use of proprioceptive feedback -hypo responsiveness to proprioception Poor motor control -Decreased intrinsic muscle strength
Observation in the classroom: *made a high-pitched sound and waved hands when finger paint is presented.*	Hyperresponsive to touch

(*Continued*)

First Phase: Data (Issues in participation, observations, other available information)	Second Phase: Hypotheses Generation/ Interpretations
Observation in the classroom: *when children talk loudly at school, the child put hands over ears.*	Hyperresponsive to auditory input
Observation in the classroom: did not talk to other children.	Decreased social interaction
Observation in specialized setting: *unable to copy circle, square or triangles*	Motor planning difficulties Visual perception difficulties
Observation in the playground: stood in the corner touching/ playing with leaves	Decreased social interaction Hyperresponsive to sensory input Decreased ideation
Observation in the specialized setting: *was not observed to use appropriate pressure with crayon.*	Decreased proprioceptive processing Decreased intrinsic muscle strength
Observation in the specialized setting: *difficulty jumping and hopping, climbing over objects*	Motor planning difficulties Decreased postural control
Observation in the specialized setting: *moves from one object to another without engaging, has a limited play repertoire*	Motor planning difficulties Decreased ideation
Observation in the specialized setting: increased vocalizations when she chooses to swing	Hyporesponsiveness to vestibular input
Standardized testing: *not able to complete performance-based assessment*	Motor planning difficulties Decreased attention Behavioral regulation
Standardized testing (Short Sensory Profile): *scored clinically significant in tactile sensitivity, sensory seeking, low energy/weak, and below average in visual/auditory sensitivity: She is a picky eater; does not like to wear socks and does not like having her hair washed or cut.*	Hyperresponsiveness to touch Decreased proprioceptive processing/ seeking Auditory sensitivity

Third Phase: Counting Data points and Conclusion

Most often Observed Signs
Decreased motor planning (7)
Decreased postural control (3)
Decreased attention (5)
Hyper responsiveness to touch (5)
Decreased proprioceptive feedback/seeking (5)

ASD Related Signs
Decreased regulation
Arousal level
Increased stress

(*Continued*)

Table 4.4 (Continued)

First Phase: Data (Issues in participation, observations, other available information)	Second Phase: Hypotheses Generation/ Interpretations
Decreased social interaction Decreased ideation Possible physical ailment	

Other Possible Explanations that Need Further Exploration
Fluctuating responsiveness to auditory input
Overall sensitivity to input
Seeking proprioceptive input to regulate behavior
Vestibular processing
Oral-motor and feeding

Box 4.2   Hypothesis Generation

Jenny has a motor planning problem, which affects her participation in functional activities. She has a limited play repertoire and difficulty initiating, planning and executing novel movement sequences. These behaviors may be related to proprioceptive and tactile processing; vestibular, visual and auditory processing needs to be further explored.

---

observations made about motor planning, postural control, and modulation difficulties are also weighed in the conclusion.

Fourth Phase: Relating the Identified Difficulties to the Reason for Referral or to Participation

Finally, the evaluator links the conclusion with the reason for referral or the participation issues. Jenny's therapist reports that:

- The aggressive behavior may be due to not only motor planning difficulties but also challenges in sensory processing affecting participation in daily activities supported by the observations and standardized testing from parental report.
- Difficulty with communication may contribute to her emotional responses and behavioral regulation.
- Self-helps skills may be related to poor motor planning skills related to difficulty receiving and interpreting tactile and proprioceptive input.
- The clinician needs to further determine to what extent executive functions and other ASD symptoms impact her performance

---

Box 4.3   Relationship to Participation

Jenny's challenges in her participation in daily activities may relate to sensory processing issues. She exhibits hyperresponsiveness to certain tactile and auditory input, particularly when the input is unexpected, imposed, or when in a multisensory environment. Feeding issues may be related to sensory processing, but this area will need to be further assessed. She may also respond negatively to situations that are stressful. Difficulty with communication may contribute to her emotional response.

Decreased postural control and motor planning abilities and her need to seek out proprioceptive input throughout the day results in disorganized behavior, which may increase in stressful situations. Sensory related as well as other ASD related challenges (executive functions, ideation, attention) impact this child's overall participation in daily occupations.

Step 3: Intervention

Given that individuals diagnosed with ASD present distinct issues in many areas of development, interventions may require using multiple approaches. Although the evidence with children with ASD is constantly changing, certain ingredients are part of the most successful intervention programs, supported by evidence and recommended in practice guidelines. These ingredients include: a combination of carefully measured evidence-based interventions; the consideration of the impact of sensory processing, contexts, and executive functions on participation, the development of meaningful partnerships with caregivers and the systematic measurement of outcomes. These ingredients are further described later.

Successful Intervention Programs Require More Than One Frame of Reference and Blending Various Approaches

Most intervention programs for children with ASD that demonstrate effectiveness, include more than one method of intervention. Generally, they include behavioral intervention principles emanating from an understanding of ABA, social interactive functions, self-regulation (Dawson & Burner, 2011; Prizant et al., 2003) and adaptive behavior (Zwaigenbaum et al., 2015). Subgroups of children with ASD may respond differently to intervention approaches – there is a need for interventions that take into consideration the child's and family's individual characteristics rather than the diagnosis.

The Center for Disease Control (2019) classifies the current interventions for individuals with ASD as: Behavioral and communication approaches, dietary approaches, medication, and complementary and alternative medicine. The organization identifies the following interventions as behavioral and communication approaches including a) ABA (Applied Behavioral Analysis) and its different types, such as Discrete Trial Training (DTT), Early Intensive Behavioral Intervention (EIBI), Pivotal Response Training (PRT), Verbal Behavior Intervention (VBI); b) Floor time/DIR (Developmental, Individual Differences, Relationship-Based Approach); c) TEACH (Treatment and Education of Autistic and Related Communication/handicapped Children); d) Occupational Therapy & Sensory Integration; e) Speech and Language Therapy and f) PECS (Picture Exchange Communication System).

The most up-to-date evidence-based practice guideline was recently published by Steinbrenner et al. (2020) and included 567 intervention studies with positive results in at least one outcome of interest. Specific outcomes included academic/pre-academic, adaptive/self-help, challenging behaviors, cognitive, communication, joint attention, mental health, motor, play, self-determination, school readiness, social and vocational areas of functioning and participation. Response to consumers' needs and choice is also considered part of the evidence (Sackett et al., 1996; Sackett, 1997).

Often combined in several intervention programs are principles of Applied Behavioral Analysis (ABA) which includes several forms and techniques (e.g., early intensive behavioral intervention), the Developmental, Individual-Difference, Relationship-Based approach (DIR) commonly referred to as "Floor time approach"; and Sensory Integration (SI). For more in depth information on these approaches, please refer to the Appendix B and references provided.

Combining Approaches

Sensory integration principles may be beneficial with a young child with emotional regulation issues. However, if the child presents behavioral issues not related to sensory processing, then a behavioral approach may be the choice of intervention. Developmental capacities, which are considered foundations for relating, thinking, and communicating, may be treated with DIR. The motor difficulties of children with ASD are widely documented (Matson et al., 2011; Fournier et al., 2010) and in current research literature there is an increasing emphasis on defining the motor constellation of problems of children with ASD as the same as those diagnosed with DCD (see Chapter 6, DCD/Dyspraxia, ASD/DCD dual diagnosis.). A comprehensive assessment contributes to the working hypothesis for the motor difficulty and its functional and participation implications. Thus, before initiating intervention, it should be determined if the child's presenting motor difficulty relates to ideation, motor planning, motor skill or to a specific body structure issue. New assessments such as the COP-R and clinical reasoning may help tease out these difficulties (Blanche et al., 2021). Examples of the differential aspects of clinical reasoning and intervention strategies are outlined in Tables 4.5 and 4.6.

Table 4.5 Clinical Reasoning of Motor Challenges for Intervention Planning

Hypothesized motor difficulty	Clinical reasoning	Interventions targets
Praxis	– Determine if related to sensory processing – Planning, arranging and sequencing motor acts during physical interactions with the environment	Opportunities for novel and unstructured play. Use of equipment, toys, and possibilities for environmental arrangement. Particular emphasis on imitation, as well as actions that utilize the whole body, oral structures, and dramatic elements of play.
Motor skills	– Consider data related to knowledge of the skill as well as previous learning and practice in various contexts – Consider the task, specific feedback, and a teaching model	Provide opportunities for acquiring specific motor skills followed by appropriate instruction and feedback. Consider the context, task complexity and the immediate need to work on transferring the learned skills to different contexts
Physical components	-Consider if function and participation are significantly impaired by factors such as strength, fatigue, postural control, range of motion, etc.	Utilize principles of neurodevelopmental treatment (NDT) and strength training. Carefully provide opportunities for play during designed challenges that include antigravity, resistance, co-contraction, weight bearing and weight shifting during aligned, stable and moving conditions.

Table 4.6 Example Interpreting and Addressing Behaviors: Emotional Outburst

Interpretations/ **Triggers**	Potential Solutions
Ideation Challenges	Start with a choice of purpose or tasks; if the child does not choose, choose for him/her and simultaneously work on joint attention while choosing and moving towards the object.

(Continued)

Table 4.6 (Continued)

Interpretations/ **Triggers**	Potential Solutions
	Provide opportunities for symbolic play with adaptive behaviors that relate to labeling objects, purposeful use of play materials, demonstrating a sense of having a goal in mind to achieve a specific purpose.
Novelty in the environment	At first, do not alter the environment. Slowly introduce change. Help the child maintain a regulated state while sensory experiences are increased in the environment.
Stereotyped behaviors	Child has been identified as presenting proprioceptive processing issues, determine if providing proprioception in the way of weight bearing, pushing, pulling, or moving equipment reduces the presence of waving and helps the child regulate his/her behavior
Task has become too challenging	Respond by reducing the challenge, break down the steps of the activity and slowly increase the challenge. Address motor planning, copying and imitation in different contexts.
Hyperresponsive to touch and other sensory input	Reduce all sensory input in the environment, then test the child's response to touch and other sensory input. Provide tactile experiences that the child can control, include deep pressure and proprioception while receiving touch.
Physical ailment	Children with ASD often experience gastric and sleep problems. A referral to a primary care physician should be completed

Addressing sensory processing issues affecting regulation and motor performance requires careful consideration of how sensory processing affects function and participation (Case-Smith et al., 2015; Watling & Hauer, 2015). Sensory integration may be a choice for intervention if the child's sensory processing difficulties impact motor planning and postural control. Other interventions such as motor task training based on motor learning and NDT may also be beneficial (see approaches table in Appendix B).

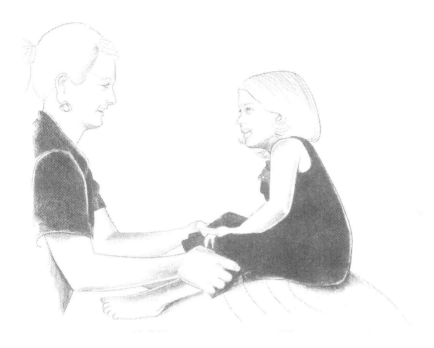

Figure 4.1 Sensory Integration and Processing

In this picture the therapist is blending at least 3 intervention approaches while the child is sitting on a ball: Sensory integration by increasing the amount of vestibular and proprioceptive input provided (bouncing), NDT by facilitating postural reactions, and DIR by facilitating interaction with the child. Increased vestibular input also facilitates expressive language and eye contact.

Parents Need to be Part of the Intervention Program

Parent education and parent-implemented interventions are crucial when working with children and adolescents with ASD. Several approaches and manualized interventions include a parental component (Ingersoll, 2010; Ingersoll & Dvortcsak, 2019; Solomon et al., 2014; Turner et al., 2010). Parents of children with autism are often exposed to conflicting information regarding intervention options, which adds a layer of confusion when making decisions about their child (Levy et al., 2016). Therefore, it is critical that families of children with ASD are involved in a shared decision-making process when selecting approaches and measuring their effectiveness. Some of the most effective intervention programs for young children with ASD include the parents not only as decision makers, but also as interveners (Hardan et al., 2014; Ingersoll, 2010; Kasari et al., 2006, 2015).

Problems in Executive Functions Are Part of the Diagnosis

Daily routine of activities has shown to be beneficial (Knüppel et al., 2019). Problems in executive functions are part of the ASD diagnosis. Executive functions include attention to task, regulation of behavior and flexibility; issues in these areas are often encountered when treating children with ASD. If the assessment indicates a link between sensory processing and attention to tasks and regulation of behavior in a child, then treatment using a SI approach is warranted. Decreased attention and regulation can be linked to hypo and hyper responsiveness to vestibular input. These sensory areas can be targeted while working on attention and purposeful interaction with the environment. Simultaneously promoting behavioral flexibility needs a combination of treatment approaches as tolerance to changes needs to be encouraged and monitored. For example, a daily routine of activities has shown to be beneficial (Knüppel et al., 2019).

The Context of the Intervention

The context of the intervention for children with ASD often depends on the funding source. Most children receive services through early intervention services, public school systems and private funding. The services are provided individually and in groups; in the home, the community, or specialized clinics. Thus, service provision varies greatly from state to state and across different countries.

The goals of the intervention will vary according to the context of the intervention. The goals of children seen in groups often focus on the development of social skills, while the goals established for children seen individually in a specialized setting focus on the development of specific skills such as speech, motor planning, and specific adaptive skills related to daily tasks and occupations.

Systematic Measurement of Performance Is Pivotal

Systematic measurement of the presenting problems and the outcomes of the intervention are pivotal. Interpretation of specialized assessment requires clinical reasoning to determine the variety of intervention approaches. The treating therapist examines the available evidence, including the individual characteristics and needs of the client to provide the context for generalization of that evidence. Systematic measurements of performance can include standardized assessments, single subject design, and Goal Attainment Scales (GAS). Standardized assessments are used pre and post intervention to measure effectiveness of the intervention. Single subject design has been used in multiple studies supporting the use of sensory integration or sensory experiences (Case-Smith & Bryan, 1999; Watling & Dietz, 2007). Goal Attainment Scales

(GAS) methodology, originally described by Kiresuk and Sherman (1968), has been adopted in intervention studies for families of children with autism (Schaaf et al., 2014; Pfeiffer et al., 2011).

Although well designed controlled studies can deal with the inherent issues of reliability (the therapist judging the overall impact of his/her own intervention) and construct validity (the measure utilized may not adequately address the construct being measured), therapists should exercise caution and use additional measures to capture the outcomes of their intervention such as video reviews and information from professionals observing and/or working with the child in context (aides, teachers, and community partners [yoga instructors, horseback riding, swimming lessons, etc.]).

Jenny's Intervention Guided by Best Practice

Jenny's therapist carefully evaluated Jenny and used the gathered information and current literature on best practice to guide the best selection of interventions strategies. The therapist discovered that sensory related as well as other ASD related challenges (executive functions, ideation, attention) impact Jenny's overall participation in daily occupations. See Table 4.4, which outlines the clinical reasoning model. The therapist's goals focused on Jenny's participation in daily tasks such as eating and dressing, as well as increasing her participation in academic environments. The specific impairments to be targeted include hyperresponsiveness to touch and auditory input and the ability to imitate and copy.

Jenny's therapist initially combined DIR with a SI approach to develop a rapport and start where the child was at developmentally, while providing calming sensory input for modulation. For example, the therapist incorporated Jenny's favorite toy and imitated what Jenny was doing with this toy to establish a rapport and become her play partner. Then, the therapist expanded the play repertoire to improve developmental capacities. The therapist also included parent engagement, coaching the parents how to be a play partner with Jenny during shared play interactions to also expand Jenny's capacities. Because proprioceptive processing impacts both motor planning and modulation, the intervener starts the intervention by offering activities that provide this type of input, paired with simple imitation of gestures and slowly adding sound and touch to increase tolerance. The therapist also offers therapeutic play activities which incorporate deep touch for modulation. As the session continues, the intervener offers a number of activities that the child needs to choose from by pointing, looking, or approaching them. Once the choice has been made, the therapist ensures that the activity is carried through, thus working on ideation, organization, motor planning or any other identified challenges.

Sensory integration intervention approaches are used to address motor planning and hyper responsiveness to touch and auditory as well as to decrease the need for large amounts of proprioception to help the child regulate her level of arousal and cope with the environmental demands. Behavioral interventions are used to help chaining/scaffolding the challenges presented to the child and the use of appropriate reinforcements when the child meets the challenge; and a focus on executive functions as impacting goal directed behaviors, short term memory and ideation is added to the intervention. Jenny's clinician also may use behavioral strategies such as a picture schedule and a visual timer. Jenny's mother began to see increased participation in Jenny's daily occupations and her teacher reported increased participation at school. In addition, Jenny appeared happier and more willing to try novel tasks and interact with her peers.

Conclusion

Autism is a heterogeneous disorder with each child presenting a unique occupational profile. Practitioners need to evaluate children with ASD by choosing the best, most comprehensive methods to gather information to identify the child's unique strengths, functional problems, and participation issues. The clinician uses clinical reasoning and the best available evidence to analyze the evidence and generate hypotheses about the link between problematic behaviors, sensory processing, and other areas of development. In this chapter a detailed case study utilizing this clinical reasoning model is presented. Through this careful analytical process, the clinician designs evidence-based intervention programs using a variety of approaches to ultimately improve the child's overall participation in daily occupations.

References

American Psychiatric Association [APA] 2013 DSM-V.

Ashburner, J., Ziviani, J., & Rodger, S. (2008). Sensory processing and classroom emotional, behavioral, and educational outcomes in children with autism spectrum disorder. *American Journal of Occupational Therapy, 62*(5), 564–573. https://doi.org/10.5014/ajot.62.5.564

Ausderau, K. K., Sideris, J., Little, L. M., Furlong, M., Bulluck, J. C., & Baranek, G. T. (2016). Sensory subtypes and associated outcomes in children with autism spectrum disorders. *Autism Research, 9*(12), 1316–1327. https://doi.org/10.1002/aur.1626

Autism Society of America. (2012, January 3). *About autism.* http://autism-society.org

Baker, A. E. Z., Lane, A., Angley, M. T., & Young, R. L. (2008). The relationship between sensory processing patterns and behavioural responsiveness in autistic disorder: A pilot study. *Journal of Autism and Developmental Disorders, 38*(5), 867–875. https://doi.org/10.1007/s10803-007-0459-0

Baranek, G. T., David, F. J., Poe, M. D., Stone, W. L., & Watson, L. R. (2006). Sensory experiences questionnaire: Discriminating sensory features in young children with autism, developmental delays, and typical development. *Journal of Child Psychology and Psychiatry, 47*(6), 591–601. https://doi.org/10.1111/j.1469-7610.2005.01546.x

Baranek, G. T., Foster, L. G., & Berkson, G. (1996). Tactile defensiveness and stereotyped behaviors. *The American Journal of Occupational Therapy, 51*(2), 91–95. https://doi.org/10.5014/ajot.51.2.91

Baranek, G. T., Woynaroski, T. G., Nowell, S., Turner-Brown, L., DuBay, M., Crais, E. R., & Watson, L. R. (2018). Cascading effects of attention disengagement and sensory seeking on social symptoms in a community sample of infants at-risk for a future diagnosis of autism spectrum disorder. *Developmental Cognitive Neuroscience, 29,* 30–40. doi:10.1016/j.dcn.2017.08.006. Epub 2017 Aug 14

Blanche, E. I., Reinoso, G., & Blanche Kiefer, D. (2021). *Structured observations of sensory integration-motor (SOSI-M) & comprehensive observations of proprioception (COP-R).* Administration Manual. Academic Therapy Publications (ATP).

Bölte, S., Mahdi, S., de Vries, P. J., Granlund, M., Robison, J. E., Shulman, C., Swedo, S., Tonge, B., Wong, V., Zwaigenbaum, L., Segerer, W., & Selb, M. (2019). The Gestalt of functioning in autism spectrum disorder: Results of the international conference to develop final consensus international classification of functioning, disability and health core sets. *Autism, 23*(2), 449–467. https://doi.org/10.1177/1362361318755522

Case-Smith, J., & Bryan, T. (1999). The effects of occupational therapy with sensory integration emphasis on preschool-age children with autism. *American Journal of Occupational Therapy, 53,* 489–497. https://doi.org/10.5014/ajot.53.5.489

Case-Smith, J., Weaver, L. L., & Fristad, M. A. (2015). A systematic review of sensory processing interventions for children with autism spectrum disorders. *Autism, 19*(2), 133–148. https://doi.org/10.1177%2F1362361313517762

Center for Disease Control and Prevention. (2019, January 3). *Data and statistics.* www.cdc.gov/ncbddd/autism/data.html

Constantino, J. N., & Gruber, C. P. (2012). *Social responsiveness scale: SRS-2.* Western Psychological Services.

Dawson, G., & Burner, K. (2011). Behavioral interventions in children and adolescents with autism spectrum disorder: A review of recent findings. *Current Opinion in Pediatrics, 23*(6), 616–20. https://doi.org/10.1097/MOP.0b013e32834cf082

Estes, A., Zwaigenbaum, L., Gu, H., St. John, T., Paterson, S., Elison, J. T., Hazlett, H., Botteron, K., Dager, S. R., Schultz, R. T., Kostopoulos, P., Evans, A., Dawson, G., Eliason, J., Alvarez, S., Piven, J., & IBIS network. (2015). Behavioral, cognitive, and adaptive development in infants with autism spectrum disorder in the first 2 years of life. *Journal of Neurodevelopmental Disorders, 7*(1), 24. https://doi.org/10.1186/s11689-015-0117-6

Flanagan, J. E., Landa, R., Bhat, A., & Bauman, M. (2012). Head lag in infants at risk for autism: A preliminary study. *American Journal of Occupational Therapy, 66*(5), 577–585. https://doi.org/10.5014/ajot.2012.004192

Foss-Feig, J. H., Heacock, J. L., & Cascio, C. J. (2012). Tactile responsiveness patterns and their association with core features in autism spectrum disorders. *Research in Autism Spectrum Disorders, 6*(1), 337–344. https://doi.org/10.1016/j.rasd.2011.06.007

Fournier, K. A., Hass, C. J., Naik, S. K., et al. (2010). *Journal of Autism Developmental Disorder, 40,* 1227. https://doi.org/10.1007/s10803-010-0981-3

Gilliam, J. E. (2014). *Gilliam autism rating scale* (3rd ed.) (GARS-3). Pro-Ed.

Hallmayer, J., Cleveland, S., Torres, A., Phillips, J., Cohen, B., Torigoe, T., Miller, J., Fedele, A., Collins, J., Smith, K., Lotspeich, L., Croen, L. A., Ozonoff, S., Lajonchere, C., Grether, J. K., & Risch, N. (2011). Genetic heritability and shared environmental factors among twin pairs with autism. *Archives of General Psychiatry, 68*(11), 1095–1102. https://doi.org/10.1001/archgenpsychiatry.2011.76

Hardan, A. Y., Gengoux, G. W., Berquist, K. L., Libove, R. A., Ardel, C. M., Phillips, J., & Minjarez, M. B. (2014). A randomized controlled trial of pivotal response treatment group for parents of children with autism. *Journal of Child Psychology and Psychiatry, 56,* 884–892. doi:10.1111/jcpp.12345

Hilton, C. L., Crouch, M. C., & Israel, H. (2008). Out-of-school participation patterns in children with high-functioning autism spectrum disorders. *American Journal of Occupational Therapy, 62*(5), 554–563. https://doi.org/10.5014/ajot.62.5.554

Ingersoll, B. (2010). Brief report: Pilot randomized controlled trial of reciprocal imitation training for teaching elicited and spontaneous imitation to children with autism. *Journal of Autism and Developmental Disorders, 40,* 1154–1160. doi:10.1007/s10803-010-0966-2.

Ingersoll, B., & Dvortcsak, A. (2019). *The project ImPACT manual for parents.* Guilford.

Kasari, C., Freeman, S., & Paparella, T. (2006). Joint attention and symbolic play in young children with autism: A randomized controlled intervention study. *Journal of Child Psychology and Psychiatry, 47*(6), 611–620. https://doi.org/10.1111/j.1469-7610.2005.01567.x

Kasari, C., Gulsrud, A., Paparella, T., Hellemann, G., & Berry, K. (2015). Randomized comparative efficacy study of parent-mediated interventions for toddlers with autism. *Journal of Consulting and Clinical Psychology, 83,* 554–563. doi:10.1037/a0039080.

Kiresuk, T. J., & Sherman, R. E. (1968). Goal attainment scaling: A general method for evaluating comprehensive community mental health programs. *Community Mental Health Journal, 4,* 443–453.https://doi.org/10.1007/BF01530764

Knüppel, A., Telléus, G. K., Jakobsen, H., & Lauritsen, M. B. (2019). Characteristics of young adults with autism spectrum disorder performing different daytime activities. *Journal of Autism and Developmental Disorders, 49*(2), 542–555. https://doi.org/10.1007/s10803-018-3730-7.

Kogan, M. D., Vladutiu, C. J., Schieve, L. A., Ghandour, R. M., Blumberg, S. J., Zablotsky, B., . . . Lu, M. C. (2018). The prevalence of parent-reported autism spectrum disorder among US children. *Pediatrics, 142*(6), e20174161. https://doi.org/10.1542/peds.2017-4161.

Lane, A. E., Young, R. L., Baker, A. E. Z., & Angley, M. T. (2010). Sensory processing subtypes in autism: Association with adaptive behavior. *Journal of Autism and Developmental Disorders, 40*(1), 112–122. https://doi.org/10.1007/s10803-009-0840-2

Le Couteur, A., Lord, C., & Rutter, M. (2003). *The autism diagnostic interview – Revised (ADI-R).* Western Psychological Services.

Levy, S. E., Frasso, R., Colatonio, S., Reed, H., Stein, G., Brag, F. K., . . . Fiks, A. G. (2016). Shared decision making and treatment decisions for young children with autism spectrum disorder. *Academic Pediatric Association, 16*(6), 571–578. doi:10.1016/j.acap.2016.04.007

Liss, M., Saulnier, C., Fein, D., & Kinsbourne, M. (2006). Sensory and attention abnormalities in autistic spectrum disorders. *Autism, 10*(2), 155–172. https://doi.org/10.1177/1362361306062021

Lord, C., Rutter, M., DiLavore, P., Risi, S., Gotham, K., & Bishop, S. L. (2012). *ADOS-2, autism diagnostic observation schedule* (2nd ed.), Part 1: Modules 1–4. Western Psychological Services.

Maddox, B. B., Cleary, P., Kuschner, E. S., Miller, J. S., Armour, A. C., Guy, L., Kenworthy, L., Schultz, R. T., & Yerys, B. E. (2018). Lagging skills contribute to challenging behaviors in children with autism spectrum disorder without intellectual disability. *Autism, 22*(8), 898–906. https://doi.org/10.1177/1362361317712651

Maenner, M. J., et al. (2020). Prevalence of autism spectrum disorder among children aged 8 years – Autism and developmental disabilities monitoring network, 11 Sites, United States, 2016. *MMWR. Surveillance Summaries, 69.*

Matson, M. L., Matson, J. L., & Beighley, J. (2011). Comorbidity of physical and motor problems in children with autism. *Research in Developmental Disabilities, 32*(6), 2304–2308. https://doi.org/10.1016/j.ridd.2011.07.036.

Nickel, L. R., Thatcher, A. R., Keller, F., Wozniak, R. H., & Iverson, J. M. (2013). Posture development in infants at heightened versus low risk for autism spectrum disorders. *Infancy, 18*(5), 639–661. https://doi.org/10.1111/infa.12025.

Orsmond, G. I., & Kuo, H.-Y. (2011). The daily lives of adolescents with an autism spectrum disorder: Discretionary time use and activity partners. *Autism, 15*(5), 579–599. https://doi.org/10.1177/1362361310386503

Ozonoff, S., Young, G. S., Carter, A., Messinger, D., Yirmiya, N., Zwaigenbaum, L., . . . Hutman, T. (2011). Recurrence risk for autism spectrum disorders: A baby siblings research consortium study. *Pediatrics, 128*(3), e488–e495. https://doi.org/10.1542/peds.2010-2825

Perrot-Beaugerie, A., Hameury, L., Adrien, J. L., Garreau, B., Pepe, M., & Sauvage, D. (1990). Autism in infants and young children. The value of early diagnosis. *Annals of Pediatrics, 37*(5), 287–293.

Pfeiffer, B. A., Koenig, K., Kinnealey, M., Sheppard, M., & Henderson, L. (2011). Effectiveness of sensory integration interventions in children with autism spectrum disorders: A pilot study. *American Journal of Occupational Therapy, 65*(1), 76–85. https://doi.org/10.5014/ajot.2011.09205

Potvin, M.-C., Snider, L., Prelock, P., Kehayia, E., & Wood-Dauphinee, S. (2013). Recreational participation of children with high functioning autism. *Journal of Autism and Developmental Disorders, 43*(2), 445–457. https://doi.org/10.1007/s10803-012-1589-6

Prizant, B. M., Wetherby, A. M., Rubin, E., & Laurent, A. C. (2003). The SCERTS model: A transactional, family-centered approach to enhancing communication and socioemotional abilities of children with autism spectrum disorder. *Infants & Young Children, 16*(4), 296–316.

Robins, D. L., Fein, D., & Barton, M. (2009). The modified checklist for autism in toddlers, revised with follow-up (M-CHAT-R/F). *Pediatrics, 133*, 37–45. https://doi.org/10.1542/peds.2013-1813

Sackett, D. L. (1997, February). Evidence-based medicine. In *Seminars in perinatology* (Vol. 21, No. 1, pp. 3–5). WB Saunders. https://doi.org/10.1016/s0146-0005(97)80013-4

Sackett, D. L., Rosenberg, W. M. C., Gray, J. A. M., Haynes, R. B., & Richardson, W. S. (1996). Evidence based medicine. *BMJ: British Medical Journal, 313*(7050), 170–171. https://doi.org/10.1136/bmj.312.7023.71

Schaaf, R. C., Benevides, T., Mailloux, Z., Faller, P., Hunt, J., van Hooydonk, E., . . . Kelly, D. (2014). An intervention for sensory difficulties in children with autism: A randomized trial. *Journal of autism and developmental disorders, 44*(7), 1493–1506. doi:10.1007/s10803-013-1983-8

Schoen, S. A., Miller, L. J., Brett-Green, B. A., & Nielsen, D. M. (2009). Physiological and behavioral differences in sensory processing: A comparison of children with autism spectrum disorder and sensory modulation disorder. *Frontiers in Integrative Neuroscience, 3,* 29. https://doi.org/10.3389/neuro.07.029.2009

Schopler, E., Reichler, R. J., & Renner, B. R. (2010). *The childhood autism rating scale (CARS).* WPS.

Solomon, R., Van Egeren, L. A., Mahoney, G., Quon Huber, M. S., & Zimmerman, P. (2014). PLAY project home consultation intervention program for young children with autism spectrum disorders: A randomized controlled trial. *Journal of Developmental and Behavioral Pediatrics, 35,* 475–485. doi:10.1097/DBP.0000000000000096

Steinbrenner, J. R., Hume, K., Odom, S. L., Morin, K. L., Nowell, S. W., Tomaszewski, B., Szendrey, S., McIntyre, N. S., Yücesoy-Özkan, S., & Savage, M. N. (2020). *Evidence-based practices for children, youth, and young adults with autism.* The University of North Carolina at Chapel Hill, Frank Porter Graham Child Development Institute, National Clearinghouse on Autism Evidence and Practice Review Team. https://doi.org/10.1007/s10803-020-04844-2

Stone, W. L., Coonrod, E. E., & Ousley, O. Y. (2000). Brief report: Screening tool for autism in two-year-olds (STAT): Development and preliminary data. *Journal of Autism and Developmental Disorders, 30*(6), 607. https://doi.org/10.1023/a:1005647629002

Strang, J. F., Kenworthy, L., Daniolos, P., Case, L., Wills, M. C., Martin, A., & Wallace, G. L. (2012). Depression and anxiety symptoms in children and adolescents with autism spectrum disorders without intellectual disability. *Research in Autism Spectrum Disorders, 6*(1), 406–412. https://doi.org/10.1016/j.rasd.2011.06.015

Thye, M. D., Bednarz, H. M., Herringshaw, A. J., Sartin, E. B., & Kana, R. K. (2018). The impact of atypical sensory processing on social impairments in autism spectrum disorder. *Developmental Cognitive Neuroscience, 29,* 151–167. https://doi.org/10.1016/j.dcn.2017.04.010

Tomchek, S. D., Little, L. M., & Dunn, W. (2015). Sensory pattern contributions to developmental performance in children with autism spectrum disorder. *American Journal of Occupational Therapy, 69*(5), 6905185040p1–6905185040p10. https://doi.org/10.5014/ajot.2015.018044

Turner, K. M., Markie-Dadds, C., & Sanders, M. R. (2010). *Practitioner's manual for primary care triple P.* Triple P International Pty.

Watling, R. L., & Dietz, J. (2007). Immediate effect of Ayres's sensory integration – based occupational therapy intervention on children with autism spectrum disorders. *American Journal of Occupational Therapy, 61,* 574–583. https://doi.org/10.5014/ajot.61.5.574

Watling, R. L., & Hauer, S. (2015). Effectiveness of ayres sensory integration® and sensory-based interventions for people with autism spectrum disorder: A systematic review. *American Journal of Occupational Therapy, 69*(5), 6905180030p1–6905180030p12. https://doi.org/10.5014/ajot.2015.018051

Watling, R. L., Tomchek, S., & LaVesser, P. (2005). The scope of occupational therapy services for individuals with autism spectrum disorders across the lifespan. *The American Journal of Occupational Therapy, 59*(6), 680. https://doi.org/10.5014/ajot.59.6.680

White, S. W., Simmons, G. L., Gotham, K. O., Conner, C. M., Smith, I. C., Beck, K. B., & Mazefsky, C. A. (2018). Psychosocial treatments targeting anxiety and depression in adolescents and adults on the autism spectrum: Review of the latest research and recommended future directions. *Current Psychiatry Reports, 20*(10), 82. https://doi.org/10.1007/s11920-018-0949-0

Zetler, N. K., Cermak, S. A., Engel-Yeger, B., & Gal, E. (2019). Somatosensory discrimination in people with autism spectrum disorder: A scoping review. *American Journal of Occupational Therapy, 73*(5), 7305205010p1–7305205010p14. https://doi.org/10.5014/ajot.2019.029728

Zwaigenbaum, L., Bauman, M. L., Stone, W. L., Yirmiya, N., Estes, A., Hansen, R. L., . . . Wheterby, A. (2015). Early identification of autism spectrum disorder: Recommendations for practice and research. *Pediatrics, 136*(1), 10–40. https://doi.org/10.1542/peds.2014-3667C

5 Combining Approaches
Cerebral Palsy

*Mary Hallway, Eirini V. Liapi,
and Anna Sampsonidis*

Objectives

1. To define Cerebral Palsy (CP) using evidence-based practice guidelines and research
2. To describe the evaluation process for children with CP, highlighting measures utilized in clinical practice and research with children with CP
3. To identify primary outcomes and interventions utilized when treating children with CP
4. To illustrate using the RAM, a case of a child with CP, from initial referral through the blending of treatment approaches in a therapy session.

Cerebral Palsy (CP) is one of the most common causes of physical disability in early childhood, occurring worldwide in two of 1000 births (Blair et al., 2018; Novak et al., 2020). Considered a non-progressive disorder, CP affects posture, movement, and functional performance throughout the lifetime. Despite the static nature of the lesion associated with CP, the clinical manifestation of a child's motor profile can change over time due to maturation of the central nervous system, internal processes, and the impact of personal and environmental factors. Rosenbaum et al., 2007 defines CP as a group of permanent developmental disorders of movement and posture, causing activity limitation. The motor disorder although a hallmark to CP are often accompanied by disturbances in sensory, perceptual, and cognitive systems which can affect functional performance as much as the motor disorder (Rosenbaum et al., 2007; Phipps & Roberts, 2012).

More recently, Blair et al. (2018) added to the definition that clinical signs of CP might change with the child's development, although the cerebral abnormalities neither resolve nor deteriorate.

These definitions highlight the primary motor challenges presented by this population and emphasize difficulties in other areas, including sensory processing. Although CP is a disorder of posture and movement,

DOI: 10.4324/9781003050810-7

therapists cannot treat children with CP with interventions exclusively targeting motor performance but also need to consider interventions addressing other areas. This chapter describes the multisystem impairments in children with CP, the impact on the child's function and the need to integrate multiple therapeutic perspectives.

Classifications of CP

Historically, CP has been classified by motor type and limb distribution (i.e., hemiplegia, diplegia, etc.). While helpful, it does not inform our understanding of the functional abilities of individuals with CP. More recently developments in classification systems used internationally and based on both the heterogeneity and the severity of CP, group individuals with CP based on functional abilities. Table 5.1 describes current systems covering various domains.

Table 5.1 Classification Scales for Children with CP

Classification scale (age range)	Description	Reference
The Gross Motor Function Classification System Expanded and Revised (GMFCS-E&R) (1–18 years)	Classifies systematically gross motor functional abilities and limitations in everyday life. Emphasizes mobility, sitting and transfers with focus on self-initiated movements. Has predictive value at 1–2 years for walking at 12 years.	Palisano, Rosenbaum, Bartlett et al., 2008; Palisano, Rosenbaum, Walter et al., 2008; Paulson & Vargus-Adams, 2017; Rosenbaum et al., 2008
Manual Ability Classification System (MACS) (4–18 years) Mini-MACS (1–4 years)	Classifies how well children use both hands to handle objects in daily activities and the amount of assistance needed to manipulate objects.	Eliasson et al., 2007, 2017
Communication Function Classification System (CFCS) (2–18 years)	Classifies how communication is expressed and received and includes all communication methods, i.e., Assistive Augmented Communication (AAC) systems, etc.	Hidecker et al., 2011; Paulson & Vargus-Adams, 2017

(Continued)

Table 5.1 (Continued)

Classification scale (age range)	Description	Reference
Eating and Drinking Ability Classification System (EDACS) (3 years and up)	Measures eating and drinking and assistance required	Sellers et al., 2013, 2019

Clinicians can use these functional classification systems to identify performance changes over time that are due to maturation or intervention (Reddihough, 2009). They help clinicians and researchers define a level of functional performance in children with CP, based on an ordinal scale ranging from one to five. The higher GMFCS and MAC levels (4–5) correlate with less functional independence, i.e., mobility, daily living skills and social participation (Kuijiper et al., 2010; Palisano, Rosenbaum, Bartlett et al., 2008; Phipp s & Roberts , 2012; Voorman et al., 2006) and the lower levels (1–2) with the highest functional performance. Based on the GMFCS, more significant sensory processing issues and their behavioral outcomes correlate with less functional mobility and less functional independence, i.e., self-care and social (Mishra, 2020; Pavão et al., 2020). The following section describes impairments and activity-participation restrictions present in children with CP.

Impairments, Activity Limitation, and Participation Issues Associated With CP

Unlike the CP classification systems focused on specific functional domains, the 2014 Comprehensive and Common Brief International Classification of Function (ICF) Core Sets for Children and Youth with CP delineates the importance of measuring or addressing individuals' abilities at all levels (Schiariti et al., 2015). The comprehensive core set for children with CP from birth to 18 years contains 135 ICF categories which comprehensively describe the array of problems specific to CP. Brief core sets are a selection of ICF categories drawn from the comprehensive core sets broken down into age ranges.

The Brief ICF Core Set for Children and Youth with CP (Schiariti et al., 2015) identifies the most common multisystem impairments in body functions; intellectual functions, sleep, motivation, mental functions of language, higher-level cognitive functions, seeing/hearing, sensation of pain, mobility of joints, muscle tone, and control of voluntary movement (Schiariti et al., 2018). However, sensory impairments co-exist with these impairments. For example, somatosensory deficits appear

Table 5.2 Sensory Features in Children With CP According to ICF

Body Function Sensory System	Body Function Movement Performance, Postural Control	Activity-Participation Skills, Self-Care Life Situations
Difficulties with somatosensory processing including: • tactile localization • 2-point discrimination • stereognosis • vibration • proprioception – joint position sense	Associated with: • Greater deviations in trunk and upper limb kinematics in wrist and elbow • Deficits in the temporal coordination of placing and releasing objects • Reduced ankle plantarflexion muscle force production and strength • Impairments in postural responses and balance • Difficulties with extremity movements • Difficulties with motor planning	Associated with: • Non-use of the affected extremity. • Decreased fine motor control and hand function • Difficulties with gait; walking speed and step length • Difficulties with lower body dressing
Inefficient sensory integration of visual and vestibular inputs Difficulties with multisensory information and modulation of sensory information	Associated with: • Decreased postural control and postural stability • Visual-vestibular impairments contributing to body position in space and postural control deficits	Associated with: • Poor fine motor coordination • Difficulties with activity level, attention and emotional responses

Source: Bleyenheuft & Gordon, 2013; de Campos et al., 2014; Gupta et al., 2017; Kinnucan et al., 2010; Klingels et al., 2012; Kurz et al., 2015; Mailleux et al., 2017; McLaughlin, 2005; Pavão et al., 2014; Pavão & Rocha, 2017; Riquelme & Montoya, 2010; Saavedra & Goodworth, 2019; Zarkou et al., 2020

in 31–97 percent of children with CP, including deficits in both upper extremities (UE) in unilateral CP (Auld et al., 2012a; Taylor et al., 2017). Furthermore, compared to typical children, differences in vestibular system functions (peripheral and central) can co-occur with motor control issues (Akbarfahimi et al., 2016; Almutairi et al., 2020) and oculomotor difficulties such as saccades and smooth pursuits influence participation (Almutairi et al., 2018). Evidence included in Table 5.2 integrates sensory and motor features of children with CP and their relation to activity and participation.

The complexity of issues observed in children with CP supports the need for a comprehensive assessment, which we describe next.

Gathering Information on the Child's Functional Problems and Diagnostic Considerations

An assessment process for children with CP needs to include information obtained from caregivers and referral sources, observations of posture and movement during performance of functional activities, and performance-based standardized assessment (Stammer, 2016). Furthermore, clinicians need to identify qualitative differences in movement and outcome measures that detect change in functional skills and performance.

Assessment of Sensory Processing

Identifying sensory impairments in children with CP is equally important to identifying movement issues (see Table 5.2). The challenge is that many assessment tools designed to identify sensory processing disorders and praxis in other populations have not been designed for children with CP and have decreased validity with this population (Imperatore Blanche & Nakasuji, 2001). For example, sensory histories for children with CP can be guided with caution by using the Sensory Profile-2. One can use a sensory questionnaire modified by Imperatore Blanche and Nakasuji (2001) designed specifically for children with CP. Table 5.3 includes a revised version of this questionnaire that can be used to guide the observation of sensory processing; such observations also need to be included in the evaluation. Clinicians can use both formal and informal tactile registration test such as the Semmes Weinstein monofilament kit, and discrimination tests such as those measuring tactile localization, two-point discrimination (static and moving), and stereognosis of familiar objects (Auld et al., 2011, 2012b; Krumlinde-Sundholm, 2007). The Sense_Assess© Kids, a standardized, norm-referenced assessment for children 6–15 years, assesses UE somatosensory processing in children with CP (Taylor et al., 2017).

Recommendations to consider in the evaluation of sensory processing:

- Don't assume a child with a head tilt has a motor issue. It could relate to a vestibular or visual issue.
- Don't assume that difficulties with head control against gravity, low postural tone and other postural problems are solely motor issues; assess vision, vestibular, and proprioceptive processing.
- Don't assume that difficulties with LE placing, weight-bearing/weight shifting during transitions or when using a walker are solely neuromuscular and musculoskeletal system issues; consider proprioception.
- Don't assume that motor coordination issues in children with hemiplegia are solely motor issues; consider somatosensation and motor planning.
- Don't assume that pocketing food in the cheeks after chewing is solely an oral motor control issue; consider somatosensation.

Table 5.3 Signs of Sensory Processing Questions in Children With CP

Tactile Processing

Hyperresponsiveness to Tactile Input

Does the child:

1. Object to therapeutic handling when not wearing clothes?
2. Avoid touching or playing with messy materials such as sticky, wet, gooey, slimy, textured objects?
3. Dislike tactile based grooming activities i.e., haircut, brushed/combed, washed, face washed? (Dunn, 2014)
4. Push therapist hand away from his or her body?
5. Show an emotional or aggressive response to touch i.e., biting, hitting. (Dunn, 2014)
6. Show increased response to pain? (Riquelme & Montoya, 2010)

Hyporesponsiveness to Tactile Input or Poor Tactile Discrimination

Does the child:

1. Fail to localize/respond when touched?
2. Seek out messy play i.e., sand, dirt, playdoh, glue?
3. Fail to notice when walking across different textured surfaces with bare feet?
4. Fail to notice when objects are placed in the hand?
5. Fail to notice messy hands or face? (Dunn, 2014)
6. Fail to notice when food is left in the mouth after chewing?
7. Fail to notice clothing twisted or not in the correct position on the body?

Proprioceptive Processing

Does the child:

1. Lean into the therapist's hands during therapeutic handling techniques?
2. Fail to adjust the body in response to changes in position?
3. Show difficulties placing and weight shifting through their lower extremities while walking and has a short step length if they are a child with hemiplegia or diplegia? (Kurz et al., 2015)
4. Grasp with too much or too little force i.e., holds object firmly or to light?
5. Show difficulties when pushing/pulling extremities in and out of the sleeve or pant leg during dressing?
6. Push firmly on the surface to release objects?

Vestibular Processing

Hyperresponsiveness to Gravity and/or Vestibular

Does the child:

1. Object to being moved backward in space even when the trunk and head are supported?
2. Express fear/anxiety when placed on a bench or large treatment ball with feet off the ground?
3. Dislike having the feet leave the supporting surface or the ground?
4. Become anxious in open spaces or looking down such as when descending stairs?

Hyporesponsive to Vestibular

Does the child:

1. Fail to notice or react when moved in space?
2. Seek out opportunities for movement i.e., bouncing, jumping, running around in circles, swinging?
3. If the child has the motor abilities, does the child like to twirl and spin? Or does the child like to be twirled and spun passively?

(Continued)

Table 5.3 (Continued)

4. Seek opportunities to throw self-backwards when held in sitting on a therapeutic ball?
5. Fail to activate neck and trunk extensor muscles when linear movement is provided?

Yes, answers to more than one question in a section may be suggestive of sensory process-
ing deficits that need further attention.
Source: Unless otherwise noted, questions in this list are adapted from Imperatore
Blanche, E. & Nakasuji, B. (2001). Sensory Integration and the Child with Cerebral Palsy
(pp. 3–6) in Smith Roley et al., Eds. *Sensory Integration with Diverse Populations*. Therapy Skill
Builders. Adapted with permission

Assessment of Posture and Movement

Examining all systems influencing postural control and functional movement is essential with this population. For example, vestibular processing impacts the ability to detect changes in relation to gravity, and hence
impacts postural responses. The evaluation of posture and movement
includes range of motion, skeletal alignment, force production, muscle
tone, muscle recruitment, timing and sequencing, selective voluntary
motor control and sensory processing (Stammer, 2016).

Based on the neurodevelopmental treatment (NDT) Contemporary
Practice Model™, examining posture and movement requires visual obser-
vation/analysis of movement and handling (Stammer, 2016). Movement
analysis occurs while a child engages in functional activities and includes
observations of biomechanical and kinesiological components (i.e., the
base of support), alignment and planes of movement, and components
of postural control (i.e., active, anticipatory, reactive) (Saavedra & Goodworth, 2019; Stammer, 2016) The influence of sensory systems on postural responses also needs to be considered. Handling during functional
activities allows clinicians to observe the child's responses to changes in
alignment and base of support, and to confirm previously observed neuromuscular and musculoskeletal impairments (Stammer, 2016).

Evaluating the impact of the environment on movement performance
and modifying it to observe a child's response is also an essential assessment component.

Performance-Based Standardized Assessments of Motor Performance

The most commonly utilized tools with this population are presented on
Table 5.4.

See the assessment table in Appendix A for further details on these
assessments and the evidence supporting their use with children with
CP. The Canadian Occupational Performance Measure (COPM) (Law
et al., 2019), although not specifically designed to measure outcomes for
children with CP, is also an effective tool.

Table 5.4 Assessment of Motor Performance for Children with CP

Activities – Participation	Body Functions		
	UE Activity	Bimanual performance	Balance Measures
Pediatric Evaluation of Disability Inventory-Computer Adaptive Test (PEDI-CAT) (Haley et al., 2020)	Melbourne Unilateral Upper Limb Assessment-2 (Randall et al., 2012)	Assisting Hand Assessment (AHA) (Krumlinde-Sundholm et al., 2014)	The Pediatric Balance Scale (Yi et al., 2012)
ACTIVLIM-CP (Bleyenheuft et al., 2017)		Hand Assessment for Infants (Krumlinde-Sundholm et al., 2017)	
Gross Motor Function Measurement (GMFM) (Russell et al., 2013)		Both Hands Assessment (BoHA) (Elvrum et al., 2017)	

Blending Intervention Approaches in Children with CP

Multisystem impairments influencing activities and participation in children with CP support the need for multiple therapeutic approaches. Treatment approaches utilized with children with CP include neurodevelopmental treatment (NDT), sensory integration, strength and endurance training, electrical stimulation and constraint-induced movement therapy (CIMT) (Anttila et al., 2008; Novak et al., 2020). Appendix B describes some of these treatment approaches. The combination of therapeutic approaches and their provision at the right time is essential to improving outcomes in children with CP (Pape, 2016). This section discusses how motor control approaches commonly blend with sensory integration principles in the treatment of children with CP.

Sensory Based Interventions and Sensory Integration

Sensory impairments in children with CP impact behavior or motor function (Pavão et al., 2014). Although research on the sensory impairments in various types of CP exists, there is limited evidence supporting effective interventions addressing sensory issues (Bleyenheuft & Gordon, 2013; Cascio, 2010; de Campos et al., 2014; Pavão & Rocha, 2017). Research using principles or elements of SI with children with CP supports positive outcomes in attention, motor performance, and daily living activities (Bumin & Kayihan, 2001; Kashoo & Ahmad, 2019; Shamsoddini & Hollisaz, 2009; Tahir et al., 2019).

Furthermore, several approaches developed to target motor performance use sensory input as a secondary aid without it being the main focus of the intervention. Proprioceptive and tactile inputs are provided through resistance and pressure in suit therapies, universal exercise units, kinesiotaping, and NDT facilitation of weight-bearing/ shifting. By increasing the amount of input provided, these interventions focusing on motor performance can also target somatosensory issues in children with low registration. Whole body vibration may also provide limited evidence for producing changes in motor performance (Novak et al., 2020), but may impact somatosensory processing. Also, using elements of sensory integration treatment (SIT) such as the use of a sensory-rich environment, attention to sensory modulation issues, and tapping into the child's intrinsic motivation and sensory preferences can help modify the conditions in a therapy session so that children can tolerate handling and increase engagement.

For example, interventions that specifically target impaired somatosensory processing in children with hemiplegic CP (HCP) have been found to be most effective when focusing on active sensory discrimination instead of using passive movement and exposure to non-specific sensations (McLean et al., 2017). Pairing tasks requiring sensory discrimination with functional UE motor activities seems to improve UE somatosensory processing and motor functions (Barati et al., 2020; McLean et al., 2017; Salkar et al., 2017). There is limited evidence for using vestibular input with children with CP, however a program combining exercise-based vestibular stimulation with NDT with children with CP identified improvements in individualized goals (Topley et al., 2020; Tramontano et al., 2017).

Recommendations for using elements of SIT with children with CP (Auld & Johnston, 2017; Barati et al., 2020; Imperatore Blanche & Nakasuji, 2001; Hosseini et al., 2015; McLean et al., 2017; Nanawati et al., 2020; Salkar et al., 2017; Topley et al., 2020; Tramontano et al., 2017):

- Children with hemiplegia often present signs of somatosensory discrimination issues and decreased motor planning; therefore, utilize active tactile discrimination activities, visual attention, and active self-initiated motor planning activities after acquiring the essential movement components.
- Children with severe motor disorders and tactile hyperresponsiveness who require intense handling benefit from being allowed to wear a compression vest or suit and provide deep pressure rather than light touch during handling.
- Children with decreased tone, low arousal, and hyporesponsiveness to sensory input benefit from more intense forms of vestibular and proprioceptive input.

- Children with diplegia with deficits in LE somatosensory processing benefit from SIT-enhancing tactile registration and discrimination, and proprioception.
- Children with ataxia presenting with deficits in proprioception, visual and vestibular processing benefit from activities that combine proprioception with vision and self-initiated movement.

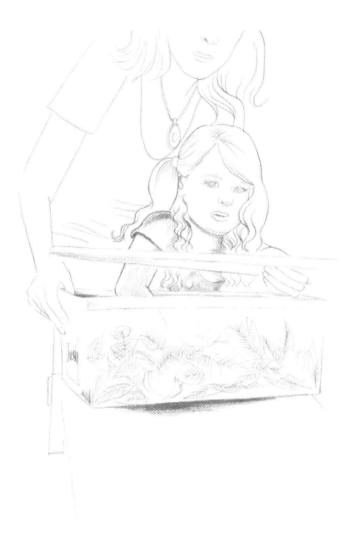

Figure 5.1 Actively searching for different objects in a container of feathers with the child's more affected UE and less affected UE to address tactile discrimination. This activity can be graded up by having the child find the object without using vision or graded down by allowing the child to use vision with tactile discrimination to locate objects.

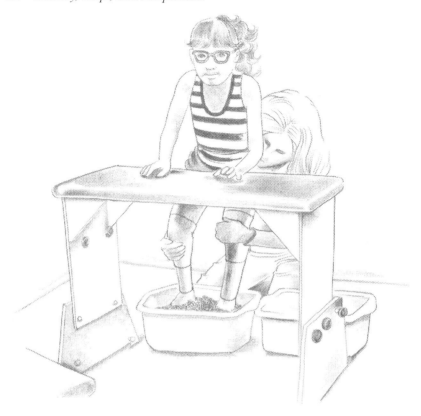

Figure 5.2 Enhancing tactile registration and proprioception while facilitating lower extremity alignment as the child actively marches with bare feet in a tactile bin filled with dry beans, rice or other textures.

Neurodevelopmental Treatment

The updated NDT Contemporary Practice Model™ emphasizes the performance of functional tasks and recognizes the importance of repetition and practice in learning new movement skills and in active participation in the execution of movement during therapeutic handling (Howle, 2016).

Studies indicate that NDT is effective for children with CP, depending on various factors utilized in its therapeutic application (Lee et al., 2017; Park & Kim, 2017; Sah et al., 2019). Factors that contribute to treatment effectiveness related to the updated definition of NDT include dosage (intensive versus conventional) and emphasis on task-oriented intervention with resulting changes noted in balance, gross motor function, and reduced spasticity in children with CP. NDT therapeutic handling can support a child in learning efficient and effective movements when functional task acquisition and individualized goals are the focus (Kalisperis et al., 2019; Sakzewski et al., 2009). NDT has traditionally used sensory feedback to elicit motor responses; thus it is imperative clinicians understand the role of sensory processing in movement performance. It is also evident that SIT cannot be used without having an understanding of motor performance. Analyzing movement components and using therapeutic handling based on NDT may provide the necessary tools to use SIT when intervening with children with CP.

Table 5.5 describes other interventions used with children with CP and their relationship to sensory processing.

Table 5.5 Motor Interventions and Their Relationship to SI

Approach	*Purpose and Evidence*	*Relationship to sensory*
Strength Training	Interventions involve effort against progressive resistance, which can improve motor outcomes. It helps increase muscle strength and improve motor function, i.e., walking, stair climbing, range of motion at the hip (Liao et al., 2007).	Can be blended with SI in that by its very nature, the use of active resistance provides proprioceptive feedback to muscles and joints, which could be coupled with an adaptive motor response targeting motor planning.
Electrical Stimulation NMES/FES	Can potentially improve ROM, selective motor control, strength in both LE and UE, gait, locomotor efficiency, balance, and core strengthening while being minimal to non invasive, painless and with minimal side effects (Bosques et al., 2016; Johnston et al., 2004; Moll et al., 2017; Van der Linden et al., 2008; Wright & Granat, 2000).	NMES/FES increases the sensory input to a specific muscle group helping children with CP localize the necessary muscles to perform a movement, i.e., wrist extension (Mäenpää et al., 2004). Simultaneously blending it with elements of SI can enhance distal UE proprioceptive feedback, for example, engaging in a task that requires active wrist extension against resistance, i.e., using a weighted rolling pin to roll out playdoh.

(Continued)

Table 5.5 (Continued)

Approach	Purpose and Evidence	Relationship to sensory
Constraint-Induced Movement Therapy (CIMT)	CIMT is used with children with HCP and involves two key features: (1) restraint of the less-involved UE, and (2) intensive structured practice with the involved UE (Eliasson et al., 2013). Variations on CIMT include; • Modified constraint-induced movement therapy (mCIMT), which varies in the type of restriction, practicing and duration • Hybrid CIMT where bimanual training (BT) is added • Forced use where practice is unstructured during UE restraint Improves UE manual ability, bimanual performance, daily activity performance, movement patterns, and participation (Eliasson et al., 2013; Gelkop et al., 2014; Ganesh & Das, 2019; Novak et al., 2020). Blending CIMT, BT and NDT improves postural symmetry in sitting and standing (Holland et al., 2019). Baby-CIMT, mCIMT and bimanual motor training have been more recently applied to infants with HCP with positive outcomes (Chamudot et al., 2018, Eliasson et al., 2018).	SI can be integrated with any variation of CIMT by having the child engage in unimanual tasks requiring enhanced somatosensory input, i.e., throwing a weighted ball, playing with sand, finding objects without vision (Maitre et al., 2020). NDT can be blended with CIMT and SI by addressing optimal trunk and UE alignment during task performance. Refer to Chapter 15, Program 4 for an example of blending SI, forced use and bimanual training.
Bimanual Training (BT)	UE bimanual training for children with HCP based on motor learning principles and includes intense practice of structured bimanual tasks to increase UE use and function.	Intensive BT can improve stereognosis and manual abilities however doesn't improve tactile spatial discrimination (Saussez et al., 2018); therefore, blending BT with elements of SI can

(Continued)

Approach	Purpose and Evidence	Relationship to sensory
	Improves UE movement quality and efficiency and bimanual performance during activities of daily living (Klepper et al., 2017; Novak et al., 2020).	enhance other areas of UE tactile discrimination i.e., localization, spatial discrimination, etc. (Kuo et al., 2016)
Motor Task Training: Principles from Motor Learning Theory	Focuses on practicing context-specific tasks using principles from motor learning (refer to Appendix B). Clinicians can incorporate these principles into other treatment approaches for children with CP, i.e., CIMT, NDT, SI. Evidence supports the use of training based interventions focusing on goal-directed functional tasks using self-initiated movements with children with CP (Novak et al., 2020).	In SI, motor learning theories are used to describe motor planning (see Figure 2.4). They can assist in the retention and generalization of new motor tasks in slightly altered contexts, i.e., throwing different size beanbags into containers.
Adeli / Therasuit as an example of an adjunct intervention	A dynamic garment that provides alignment of segments, resistance for muscle strengthening and enhanced proprioceptive feedback while the child performs active movements and can be used with the Universal Exercise Unit/Cage (Martins et al., 2015) Improves proximal stability, gross motor function, gait (Karadağ-Saygı & Giray, 2019). Combined with NDT improves spatial temporal aspect of gait (Kim et al., 2016)	Blending the Adeli/Therasuit with SI can enhance proprioceptive feedback while the child performs motor tasks (Yardımcı-Lokmanoğlu et al., 2019).

Blending Approaches when Treating a Child with CP

A thorough evaluation of the child's impairments impacting partici-pation guides a clinician's choice of treatment approaches. Blend-ing treatment approaches with children with CP can occur within a treatment session or overtime. Within a treatment session, combining approaches occurs simultaneously or with one approach playing a primary role and another a complementary role. For example, when blending NDT and SI simultaneously with a child who is hyporesponsive to vestibular input and has a low arousal level, it is recommended to use moving equipment while handling the child to increase the level of arousal and antigravity trunk extension while simultaneously facilitating trunk alignment, postural control, and muscle activation. Over time the child's needs and goals will determine which approaches to use and how they are blended.

The following case study depicts using the RAM to guide the decision-making process when blending approaches with a child with CP. Table 5.6 summarizes the assessment data and hypothesis.

Box 5.1   Case Study

George was diagnosed with diplegia (CP) and left UE involvement. He began weekly physical therapy at three months old and occupational therapy at fourteen months. At five years, mCIMT was utilized to increase left UE function. At 7 years old, a parent interview was conducted to identify the family's functional concerns and needs. Their concerns included lack of independence at school, like school-related self-care, handwriting and mobility, which the clinicians corroborated. George's evaluation included the following assessment tools; GMFM, Berg Balance Scale (BBS), AHA and Berry-Buktenica Test of Visual Motor Integration (VMI). Subtests from the Sensory Integration and Praxis Test (SIPT) were also utilized; Localization of Tactile Stimuli (LTS), Manual Form Perception (MFP) and Finger Identification (FI). This included skilled observations of movement, sensory responsiveness, and behavior. George was observed in his natural environments to track any possible barriers affecting his participation in his preferred activities, i.e., bike riding, basketball and soccer, chess.

George scored the following on standardized tests:

GMFM: Moderately low scores in standing, lower scores in walking, running & jumping

Pediatric BBS: lower scores in items related to dynamic balance

VMI: Scored below the mean in all categories; lowest scores in subtests Visual Motor Integration (copying) and Motor Coordination.

Table 5.6 Summary of Data, Hypothesis, and Interpretation

First Phase: Data (Issues in participation, observations, other available information)	*Second Phase: Hypotheses Generation/ Interpretations*
Reason for referral and parent interview: • Appears anxious when walking on sand, uneven dirt • Holds onto rail or hand when walking downstairs and going up/ down curbs	• Decreased postural control and balance • Limited LE range of motion (ROM) • Increased muscle tone in LE • Gravitational insecurity
Reason for referral: • Has difficulties pulling pants up	• Decreased postural control and balance • Decreased strength in trunk and LE musculature • Decreased tactile discrimination • Poor motor planning • Poor proprioception
Reason for referral: • Difficulty wiping using toilet paper	• Decreased tactile discrimination • Poor motor planning
Reason for referral: • Difficulties copying from the board,	• Decreased visual perception • Poor motor planning • Hypo responsive to vestibular processing impacting oculomotor control
Observation in a natural environment: • On the playground, leans on others and pulls on them for support, prefers to watch instead of joining play activities	• Poor proprioception • Poor motor planning • Decreased postural control and balance
Observations in a natural environment: • Difficulties kicking a moving ball	• Poor motor planning (anticipatory/ feedforward) • Decreased strength in trunk and LE musculature • Decreased postural control and balance (anticipatory)
Observations during testing: **Maintains head tilted to the right**	• Poor postural control • Visual Impairment • Hyporesponsive to vestibular input
Observations during testing: Difficulties alternate stepping when descending and ascending stairs	• Decreased postural control and balance • Decreased strength in trunk and LE musculature • Limited LE ROM • Increased muscle tone in LE

(Continued)

Table 5.6 (Continued)

First Phase: Data (Issues in participation, observations, other available information)	Second Phase: Hypotheses Generation/ Interpretations
Standardized Testing: AHA – Moderately neglects his left (L) UE during everyday functional tasks.	• Poor proprioception • Increased muscle tone in LUE • Decreased LUE motor coordination
**Subtests from the SIPT *not validated for children with CP used items for structured observations; **LTS and FI subtests.	• Decreased tactile discrimination in both UE • Decreased LUE motor coordination

Third Phase: Counting data points and conclusion

Most often observed signs:
Poor motor planning (5)
Decreased postural control and balance (6)
Increased muscle tone in LE and LUE (3)
Poor proprioception (3)
Decreased tactile discrimination (3)
Decreased strength in trunk and LE musculature (3)
Limited LE ROM (2)
Decreased LUE motor coordination (2)

Other Possible Explanations that Need Further Exploration:
Hyporesponsive to vestibular (1)
Hypo responsive to vestibular processing impacting oculomotor control (1)
Visual Impairment (1)
Visual perception (1)
Gravitational Insecurity (1)

Box 5.2   Case Study Hypothesis Generation

Based on data collection, George demonstrates the following: decreased strength in the trunk and LE musculature, increased LE muscle tone, decreased range of motion and difficulties with postural control and balance for mobility over uneven terrain, curbs and stairs and pulling up his pants. Decreased tactile discrimination and proprioception contribute to moderate neglect of the left UE, motor planning and execution deficits impacting toileting, copying from the board, and play. Deficits in postural control and feedforward motor planning impacted kicking a moving ball.

George's Interventions

Based on the clinical findings of George's strengths and areas of needs, his therapists determined his goals would include: managing curbs and stairs, kicking a ball, pulling up pants, copying from the board and participating during play with peers. Impairments targeted include LE ROM, trunk and LE strength, postural control, tactile discrimination and proprioception, motor planning and execution. George's therapists chose to simultaneously blend NDT and SI as primary interventions while including motor learning theory principles for retention and generalization of new motor skills. George's treatment plan includes the use of the Therasuit, where he receives an intensive therapy model, three hours per day, five days per week, over four weeks. Parent and school staff collaboration focuses on carry over in all environments.

During the session, all activities are implemented while wearing a Therasuit to increase trunk and LE muscle strength and proprioception during movement. The therapist uses NDT therapeutic handling to improve LE range of motion, alignment and strength and activate trunk musculature in all planes while facilitating gait. SI addresses tactile discrimination and proprioception, feedback and feedforward motor planning, and sequencing and timing of new motor tasks while changing parameters in familiar activities. For example, George collaborates in choosing and setting up a new activity. He walks up an inclined ramp pushing a weighted ball with both UE as the therapist facilitates increased stride length by having George step onto textured squares. At the top of the incline, he places the ball into a box. Walking through a Lycra bridge hung on an incline requires George to use both UE for support and motor planning. Tactile – proprioceptive feedback is provided through the resistance and touch pressure offered by the Lycra material. Walking on an uneven surface challenges postural adjustment. Transitioning from the Lycra bridge to a higher platform requires George to recruit trunk rotation, lateral flexion, LE dissociation, and motor planning. At the same time, his therapist facilitates LE dissociation and alignment. George is then required to ascend and descend stairs. George repeats the entire sequence with minor changes to enhance motor learning. Finally, George plays a soccer game with other children to increase feedforward motor planning and spatial organization. Temporal organization/ feedforward is addressed by kicking a stationary ball while standing, followed by walking/running to kick the stationary ball, and finally by running to kick a moving ball. Variability is addressed by using balls with different properties (i.e., weight, size, texture).

Conclusion

Given the multisystem challenges present in children with CP, clinicians need to choose the most comprehensive data gathering methods to identify the strengths, impairments, activity, and participation issues facing each child. The clinical reasoning process leads the clinician to determine which therapeutic approaches should be blended during clinical practice to meet the child's therapeutic goals best and improve participation.

References

Akbarfahimi, N., Hosseini, S., Rassafiani, M., Rezazadeh, N., Shahshahani, S., Ghomsheh, F., & Karimlou, M. (2016). Assessment of the saccular function in children with spastic cerebral palsy. *Neurophysiology, 48*(2), 141–149. https://doi.org/10.1007/s11062-016-9580-z

Almutairi, A., Christy, J., & Vogtle, L. (2018). Vestibular and oculomotor function in children with cerebral palsy: A scoping review. *Seminars in Hearing, 39*(3), 288–304. https://doi.org/10.1055/s-0038-1666819

Almutairi, A., Christy, J., & Vogtle, L. (2020). Psychometric properties of clinical tests of balance and vestibular-related function in children with cerebral palsy. *Pediatric Physical Therapy, 32*(2), 144–150. https://doi:10.1097/PEP.0000000000000682

Anttila, H., Autti-Rämö, I., Suoranta, J., Mäkelä, M., & Malmivaara, A. (2008). Effectiveness of physical therapy interventions for children with cerebral palsy: A systematic review. *BMC Pediatrics, 8*(1). https://doi.org/10.1186/1471-2431-8-14

Auld, M., Boyd, R., Moseley, G., & Johnston, L. (2011). Tactile assessment in children with cerebral palsy: A clinimetric review. *Physical & Occupational Therapy in Pediatrics, 31*(4), 413–439. https://doi.org/10.3109/01942638.2011.572150

Auld, M., Boyd, R., Moseley, G., Ware, R., & Johnston, L. (2012a). Impact of tactile dysfunction on upper-limb motor performance in children with unilateral cerebral palsy. *Archives of Physical Medicine and Rehabilitation, 93*(4), 696–702. https://doi.org/10.1016/j.apmr.2011.10.025

Auld, M., & Johnston, L. (2017). Perspectives on tactile intervention for children with cerebral palsy: A framework to guide clinical reasoning and future research. *Disability And Rehabilitation, 40*(15), 1849–1854. https://doi.org/10.1080/09638288.2017.1312571

Auld, M., Ware, R., Boyd, R., Moseley, G., & Johnston, L. (2012b). Reproducibility of tactile assessments for children with unilateral cerebral palsy. *Physical & Occupational Therapy in Pediatrics, 32*(2), 151–166. https://doi.org/10.3109/01942638.2011.652804

Barati, A., Rajabi, R., Shahrbanian, S., & Sedighi, M. (2020). Investigation of the effect of sensorimotor exercises on proprioceptive perceptions among children with spastic hemiplegic cerebral palsy. *Journal of Hand Therapy, 33*(3), 411–417. https://doi.org/10.1016/j.jht.2019.12.003

Blair, E., Cans, C., & Sellier, E. (2018). Epidemiology of the cerebral palsies. In C. Panteliadis (Eds.), *Cerebral palsy*. Springer. https://doi.org/10.1007/978-3-319-67858-0_3

Bleyenheuft, Y., & Gordon, A. (2013). Precision grip control, sensory impairments and their interactions in children with hemiplegic cerebral palsy: A systematic review. *Research in Developmental Disabilities, 34*(9), 3014–3028. https://doi.org/10.1016/j.ridd.2013.05.047

Bleyenheuft, Y., Paradis, J., Renders, A., Thonnard, J. L., & Arnould, C. (2017). ACTIVLIM-CP a new Rasch-built measure of global activity performance for children with cerebral palsy. *Research in Developmental Disabilities, 60*, 285–294. https://doi.org/10.1016/j.ridd.2016.10.005

Bosques, G., Martin, R., McGee, L., & Sadowsky, C. (2016). Does therapeutic electrical stimulation improve function in children with disabilities? A comprehensive literature review. *Journal of Pediatric Rehabilitation Medicine, 9*(2), 83–99. https://doi.org/10.3233/prm-160375

Bumin, G., & Kayihan, H. (2001). Effectiveness of two different sensory-integration programmes for children with spastic diplegic cerebral palsy. *Disability and Rehabilitation, 23*, 394–399. https://doi.org/10.1080/09638280010008843

Cascio, C. (2010). Somatosensory processing in neurodevelopmental disorders. *Journal of Neurodevelopmental Disorders, 2*(2), 62–69. https://doi.org/10.1007/s11689-010-9046-3

Chamudot, R., Parush, S., Rigbi, A., Horovitz, R., & Gross-Tsur, V. (2018). Effectiveness of modified constraint-induced movement therapy compared with bimanual therapy home programs for infants with hemiplegia: A randomized controlled trial. *American Journal of Occupational Therapy, 72*(6), 7206205010p1. https://doi.org/10.5014/ajot.2018.025981

de Campos, A., Kukke, S., Hallett, M., Alter, K., & Damiano, D. (2014). Characteristics of bilateral hand function in individuals with unilateral dystonia due to perinatal stroke. *Journal of Child Neurology, 29*(5), 623–632. https://doi.org/10.1177/0883073813512523

Dunn, W. (2014). *Sensory Profile™2*. Pearson.

Eliasson, A. C., Krumlinde-Sundholm, L., Gordon, A., Feys, H., Klingels, K., & Aarts, P., et al. (2013). Guidelines for future research in constraint-induced movement therapy for children with unilateral cerebral palsy: An expert consensus. *Developmental Medicine & Child Neurology, 56*(2), 125–137. https://doi.org/10.1111/dmcn.12273

Eliasson, A. C., Krumlinde-Sundholm, L., Rösblad, B., Beckung, E., Arner, M., Öhrvall, A., & Rosenbaum, P. (2007). The manual ability classification system (MACS) for children with cerebral palsy: Scale development and evidence of validity and reliability. *Developmental Medicine & Child Neurology, 48*(7), 549–554. https://doi.org/10.1111/j.1469-8749.2006.tb01313.x

Eliasson, A. C., Nordstrand, L., Ek, L., Lennartsson, F., Sjöstrand, L., Tedroff, K., & Krumlinde-Sundholm, L. (2018). The effectiveness of Baby-CIMT in infants younger than 12 months with clinical signs of unilateral-cerebral palsy; An explorative study with randomized design. *Research in Developmental Disabilities, 72*, 191–201. https://doi.org/10.1016/j.ridd.2017.11.006

Eliasson, A. C., Ullenhag, A., Wahlstrome, U., & Kumlinde-Sundholm, L. (2017). Mini-MACS. Development of the manual ability classification system for children younger than 4 years of age with signs of cerebral palsy. *Developmental Medicine & Child Neurology, 59*, 72–78. https://doi.org/10.1111/dmcn.13162

Elvrum, A.-K. G., Zethræus, B.-M., & Krumlinde-Sundholm, L. (2017). *Both hands assessment administration and scoring manual*. Bversion 1.1 English. Handfast. https://doi.org/10.1080/01942638.2017.1318431

Ganesh, G., & Das, S. (2019). Evidence-based approach to physical therapy in cerebral palsy. *Indian Journal of Orthopaedics, 53*(1), 20. https://doi.org/10.4103/ortho.ijortho_241_17

Gelkop, N., Burshtein, D., Lahav, A., Brezner, A., AL-Oraibi, S., Ferre, C., & Gordon, A. (2014). Efficacy of constraint-induced movement therapy and bimanual training in children with hemiplegic cerebral palsy in an educational setting. *Physical & Occupational Therapy in Pediatrics, 35*(1), 24–39. https://doi.org/10.3109/01942638.2014.925027

Gupta, D., Barachant, A., Gordon, A., Ferre, C., Kuo, H., Carmel, J., & Friel, K. (2017). Effect of sensory and motor connectivity on hand function in pediatric hemiplegia. *Annals of Neurology, 82*(5), 766–780. https://doi.org/10.1002/ana.25080

Haley, S. M., Coster, W. J., Dumas, H. M., Fragala-Pinkham, M. A., & Moed, R. (2020). *Pediatric evaluation of disability inventory computer adaptive test – PEDI CAT: Administration manual*. Pearson.

Hidecker, M., Paneth, N., Rosenbaum, P., Kent, R., Lillie, J., Eulenberg, J., et al. (2011). Developing and validating the communication function classification system for individuals with cerebral palsy. *Developmental Medicine & Child Neurology, 53*(8), 704–710. https://doi.org/10.1111/j.1469-8749.2011.03996.x

Holland, H., Blazek, K., Haynes, M., & Dallman, A. (2019). Improving postural symmetry: The effectiveness of the CATCH (Combined Approach to Treatment for Children with Hemiplegia) protocol. *Journal of Pediatric Rehabilitation Medicine, 12*(2), 139–149. https://doi.org/10.3233/prm-180550

Hosseini, S. A., Ghoochani, B. Z., Talebian, S., Pishyare, E., Haghgoo, H. A., Meymand, R. M., & Zeinalzadeh, A. (2015). Investigating the effects of vestibular stimulation on balance performance in children with cerebral palsy: A randomized clinical trial study. *Journal of Rehabilitation Sciences and Research, 2*, 41–46.

Howle, J. M. (2016). Motor learning in Bierman et al., Eds. In *Neuro-developmental treatment: A guide to NDT clinical practice*. Thieme Medical Publishers Incorporated.

Imperatore Blanche, E., & Nakasuji, B. (2001). Sensory integration and the child with cerebral palsy in Smith Roley et al., Eds. In *Sensory integration with diverse populations*. Therapy Skill Builders.

Johnston, T., & Moore, S. E., Quinn, L. T., & Smith, B. T. (2004). Energy cost of walking in children with cerebral palsy: Relation to the gross motor function classification system. *Developmental Medicine & Child Neurology, 46*. doi:10.1111/j.1469-8749.2004.tb01018.x

Kalisperis, F. R., Shanline, J. M., & Styer-Acevedo, J. (2019). Neurodevelopmental treatment clinical practice model's role in the management of children with cerebral palsy. In F. Miller, S. Bachrach, N. Lennon, & M. O'Neil (Eds.), *Cerebral palsy*. Springer. https://doi.org/10.1007/978-3-319-50592-3_216-1

Karadağ-Saygı, E., & Giray, E. (2019). The clinical aspects and effectiveness of suit therapies for cerebral palsy: A systematic review. *Turkish Journal of Physical Medicine and Rehabilitation, 65*(1), 93–110. https://doi.org/10.5606/tftrd.2019.3431

Kashoo, F. Z., & Ahmad, M. 2019. Effect of sensory integration on attention span among children with infantile hemiplegia. *International Journal of Health Science (Qassim), 13*(3), 29–33.

Kim, M., Lee, B., & Park, D. (2016). Effects of combined Adeli suit and neurodevelopmental treatment in children with spastic cerebral palsy with gross motor function classification system levels I and II. *Hong Kong Physiotherapy Journal, 34*, 10–18. https://doi.org/10.1016/j.hkpj.2015.09.036

Kinnucan, E., Van Heest, A., & Tomhave, W. (2010). Correlation of motor function and stereognosis impairment in upper limb cerebral palsy. *The Journal of Hand Surgery*, 35(8), 1317–1322. https://doi.org/10.1016/j.jhsa.2010.04.019

Klepper, S., Clayton Krasinski, D., Gilb, M., & Khalil, N. (2017). Comparing unimanual and bimanual training in upper extremity function in children with unilateral cerebral palsy. *Pediatric Physical Therapy*, 29(4), 288–306. https://doi.org/10.1097/pep.0000000000000438

Klingels, K., Demeyere, I., Jaspers, E., De Cock, P., Molenaers, G., Boyd, R., & Feys, H. (2012). Upper limb impairments and their impact on activity measures in children with unilateral cerebral palsy. *European Journal of Paediatric Neurology*, 16(5), 475–484. https://doi.org/10.1016/j.ejpn.2011.12.008

Krumlinde-Sundholm, L., Ek, L., Sicola, E., Sjöstrand, L., Guzzetta, A., Sgandurra, G., Eliasson, A.- C. (2017). Development of the hand assessment for infants: Evidence of internal scale validity. *Developmental Medicine & Child Neurology*, 59(12), 1276–1283. https://doi.org/10.1111/dmcn.13585

Krumlinde-Sundholm, L., & Eliasson, A. (2007). Comparing tests of tactile sensibility: Aspects relevant to testing children with spastic hemiplegia. *Developmental Medicine & Child Neurology*, 44(9), 604–612. https://doi.org/10.1111/j.1469-8749.2002.tb00845.x

Krumlinde-Sundholm, L., Holmefur, M., & Eliasson, A. (2014). *Manual: Assisting hand assessment – Kids, 18 months to 12 years, β-version 5.0, English.* Karolinska Institutet.

Kuijiper, M. A., van der Wilden, G. J., Ketelaar, M., & Gorter, J. W. (2010). Manual ability classification system for children with cerebral palsy in a school setting and its relationship to home self-care activities. *American Journal of Occupational Therapy*, 64(4), 614–620. https://doi.org/10.5014/ajot.2010.08087

Kuo, H., Gordon, A., Henrionnet, A., Hautfenne, S., Friel, K., & Bleyenheuft, Y. (2016). The effects of intensive bimanual training with and without tactile training on tactile function in children with unilateral spastic cerebral palsy: A pilot study. *Research in Developmental Disabilities*, 49–50, 129–139. https://doi.org/10.1016/j.ridd.2015.11.024

Kurz, M., Heinrichs-Graham, E., Becker, K., & Wilson, T. (2015). The magnitude of the somatosensory cortical activity is related to the mobility and strength impairments seen in children with cerebral palsy. *Journal of Neurophysiology*, 113(9), 3143–3150. https://doi.org/10.1152/jn.00602.2014

Law, M., Baptiste, S., Carswell, A., McColl, M. A., Polatajko, H. J., & Pollock, N. (2019). *Canadian occupational performance measure (COPM) user's manual* (5th ed.). COPM Inc.

Lee, D., Pae, C., Lee, J., Park, E., Cho, S., Um, M., et al. (2017). Analysis of structure – function network decoupling in the brain systems of spastic diplegic cerebral palsy. *Human Brain Mapping*, 38(10), 5292–5306. https://doi.org/10.1002/hbm.23738

Liao, H., Liu, Y., Liu, W., & Lin, Y. (2007). Effectiveness of loaded sit-to-stand resistance exercise for children with mild spastic diplegia: A randomized clinical trial. *Archives of Physical Medicine and Rehabilitation*, 88(1), 25–31. https://doi.org/10.1016/j.apmr.2006.10.006

Mäenpää, H., Jaakkola, R., Sandström, M., Airi, T., & von Wendt, L. (2004). Electrostimulation at sensory level improves function of the upper extremities in children with cerebral palsy: A pilot study. *Developmental Medicine & Child Neurology, 46*(2). https://doi.org/10.1017/s0012162204000180

Mailleux, L., Jaspers, E., Ortibus, E., Simon-Martinez, C., Desloovere, K., Molenaers, G., et al. (2017). Clinical assessment and three-dimensional movement analysis: An integrated approach for upper limb evaluation in children with unilateral cerebral palsy. *PLoS One, 12*(7), e0180196. https://doi.org/10.1371/journal.pone.0180196

Maitre, N., Jeanvoine, A., Yoder, P., Key, A., Slaughter, J., Carey, H., et al. (2020). Kinematic and somatosensory gains in infants with cerebral palsy after a multi-component upper-extremity intervention: A randomized controlled trial. *Brain Topography, 33*(6), 751–766. https://doi.org/10.1007/s10548-020-00790-5

Martins, E., Cordovil, R., Oliveira, R., Letras, S., Lourenço, S., Pereira, I., et al. (2015). Efficacy of suit therapy on functioning in children and adolescents with cerebral palsy: A systematic review and meta-analysis. *Developmental Medicine & Child Neurology, 58*(4), 348–360. https://doi.org/10.1111/dmcn.12988

McLaughlin, J. F. 2005. Lower extremity sensory function in children with cerebral palsy. *Pediatric Rehabilitation, 8*(1), 45–52. https://doi.org/10.1080/13638490400011181

McLean, B., Taylor, S., Blair, E., Valentine, J., Carey, L., & Elliott, C. (2017). Somatosensory discrimination intervention improves body position sense and motor performance in children with hemiplegic cerebral palsy. *American Journal of Occupational Therapy, 71*(3), 7103190060p1. https://doi.org/10.5014/ajot.2016.024968

Mishra, P. D. (2020). Sensory processing/integration dysfunction affects functional mobility of children with cerebral palsy. *Neonatology and Clinical Pediatrics, 7*(1), 1–6. https://doi.org/10.24966/ncp-878x/100043

Moll, I., Vles, J., Soudant, D., Witlox, A., Staal, H., Speth, L., et al. (2017). Functional electrical stimulation of the ankle dorsiflexors during walking in spastic cerebral palsy: A systematic review. *Developmental Medicine & Child Neurology, 59*(12), 1230–1236. https://doi.org/10.1111/dmcn.13501

Nanawati, M., Rane, N., & Ansari, T. (2020). To study the effects of vestibular stimulation using the vestibulator on the muscle tone and reflex responses in children with cerebral palsy. *International Journal of Medicine and Pharmaceutical Science, 10*(2), 27–44. https://doi.org/10.18376//2012/v8i1/67600

Novak, I., Morgan, C., Fahey, M., Finch-Edmondson, M., Galea, C., Hines, A., et al. (2020). State of the evidence traffic lights 2019: Systematic review of interventions for preventing and treating children with cerebral palsy. *Current Neurology and Neuroscience Reports, 20*(2). https://doi.org/10.1007/s11910-020-1022-z

Palisano, R., Rosenbaum, P., Bartlett, D., & Livingston, M. (2008). Content validity of the expanded and revised gross motor function classification system. *Developmental Medicine & Child Neurology, 50*(10), 744–750. https://doi.org/10.1111/j.1469-8749.2008.03089.x

Palisano, R., Rosenbaum, P., Walter, S., Russell, D., Wood, E., & Galuppi, B. (2008). Development and reliability of a system to classify gross motor function in children with cerebral palsy. *Developmental Medicine & Child Neurology, 39*(4), 214–223. https://doi.org/10.1111/j.1469-8749.1997.tb07414.x

Pape, K. (2016). *The boy who could run but not walk: Understanding neuroplasticity in the child's brain.* Barlow Book Publishing.

Park, E., & Kim, W., 2017. Effect of neurodevelopmental treatment-based physical therapy on the change of muscle strength, spasticity, and gross motor function in children with spastic cerebral palsy. *Journal of Physical Therapy Science,* 29(6), 966–969. https://doi.org/10.1589/jpts.29.966

Paulson, A., & Vargus-Adams, J. (2017). Overview of four functional classification systems commonly used in cerebral palsy. *Children, 4*(4), 30. www.mdpi.com/journal/children

Pavão, S., Lima, C., & Rocha, N. (2020). Association between sensory processing and activity performance in children with cerebral palsy levels I-II on the gross motor function classification system. *Brazilian Journal of Physical Therapy.* https://doi.org/10.1016/j.bjpt.2020.05.007

Pavão, S., & Rocha, N. (2017). Sensory processing disorders in children with cerebral palsy. *Infant Behavior and Development, 46,* 1–6. https://doi.org/10.1016/j.infbeh.2016.10.007

Pavão, S., Silva, F., Savelsbergh, G., & Rocha, N. (2014). Use of sensory information during postural control in children with cerebral palsy: Systematic review. *Journal of Motor Behavior, 47*(4), 291–301. https://doi.org/10.1080/0222895.2014.981498

Phipps, S., & Roberts, P. (2012). Predicting the effects of cerebral palsy severity on self-care, mobility, and social function. *American Journal of Occupational Therapy, 66,* 422–429. https://doi.org/10.5014/ajot.2012.003921

Randall, M., Johnson, L., & Reddihough, D. (2012). *The Melbourne assessment 2: A test of unilateral upper limb function.* www.rch.org.au/melbourneassessment

Reddihough, D. (2009). Use of the gross motor function classification system in infants with cerebral palsy. *Developmental Medicine and Child Neurology, 51,* 1–5. https://doi.org/10.1111/j.1469-8749.2008.03212.x

Riquelme, I., & Montoya, P. (2010). Developmental changes in somatosensory processing in cerebral palsy and healthy individuals. *Clinical Neurophysiology, 121*(8), 1314–1320. https://doi.org/10.1016/j.clinph.2010.03.010

Rosenbaum, P., Panneth, N., Leviton, A., Goldstein, M., & Bax, M. (2007). A report: The definition and classification of cerebral palsy April 2006 in the definition and classification of cerebral palsy. *Developmental Medicine & Child Neurology, 49,* 1–44. https://doi.org/10.1111/j.1469-8749.2007.00001.x

Rosenbaum, P., Palisano, R., Bartlett, D., Galuppi, B., & Russell, D. (2008). Development of the gross motor function classification system for cerebral palsy. *Developmental Medicine & Child Neurology, 50*(4), 249–253. https://doi.org/10.1111/j.1469-8749.2008.02045.x

Russell, D. J., Rosenbaum, P., Wright, M., & Avery, L. M. (2013). *Gross motor function measure (GMFM-66 & GMFM-88) user's manual* (2nd ed.). MacKeith Press.

Saavedra, S., & Goodworth, A. (2019). Postural control in children and youth with cerebral palsy. *Cerebral Palsy,* 1–21. https://doi.org/10.1007/978-3-319-50592-3_161-1

Sah, A., Balaji, G., & Agrahara, S. (2019). Effects of task-oriented activities based on neurodevelopmental therapy principles on trunk control, balance, and gross motor function in children with spastic diplegic cerebral palsy: A single-blinded randomized clinical trial. *Journal of Pediatric Neurosciences, 14*(3), 120. https://doi.org/10.4103/jpn.jpn_35_19

Salkar, P., Pazare, S., & Harle, M. (2017). Effect of tactile stimulation on dexterity and manual ability of hand in hemiplegic cerebral palsy children. *International Journal of Therapies and Rehabilitation Research, 6*(1), 91. https://doi.org/10.5455/ijtrr.000000226

Sakzewski, L., Ziviani, J., & Boyd, R. (2009). Systematic review and meta-analysis of therapeutic management of upper-limb dysfunction in children with congenital hemiplegia. *Pediatrics, 123*(6), e1111–e1122 https://doi.org/10.1542/peds.2008-3335

Saussez, G., Van Laethem, M., & Bleyenheuft, Y. (2018). Changes in tactile function during intensive bimanual training in children with unilateral spastic cerebral palsy. *Journal of Child Neurology, 33*(4), 260–268. https://doi.org/10.1177/0883073817753291

Schiariti, V., Longo, E., Shoshmin, A., Kozhushko, L., Besstrashnova, Y., Król, M., Correia Campos, T. N., Confessor Ferreira, H. N., Verissimo, C., Shaba, D., Mwale, M., & Amando, S. (2018). Implementation of the international classification of functioning, disability, and health (ICF) core sets for children and youth with cerebral palsy: Global initiatives promoting optimal functioning. *International Journal of Environmental Research and Public Health, 15*(9), 1899. doi:10.3390/ijerph15091899

Schiariti, V., Selb, M., Cieza, A., & O'Donnell, M. (2015). International classification of functioning, disability and health core sets for children and youth with cerebral palsy: A consensus meeting. *Developmental Medicine & Child Neurology, 57*, 149–158. https://doi.org/10.1111/dmcn.12551

Sellers, D., Bryant, E., Hunter, A., Campbell, V., & Morris, C. (2019). The eating and drinking ability classification system for cerebral palsy: A study of reliability and stability over time. *Journal of Pediatric Rehabilitation Medicine, 12*(2), 123–131. https://doi.org/10.3233/prm-180581

Sellers, D., Mandy, A., Pennington, L., Hankins, M., & Morris, C. (2013). Development and reliability of a system to classify the eating and drinking ability of people with cerebral palsy. *Developmental Medicine & Child Neurology, 56*(3), 245–251. https://doi.org/10.1111/dmcn.12352

Shamsoddini, A. R., & Hollisaz, M. T. (2009). Effect of sensory integration therapy on gross motor function in children with cerebral palsy. *Iran Journal of Child Neurology, 3*(1), 43–48.

Stammer, M. (2016). Examination in Bierman et al., Eds. In *Neuro-developmental treatment: A guide to NDT clinical practice.* Thieme Medical Publishers Incorporated.

Tahir, N., Ahmed, S. I., Ishaque, F., Jawaria, S., Amir, A., & Kama, A. (2019). Effectiveness of sensory integration therapy (vestibular & proprioception input) on gross motor functioning in developmental delayed and spastic diplegic CP children. *International Journal of Research and Innovation in Social Science, 3*(6), ISSN 2454–6186.

Taylor, S., McLean, B., Blair, E., Carey, L., Valentine, J., Girdler, S., & Elliott, C. (2017). Clinical acceptability of the sense_assess© kids: Children and youth perspectives. *Australian Occupational Therapy Journal, 65*(2), 79–88. https://doi.org/10.1111/1440-1630.12429

Topley, D., McConnell, K., & Kerr, C. (2020). A systematic review of vestibular stimulation in cerebral palsy. *Disability and Rehabilitation, 1–7.* https://doi.org/10.1080/09638288.2020.1742802

Tramontano, M., Medici, A., Iosa, M., Chiariotti, A., Fusillo, G., Manzari, L., & Morelli, D. (2017). The effect of vestibular stimulation on motor functions of children with cerebral palsy. *Motor Control*, *21*(3), 299–311. https://doi.org/10.1123/mc.2015-0089

van der Linden, M., Hazlewood, M., Hillman, S., & Robb, J. (2008). Functional electrical stimulation to the dorsiflexors and quadriceps in children with cerebral palsy. *Pediatric Physical Therapy*, *20*(1), 23–29. https://doi.org/10.1097/pep.0b013e31815f39c9

Voorman, J., Dallmeijer, A., Schuengel, C., Knol, D., Lankhorst, G., & Becher, J. (2006). Activities and participation of 9- to 13-year-old children with cerebral palsy. *Clinical Rehabilitation*, *20*(11), 937–948. https://doi.org/10.1177/0269215506069673

Wright, P., & Granat, M. (2000). Therapeutic effects of functional electrical stimulation of the upper limb of eight children with cerebral palsy. *Developmental Medicine & Child Neurology*, *42*(11), 724–727. https://doi.org/10.1017/s0012162200001341

Yardımcı-Lokmanoğlu, B., Bingöl, H., & Mutlu, A. (2019). The forgotten sixth sense in cerebral palsy: Do we have enough evidence for proprioceptive treatment? *Disability and Rehabilitation*, *42*(25), 3581–3590. https://doi.org/10.1080/09638288.2019.1608321

Yi, S., Hwang, J., Kim, S., & Kwon, J. (2012). Validity of pediatric balance scales in children with spastic cerebral palsy. *Neuropediatrics*, *43*(6), 307–313. https://doi.org/10.1055/s-0032-1327774

Zarkou, A., Lee, S., Prosser, L., & Jeka, J. (2020). Foot and ankle somatosensory deficits affect balance and motor function in children with cerebral palsy. *Frontiers in Human Neuroscience*, *14*. https://doi.org/10.3389/fnhum.2020.00045

6   Combining Approaches
Developmental Coordination Disorder (DCD) and Other Motor Challenges

Clare Giuffrida and Lisa R. Reyes

Objectives

- To identify DCD, a motor disorder, according to DSM-V characteristics
- To describe challenges of children with DCD and other motor problems
- To select research to guide evidence-based evaluation and treatment
- To apply the clinical Reasoning and Action Model (RAM) to a child presenting with DCD and other motor problems
- To select evidenced-based clinical interventions and blend, as appropriate, with sensory integration treatment strategies

---

Box 6.1   Introducing Paul

Paul, a 6-year-old boy, struggles with dressing and needs help to get ready for school. He avoids climbing, running, and playing ball games with other children, trips often, and misses the ball when thrown to him. His teacher is puzzled by Paul's performance as he seems bright and eagerly participates in class discussions, although he is inattentive and disorganized at times. Paul enjoys and reads well, but he is slow to finish schoolwork, and his final products are messy and illegible. After school, Paul rides his bike but is frustrated as he still needs training wheels. Paul's parents contacted his pediatrician to investigate further if he has an underlying condition.

Paul is similar to many children referred to occupational therapy (OT) for "motor problems" with possible sensory processing problems impacting self-care, play, academic performance, and productivity. These children are ideally evaluated by a health care team consisting of a developmental pediatrician, an occupational therapist (herein referred to as "clinician"), and a physical therapist (PT), sometimes resulting in a

DOI: 10.4324/9781003050810-8

diagnosis of Developmental Coordination Disorder (DCD). In this chapter, we will focus on the literature on DCD, with an understanding that we include motor problems that are often not necessarily diagnosed as DCD.

What Is DCD?

DCD is a common, but often unrecognized, neuromotor disorder impacting 5 to 6 percent of the population (American Psychiatric Association (APA, 2013; Blank et al., 2012). Boys are 1.7 to 2.8 times more likely than girls to have this disorder (Zwicker et al., 2013). Risk factors associated with DCD include prematurity, low socioeconomic status, and possibly a genetic factor since DCD can co-occur in twins (Zwicker et al., 2013). There is a high incidence of co-occurrence with Attention Deficit Hyperactive Disorder (50 percent), Autism (79 percent), and with language impairments (70 percent) as reported in the most recent European Academy of Childhood Disabilities (EACD), international clinical practice recommendations for DCD (CPR-DCD) (Blank et al., 2019).

The Diagnostic and Statistical Manual of Mental Disorders (DSM-V) from the American Psychiatric Association (APA, 2013) identifies DCD as a motor disorder within the broader category of neurodevelopmental disorders. It describes four diagnostic criteria (A-D) for DCD as follows:

A. Given the opportunity for skill learning, a child's motor performance is below age level.
B. Motor skill deficit interferes with activities of daily living associated with age (e.g., self-care and self-maintenance) and impacts academic productivity, prevocational and vocational activities, and leisure and play.
C. Onset of symptoms is early in life; developmental history indicates delays in motor milestones such as crawling and walking and not acquired by a lesion. The current recommendation is to identify the motor delays between 3 and 5 years, as early identification and intervention are beneficial (Blank et al., 2019). However, it is not recommended to diagnose children with motor delays until 5 or 6 years, as early development varies markedly.
D. Motor skills are not associated with intellectual delay or related to a medical condition or disease (e.g., cerebral palsy, muscular dystrophy, visual impairment, or intellectual disability).

DCD deficits and other undiagnosed motor problems span sensory, neuromotor, musculoskeletal, cardiorespiratory, cognitive, and psychological systems. These children present with multisystem impairments impacting their motor planning, coordination, physical activity, skills, and emotional regulation (see Table 6.1). Secondary psychosocial consequences

Table 6.1 Features of DCD and Other Motor Problems According to ICF-CY

Body Structures and Functions	Activity-Participation
Under 60 months	
Impaired/Delayed: • Sensory processing • Motor milestones • Speech	**Restricted:** • Imitative, constructive, and interactive play • Copying for words, gestures, postures • Running after a ball, climbing onto a couch, catching bubbles
Decreased: • Muscle tone • Postural control	**Difficulty with:** • Feeding, use of utensils • Dressing/undressing • Sleep
60 months-Adolescence	
Impaired: • Executive function (e.g., working, long-term memory) and attention • Body schema • Motor control and planning • Visual, vestibular, and touch integration for postural control and balance	**Restricted:** • Slow and awkward gait, climbing stairs, travel between classrooms • Visual strategies for eye-hand coordination activities; difficulty with ball skills for sports • Oral motor skills; impacting communication in group projects interfering with academic performance and social activities
Decreased: • Movement quality, variability, initiation, and pacing • Motor competence lowering self-esteem; increasing anxiety and depression • Vision/oculomotor control impacting actions and postural stability	**Difficulty with:** • Dressing/undressing skills; impacts transitions to school and home • Simultaneous tasks; having a conversation while walking • Graphomotor skills, reading, writing, calculating; impairs school performance • Grasp of rules, gameplay, and group activities
Adolescence-Adulthood	
Impaired: • Motor control, executive function, and sensory deficits • Physical inactivity, obesity, depression, social isolation, and anxiety	**Restricted:** • Home management tasks (e.g., preparing meals, financial planning) • Driving and employment opportunities (e.g., new job skills)
Decreased: • Organization of task materials • Movement planning and execution • Motor learning of new skills	**Difficulty with:** • Mobility, prefers sedentary activities • Written and verbal communication • Participation in social activities

Source: Body Structures, and Functions (Smits-Engelsman et al., 2018; see also Dannemiller et al., 2020; Ferguson et al., 2014; Wilson et al., 2013), Activity-Participation (Smits-Engelsman et al., 2018; see also Dannemiller et al., 2020; Ferguson et al., 2014; Wilson et al., 2013), Adolescence-Adulthood (Purcell et al., 2015)

of low self-esteem, depression, emotional lability, prevocational anxiety, and poor fitness can evolve with increasing demands as the child matures further decreasing participation. Recent research shows DCD can persist into adolescence and adulthood, resulting in a complex array of difficulties impacting physical and mental health, education and vocational opportunities, life satisfaction, and quality of life (Harrowell et al., 2018; O'Dea & Connell, 2016). A host of contextual factors mediates each individual's unique challenges, both personal (e.g., age, gender) and environmental (e.g., home, play space, and equipment).

An Evolution of Terms – Coordination Problems to Developmental Dyspraxia to DCD

Early clinical research focused on examining "coordination problems" in children while describing a wide variety of motor impairments, including clumsiness, apraxia (derived from adult stroke literature), developmental dyspraxia (motor planning problems), perceptual motor difficulties, balance problems, and or sensory integrative difficulties. Developmental dyspraxia refers to an idiopathic problem occurring in a developmental context contrasted to apraxia which is the loss of the ability to plan acquired movements secondary to a neurological problem (Vaivre-Douret, 2016). Children with developmental dyspraxia may have sensory-based movement problems linked to inadequate body awareness and visual, proprioceptive, kinesthetic, vestibular, and tactile processing issues (Ayres, 1965, 1985; Bundy & Lane, 2020). Developmental dyspraxia affects motor functions with difficulties of imitating novel gestures and body movements, sequencing, and overall planning and coordinating movements. Children with developmental dyspraxia and other motor planning disorders are sometimes diagnosed with DCD. Dyspraxia is also evident in children with Autism Spectrum Disorder (ASD) (see Chapter 4).

Dr. A. Jean Ayres (Ayres, 1963), a leader in occupational therapy, was among the first to research the link between motor coordination problems and sensory processing difficulties (see Chapter 2). This relationship was evident in her frequent reminders of "see motor" but "think sensory" as reflected in her teachings (Hill-Giuffrida, USC 610 course notes, 1978) and practice throughout her life. Her ground-breaking research (Ayres, 1972) led to the Southern California Sensory Integration Tests' design, the first battery of normative, standardized tests examining the relationship between a child's sensory and motor functions, later revised in 1989 as the Sensory Integration and Praxis Tests (SIPT).

The SIPT focuses on the normative development of sensory and motor functions rather than solely on motor skills, such as the Bruininks-Oseretsky Test of Motor Proficiency-2nd Edition (BOT-2). By administering the

SIPT or more recent assessments grounded in sensory integration theory, the clinician could determine whether a child's sensory and motor functions cluster into meaningful patterns of behavioral and movement functions and dysfunctions.

Dyspraxia has been linked to sensory discrimination problems both somatosensory (tactile and proprioceptive) and vestibular/proprioceptive (Mailloux et al., 2011) as they were the ones that relate to the Kinesthesia test. These sensory processing difficulties through SIPT testing are classified as either Somatodyspraxia, Bilateral Integration and Sequencing problems (BIS), and or constructional praxis, also referred by Ayres as Visuodyspraxia. For an in-depth explanation of these disorders and sensory modulation disorders, refer to Ayres (1972, 1979, 2005); Bundy and Lane (2020); and Chapter 2 for an overview of sensory integration theory and treatment.

The terms developmental dyspraxia, sensory processing, and sensory integration continue to prevail in the clinical arena and are often used to describe children with motor problems. However, the DCD criteria are defined by DSM-V. The term, DCD, was originally derived at the international conference in Leeds in 1994 for children with motor coordination problems and is now used to guide medical diagnosis, research, and evidence-based practice. In this chapter, the term DCD encompasses dyspraxia and the contributing research (Ayres, 1985, 1989; Ayres et al., 1987; Cermak, 2011).

Motor Problems: More Than Just Motor Problems

Current research supports the impact of motor problems on self-help and school related skills, occupational engagement, and other areas of participation across all contexts. Also, there is an increasing emphasis on understanding motor problems and DCD as a co-occurring condition with Autism Spectrum Disorder (ASD) (Kilroy et al., 2019; Licari et al., 2019). There is a focus on the higher-level central nervous system functions and sensory motor impairments for DCD (Gomez & Sirigu, 2015). For example, deficits in internal modeling (IMD) of movements linked to sensory processing and spatiotemporal parameters impact feedforward movement essential for predictive motor control (Blank et al., 2019; Gomez & Sirigu, 2015). See Table 6.2 for motor problems and DCD observed characteristics in daily life with associated contemporary research about sensory motor deficits and motor control deficits.

Furthermore, sensory processing difficulties are also identified in children with DCD and ASD, see Chapter 4. Of all children diagnosed with DCD, either alone or co-occurring with ASD, 86 percent to 100 percent demonstrate (Allen & Casey, 2017) sensory processing problems related

Table 6.2 DCD and Other Motor Problems: Observed Characteristics and Related Evidence for Sensory Motor and Motor Control Deficits

Functional Issues	Sensory Motor Deficits	Motor Control Deficits
• Clumsy • Awkward and inaccurate performance with scissors, markers, utensils • Struggles with scooters, biking, hopping, jumping • Slowness and inaccuracy of skilled performance (tracing over lines, catching and throwing, or participating in sports) • Delayed handwriting and poor letter formation • Delays in daily living activities • Decreased attention, inadequate organization, planning	• Perceptual or sensory integration deficits; kinesthetic processing impacting motor control (Gubbay et al., 1965; Li et al., 2015) • Proprioceptive impairments with decreased tactile localization of tactile/double tactile stimuli (Elbasan et al., 2012) • Visual and visual spatial processing problems impairing initiation of action and sensory feedback estimation (Gomez & Sirigu, 2015) • Slower to adapt to sensory motor remapping due to inefficient sensory feedback (visual or kinesthetic) or inability to build efference copy of motor plan (Gomez & Sirigu, 2015) • In stance, atypical developmental trajectory of somatosensory, vestibular, and visual systems (Fong et al., 2013)	• Postural control, most common impairment, evident in 73% – 87% of population (Macnab et al., 2001) • Inability to take sensory feedback from handwriting and shift to feedforward control, cognitive-sensorimotor dysfunction (Gomez & Sirigu, 2015) • Deficit in efference copy or in monitoring of execution (Gomez & Sirigu, 2015) • Diminished motor imagery (Wilson et al., 2013) • Impaired internal modeling, predictive control, and rhythmic coordination (Smits-Engelsman, 2018) • Decreased motor learning and generalization (transfer) (Ferguson et al., 2014) • Decreased automaticity (Wilson et al., 2013) • Irregular muscle contraction (Fong et al., 2013)

to self-regulation and motor difficulties. It is important to incorporate these findings into the clinical reasoning process during evaluation and intervention.

Evidence-Based Evaluation of DCD

The current international clinical practice guidelines for DCD address: definition, diagnosis, assessment, intervention, and psychosocial aspects of DCD. These guidelines incorporate research focusing on multiple outcomes at different levels of the ICF. Also, they now cover research for adolescents and adults. Overall, there is increasing emphasis on examining research across ages focusing on multiple individual, task, and environmental factors impacting movement, behavior, and learning (Barnett & Hill, 2019; Blank et al., 2019).

The international guidelines for evaluation recommend multiple sources of data to obtain an overview of the child's neurological, sensory, cognitive, and motor status. These multiple data sources include parent-teacher interviews or questionnaires, skilled observations, standardized motor testing, and separate testing for handwriting/keyboarding. Table 6.3 provides a list of recommended outcome measures across ICF-CY levels.

Table 6.3 DCD Selected Outcome Measures for Children With Motor Problems Across ICF-CY Levels

ICF-CY	Outcomes	Domain
Body Structures and Functions	• Sensory Organization Test (SOT)[a]	• Balance, postural control
	• Movement Assessment Battery for Children-2nd Edition (MABC-2)[b]	• Manual dexterity
	• Bruininks-Oseretsky Test of Motor Proficiency (BOT-2)[b]	• Fine motor control
Activity and Participation	• MABC-2, BOT-2[c]	• Gross and fine motor skills
	• Developmental Coordination Disorder Daily (DCDDaily)[a, c]	• Self-care and management
	• Systematic Detection of Writing Problems (SOS)[c]	• Handwriting
	• Canadian Occupational Performance Measure (COPM)[a, c]	• Specific activity goals
	• DCD Questionnaire revised '07 (DCDQ-R) or Little DCDQ[c]	• Participation in everyday functional activities
	• MABC-2 Checklist[c]	• Home activities
	• Developmental Coordination Disorder Daily Questionnaire (DCDDaily-Q)[d]	• Self-care activities
	• Motor Observation Questionnaire-Teacher (MOQ-T)[d]	• School activities

Source: See Assessment Table in Appendix A. The SOT is not covered in the Assessment Table as more current tests are available in the market at present and are identified later in the section on sensory-motor assessments.
[a]Dannemiller et al., 2020. [b]Bieber et al., 2016. [c]Blank et al., 2019; Cancer et al., 2020. [d]Asunta et al., 2019.

Due to the heterogeneity of motor problems and DCD, there is no one recommended measure used to identify motor problems in children with DCD. However, key points from the international guidelines are emphasized below:

- Use MABC-2 or BOT-2 as a primary standardized measure of motor performance to identify DCD in children. In adolescents or adults use BOT-2.
- Consider using the Canadian Occupational Performance Measure (COPM) and the DCDDaily for clinical and research outcome studies (Heus et al., 2020).

See Motor, Think Sensory, and More

After motor performance and its impact on function is assessed, other contributing factors need to be identified through the evaluation process. The link between sensory processing disorders and motor performance originally established by Ayres (1972, 1985, 1989) is now being supported in DCD using two screening measures: the Sensory Profile-2 (SP-2) (Goyen et al., 2011; Kim, 2020; Delgado-Lobete et al., 2020; Mikami et al., 2020) and the Sensory Processing Measure (SPM) (Allen & Casey, 2017).

Research using these measures further examines the incidence, relationship between sensory problems and motor performance, and the specific sensory patterns related to motor performance. Furthermore, these studies provide a comparison between the sensory processing problems in children with DCD and children with ASD. In these studies, the sensory patterns of children with DCD are characterized as either low-threshold (behavioral tendency is hyper-responsive or avoidant) or high-threshold (behavioral tendency to act passively/miss cues) (Allen & Casey, 2017; Delgado-Lobete et al., 2020). Also, these studies further corroborate problems with proprioceptive, tactile, and visual systems. See Table 6.2. However, these caregiver/parent questionnaires only serve as a screen, indicating the need for further testing.

Structured clinical observations as developed by Ayres and standardized by different authors suggest both parent reports and observational tools need to be used when assessing motor performance and motor planning (Blanche et al., 2021). To assess sensory motor functions and motor planning problems comprehensively, consider the following observational measures and standardized tests:

- Clinical Observations of Motor and Postural Skills (COMPS) published in 2000.
- Goal-Oriented Assessment of Life Skills (GOAL) published in 2013.
- Miller Assessment for Preschoolers (MAP) published in 1983.

- Miller Function & Participation Scales (M-FUN) published in 2006.
- Sensory Integration and Praxis Test (SIPT) published in 1989.
- Structured Observations of Sensory Integration-Motor (SOSI-M) in conjunction with Comprehensive Observations of Proprioception (COP-R, published in 2021).

With the increased understanding of movement behavior and the role of the sensory and cognitive systems, further test development continues. The following measures focus on expanding the understanding of sensory and cognitive contributions to movement planning and motor control in children:

- Evaluation of Ayres Sensory Integration® (EASI) (in development)
- Sensory Processing-3 Dimensions (SP-3D) (in development)
- Test of Ideational Praxis (TIP) (ongoing development)

Interventions for Children With Motor Problems or DCD

Children diagnosed with DCD or having motor problems vary considerably in their challenges and their physical, psychological, and social well-being across ages, which factor into treatment choices (see Table 6.1). Although evaluation tools exist that help clinicians identify problems in children with DCD, there is less research on the effectiveness of interventions used to address them. A further impacting factor is that motor problems co-occur with other neurodevelopmental conditions (e.g., ASD, ADHD), requiring the need to blend approaches.

See Motor Problems – Task and Process Approaches

Earliest intervention research for motor problems was based on models of motor development and motor control (Normative Functional, General Abilities, Neurodevelopmental, Dynamical Systems Approach, and Cognitive Neuroscience). Later, motor interventions were grouped into two broad categories, task-oriented or top-down approaches and process-oriented or bottom-up approaches. Task-oriented approaches, corresponding with theoretical principles of motor control and learning, focus on skill development and problem solving with practice of skills (Barnhart et al., 2003). Process-oriented approaches, among the earliest "motor" interventions, were designed to focus on treating and improving underlying deficits (weakness, balance) or problem areas contributing to poor motor function and skill (Barnhart et al., 2003). See Appendix B for general approaches and Tables 6.4 and 6.5 for description and examples of intervention approaches for task-oriented approaches and process-oriented approaches, respectively.

Table 6.4 Contemporary, Evidence-Based, Task-Oriented Approaches for DCD

Task-Oriented Approaches	Example
Goal: Child will independently get onto bike with training wheels in 5–10 seconds.	

Motor skill training (MST)[a]
e.g., Functional Movement Training
- Contemporary OT and PT activity-based interventions emphasizing motor learning
- Establishes effective strategies to optimize participation
- Emphasizes practice, repetition with clinician feedback to the child for task performance

- Repetitive practice with feedback to the child of getting onto bike
- Getting onto bike with training wheels in different environments with weight shift in sitting and placing hands on handlebar
- Varying of simple to complex task demands (quiet environment, child carrying on a conversation with a clinician)

Cognitive Orientation to Daily Occupational Therapy Performance (CO-OP)[b]
- Requires verbal and cognitive skills as the child learns to apply different strategies
- The child identifies 3–4 meaningful goals for several practice sessions
- The clinician uses Dynamic Performance Analysis to break down performance with guided discovery
- Modeling and cognitive strategies to solve functional problems
- Four-step problem solving instructional strategy: "Goal-Plan-Do-Check"

- **Goal:** "What do I want to do?" Bike ride with friends.
- **Plan:** "How am I going to do it?" Stand next to bike, place my hand on handlebar, put foot on bike pedal and sit on bike.
- **Do:** "Carry out the plan." Practice getting on bike seat.
- **Check:** "How well did my plan work?" Child talks through difficulty encountered using problem solving strategies.

Neuromotor Task Training (NTT)[c]
- Recommended for younger child and approach efficacious for handwriting for each task
- Form end goals: what, how, when, where
- Observe and analyze child's performance
- Identify constraints limiting performance and goal attainment
- Devise adapted assessment tasks varying task demands, to identify constraints
- Design activity training providing opportunity to overcome difficulty

- **Observe:** Child (physical capacity and motor planning) getting on bike **Identify:** Child, task and environmental constraints limiting getting on bike
- **Ongoing assessment of task constraints:** Vary task and environmental demands
- **Design training activities** providing child with opportunities to learn and overcome limits.

Motor Imagery[d]
- Mental practice alone or mental practice joined with physical practice which is more effective

Strategies:
- Imagining getting on a bike
- Imagining getting on a bike and practicing getting on a bike in separate session

(Continued)

Table 6.4 (Continued)

Task-Oriented Approaches	Example
• Includes: visual imagery exercises; relaxation and mental preparation; and visual modeling of motor skills using various strategies • Completed from first- or third-person perspective • Physical imagery is more effective if it includes all the senses to be engaged • Requires self-reflection and ability to pretend	• Motor imagery guided by therapist in same session with alternating sequence of practice • Use first person perspective, imagining self-getting on bike, or third person perspective, watching self-getting on bike • Imagine getting on bike as closely matched to specific task and in environment that is most similar, such as at the park

Source: [a] Blank et al., 2019. [b] Martini et al., 2014; Polatajko & Mandich, 2004. [c] Dannemiller et al., 2020. [d] Adams et al., 2016.

Table 6.5 Contemporary, Evidence-Based, Process-Oriented Approaches for DCD

Process-Oriented Approaches	Example
Goal: Child will independently get onto bike with training wheels in 5–10 seconds.	
Kinesthetic Sensitivity Training	
• Focuses on kinesthesia as integral in skill acquisition, possible problem area for children with DCD[a] • Has inherent reward system using positive reward; presentation of activities within the scope of the child's skill level and graded[b]	• For riding a bike would focus on stationary bike or bike with training wheels • Augment kinesthetic input through resistance or added weights to leg and arm motions while biking to emphasize the "feel" of the movement
Perceptual Motor Training	
• Eclectic approach based on standardized testing for visual motor tasks, eye hand coordination, bilateral upper body coordination and balance • Provide learning through positive feedback and reinforcement, does not involve child in cognitive and problem-solving strategies	• Activity program for biking focusing on component parts such as: bilateral control and balance • Provide a wide range of experiences and opportunity to practice skill components
Sensory Integration (See Chapters 2 and 3 for definition of terms)	
• Sensory integration treatment is described as an intervention combining the necessary sensory experiences with a challenge to motor development in the context of play, the therapist-child interaction, and an enriched environment.	• Focus on integrating sensory motor responses supporting task learning such as bike riding but not necessarily focus on practice and repetition of task.

Source: [a] Blank et al., 2012. [b] Laszlo & Bairstow, 1985.

Strengths and Weaknesses of Task and Process-Oriented Approaches

In both publications of the EACD international recommendations for DCD (Blank et al., 2012, 2019; Smits-Engelsmen et al., 2013; Wilson et al., 2013), neither kinesthetic, sensitivity training, nor sensory integration was recommended as sufficient evidence was lacking. However, in the last ten years, with research studies designed more rigorously and the adoption of a fidelity measure (Parham et al., 2007), there is more contemporary evidence supporting the use of SIT in various pediatric populations (Schaaf et al., 2018; Watling & Hauer, 2015). Increasing evidence supports using sensory integrative treatment for children with ASD having sensory and motor problems and thus those with co-occurring motor planning problems (see Chapter 4). Also, in 2012 the American Academy of Pediatrics supported the judicious use of sensory integrative therapy for children as part of a comprehensive (blended) therapy program while recommending that practitioners inform and educate parents about its use and monitor functional changes in a child (AAP, 2012).

ICF Considerations

In current ICF-CY terms, process-oriented approaches focus on body, structure, and function approaches whereas task-oriented approaches focus on activities-participation approaches. Task-oriented approaches have increasingly been used in the clinic with positive recommendations in the EACD international guideline. However, a current systematic review (Miyahara et al., 2020) questioned the strength of evidence for task-oriented approaches due to the limited sample size of several studies and the need for more rigorously controlled randomized clinical trials.

Today's DCD research, EACD practice guidelines, and systematic reviews recommend using a multilevel approach to intervention and outcomes, corresponding to the child's and family's goals (Blank et al., 2019; Cabello, 2019; Preston, 2017; Yu et al., 2018). Therefore, the clinician's challenge is not to consider "what is the best evidence-based treatment approach for changing the child's motor skills?" but rather to consider "what ingredients work for the child, under what circumstances, and how to blend approaches given the child and family's goals?".

Treatment Goals

The treatment goal for children with motor problems is to enable the child to perform important activities as identified by the child and family and to participate in life situations across contexts (Blank et al., 2012, 2019; Dannemiller et al., 2020). Interventions can provide skills, strategies, psychosocial supports, and environmental accommodations to make it easier for children with motor problems to execute motor tasks for daily living and school activities.

Context and Principles

Children with motor problems or DCD vary in their everyday challenges across domains (see Table 6.1). Guiding intervention principles recommended by the EACD for DCD (Blank et al., 2012, 2019) are as follows:

- Engage a child in meaningful, functional activities based on the child's and family's goals targeting the assessment results and building upon other factors such as self-esteem and self-confidence.
- Involve a child in choosing intervention activities, determining priorities, and defining targets of success.
- Account for context of family life, school, and other life circumstances.
- Use evidence-based treatment grounded in applicable theories impacting everyday activities and participation.
- Target areas including self-care, academic performance, and play/recreation.
- For a child with social participation goals, progress to group interventions of four to six for optimal effect sizes when promoting motor performance.
- When using activity-participation approaches, select similar activities comparable to the goal activity.
- To improve function within skills, incorporate the underlying deficits (e.g., balance) when performing activities (e.g., biking).
- Combine video games as adjunct to traditional activity-oriented and participation-oriented interventions in supervised group interventions.
- Include a physical fitness program as part of intervention planning.

Interventions can occur in schools, community outpatient clinics, or hospital-based outpatient departments, be delivered via group or individually, and involve parent support and education for home carryover. Guidelines for dosage, timing, scheduling, and content of interventions are not specific as comparison studies are lacking.

As mentioned, children with DCD have challenges beyond motor problems. Figure 6.1 provides a map of how to use the DCD literature to support intervention.

Sensory Based Interventions, Think Sensory

In addition to determining if a child with motor problems has DCD, it is also necessary to consider other factors impacting performance such as sensory processing problems, motor planning, and ideation (executive

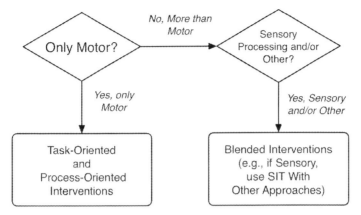

Figure 6.1 Evidence-Based Treatment for Children with Motor Problems

A flow chart depicting a clinician's decision making and choices when considering different evidence based interventions for children with only motor problems and children with motor problems plus other contributing factors impacting function

functioning). A child with DCD may require a blended approach when considering multiple factors. Guidelines for assessment and intervention when blending approaches are as follows:

- Assess motor performance to establish the impact of motor issues on postural control, fine motor development, and gross motor development.
- Even if the child is referred only for motor problems, screen for deficits in cognitive, sensory, and other systems, if warranted.
- To identify how motor challenges impact functional performance and participation, use standardized assessments and observational measures targeting different levels of the ICF-CY.
- Once the motor disorders are established, identify underlying complicating factors and their links to the motor disorder. For example, assess sensory processing to identify links between behavior, motor performance, and sensory processing disorders. More specifically, if motor planning problems are present, assess sensory processing to determine if motor planning is impacted by somatosensory, proprioceptive, and visual input impacting body schema or whether ideation is a factor.
- During the intervention, blend process-oriented approaches (focusing on body structures and function) and task-oriented approaches (focusing on function and participation), evaluating outcomes with a recursive process at more than one ICF-CY level.

Paul's Case Study: Using the RAM Model to Guide the Evaluation and Treatment Process

Step 1: Gathering Information on Paul's Functional Problems and Diagnostic Considerations Specific to DCD and Motor Problems

Following the RAM (see Chapter 2), Paul's case incorporates evidence-based guidelines for a child with DCD and examines sensory

---

Box 6.2   Referral and Initial Questionnaires

See Motor

Intake. Using a teletherapy platform, the clinician discusses with Paul's parents their concerns. Paul's mother completes the DCDDaily-Q to determine Paul's ADL performance, and his teacher completes the Motor Observation Questionnaire – Teacher (MOQ – T) to identify his school performance, including handwriting. Results follow:

- The DCDDaily-Q: Decreased participation, performance, frequency, and learning of self-care, self-maintenance, fine and gross motor skills
- MOQ-T: Demonstrated difficulty across domains. The overall score indicates problems with general motor functioning and specifically with handwriting

Think Sensory and More

Clinician Reasoning. The clinician recognizes motor problems may be related to various factors and due to recent findings in research, hypothesizes sensory problems may also contribute. Using parent questionnaires, the clinician screens for sensory contributions using both the SPM-Home and SP-2, Child version as together, the questionnaires assess aspects of sensory processing, modulation, and discrimination. Results follow:

- SPM-Home and SP-2, sensory patterns: Hyporesponsive (low registration) for body position, visual processing; hyper-responsive (avoidant to touch) with some sensory basis for social-emotional problems; suggesting difficulties with somatosensory processing and body awareness, impacted motor planning and social participation.

---

contributions. Through this process, his clinician defines Pauls' strengths and challenges with everyday activities across contexts. This reflective reasoning highlights how his challenges interfere with his performance and how his strengths, adaptive strategies, and environmental supports can enable Paul to participate effectively.

Step 2: Identifying Difficulties Affecting Movement, Social Interactions, Emotional Stability, and Adaptive Behavior

Paul continues with an in-clinic evaluation beginning with a motor assessment.

Box 6.3   Clinical Evaluation

See Motor

Clinician Reasoning. The clinician chooses BOT-2 subtests and the MABC-2 to report motor performance results back to the referring physician.

- MABC-2: Paul's overall score and subsection scores (manual dexterity, throwing and catching, balance) were at the fifth percentile, the cut-off point for having significant motor coordination problems, suggests DCD.

Think Sensory and More

Clinician Reasoning. Since Paul's initial sensory motor screens suggested problems, further standardized sensory and observational measures are indicated. The Kinesthesia and tactile discrimination tests of the SIPT will be performed. The motor planning and coordination tests of the SIPT will identify if Paul's motor difficulties relate to action sequencing, timing, increasing complexity of movements and coordination. However, these tests are limited in that they have not been updated, may in the future no longer be available, and are being replaced by standardized observational tools.

With Paul, the COP-R was used to determine if proprioceptive processing difficulties impact motor planning, postural control, and proximal joint stability. Results follow:

- BOT-2: Different subtests revealed decreased bilateral motor coordination, decreased overall motor proficiency, decreased ability to copy simple designs, and decreased fine motor precision, such as when using scissors and handwriting.

- SIPT: Low scores, more than one SD below the mean, in Kinesthesia (KIN) and Somatosensory tests (Manual Form Perception [MFP], Graphesthesia [GRA], Localization of Tactile Stimuli [LTS], Finger Identification [FI], Double Tactile Stimuli [DTS]), Postural Praxis (PP), Design Copying (DC), Constructional Praxis (CP), and Bilateral Motor Coordination (BMC).
- COP-R: Below the 5th percentile suggesting decreased proprioceptive skills impacting motor planning, postural control, and joint stability.
- The SOSI-M was not available for use in this case.

Skilled Observations. Additional observations were used to assess ideation/organization, attention, interaction, and quality of motor performance, as follows:

- To unbutton his sweater, Paul pulls on his sweater. He plops down on a mat and forcefully pulls off his sneakers.
- Paul demonstrates a tight pencil grip with thumb adduction and hyperextension at the MP joint while leaning on the table with his forearms. He appears to have poor proximal joint stability and joint alignment. He makes different-sized letters, spaced unevenly on the page.
- During observation of play, Paul exhibited difficulties manipulating different-sized coins and buttons. Additionally, he was hesitant to climb on the swing, became anxious when placed on the therapeutic ball; and had difficulty standing on the mat and kicking a ball. Furthermore, when barefoot, he appeared unstable, stiff, and awkward as he walked across the mats. When the clinician approached him from behind and tapped him lightly on the back, Paul did not respond.

The clinician records relevant observations throughout testing, along with the reason for referral and sensory assessment results (see Table 6.6).

Table 6.6 Clinical Reasoning Model: Paul

First Phase: Performance Data	Second Phase: Hypotheses Generation/ Interpretations
Reason for Referral/Parent observation: struggles with dressing and needs help to get ready for school	• Decreased selective and sustained attention • Poor motor planning
Reason for Referral/Parent report: difficulty playing ball games with other children and misses the ball when thrown to him.	• Decreased postural control/balance • Poor motor planning (feedforward – upper limb)
Observations during BOT-2: Excessive sway on balance items with eyes closed on hard surface	• Decreased postural control • Inefficient proprioceptive and vestibular processing in stance
Observations during BOT-2: During catching, often missed or trapped the ball with his body.	• Difficulties with visual processing (visual motor, visual perception) • Poor motor planning (decreased feedforward control) • Poor bilateral control (upper limb)
Skilled observations: To unbutton his sweater, Paul pulls on his sweater.	• Hyporesponsive to proprioception • Hyporesponsive/decreased tactile discrimination • Poor motor planning • Poor bilateral control (upper limb) • Difficulties with visual processing (visual spatial)
Skilled observations: Plops down on the mat and forcefully pulls off his sneakers	• Hyporesponsive to proprioception (impacting midrange control) • Decreased postural control
Skilled observations: He has a tight pencil grip with thumb adduction and hyperextension at the MP joint while leaning on the table with his forearms.	• Hyporesponsive to proprioception • Low functional muscle tone
Skilled observations: He makes different sized letters, spaced unevenly on the page	• Poor motor planning • Difficulties with visual processing (visual spatial)
Skilled observations: Exhibits some difficulties moving different sized coins and buttons in his hand	• Decreased tactile discrimination • Hyporesponsive/decreased tactile discrimination • Hyporesponsive to proprioception • Decreased motor planning
Skilled observations: Hesitant climbing on the swing; became anxious when placed on the therapeutic ball.	• Gravitational insecurity • Decreased postural control
Skilled observations: Difficulty with standing and kicking a ball	• Decreased postural control • Poor motor planning

(Continued)

Table 6.6 (Continued)

First Phase: Performance Data	Second Phase: Hypotheses Generation/ Interpretations
Skilled observations: When barefoot, he is unstable, stiff, and awkward as he walked across the mats	• Decreased postural control/balance • Low functional muscle tone • Poor motor planning
Skilled observations: When tapped lightly on the back, he did not respond.	• Hyporesponsive/decreased tactile discrimination.
SIPT: Low scores, more than one SD below the mean, in Tactile discrimination tests (MFP, GRA, LTS, FI, DTS)	• Hyporesponsive/decreased tactile discrimination • Decreased proprioception
SIPT: Low scores in Kinesthesia	• Hyporesponsive to proprioception
BOT-2: Decreased performance in bilateral motor coordination and fine motor integration subtests (copying) and decreased performance on motor planning and coordination SIPT tests.	• Poor motor planning
Low scores on the COP-R	• Hyporesponsive to proprioception
SPM-Home and SP2: Some problems in body awareness; balance; and motor planning and ideas	• Hyporesponsive to proprioception • Poor motor planning and ideation • Decreased postural control • Hyper responsive to touch

Third Phase: Counting data points and Conclusions

Most Often Observed Signs:
• Poor motor planning = 10
• Hyporesponsive to proprioception = 8
• Decreased postural control = 7
• Hyporesponsive/poor tactile discrimination = 4
• Difficulties with visual processing skills = 3
• Poor bilateral control = 2
• Low functional muscle tone = 2

Strengths
• No reported language difficulties
• Enjoys reading and participating in group discussions
• Verbally advocates for self

DCD Related Signs
• Decreased motor proficiency
• Decreased postural control
• Decreased motor planning and coordination impacting gross and fine motor skills across multiple domains (home, school, play)
• Co-occurring non-motor (sensory) factors possibly impacting motor planning and motor control.

(Continued)

- Motor learning difficulties
- Secondary social-emotional consequences

Possible Explanations Needing Further Exploration
- Additional sensory and motor contributions to Paul's inefficient postural control
- Distinguish factors contributing to visual processing difficulties such as visual acuity, oculomotor control, visual perception, visual motor functions
- Ongoing surveillance of Paul's social-emotional status and its impact on his participation

The clinician feels confident with the following:

- Standardized scores (MABC-2), as well as teacher report (MOQ-T), parent report (DCDDaily-Q), and observations suggest he meets the criteria for DCD.
- Standardized scores (BOT-2) suggest difficulties with motor planning and postural control.
- Standardized scores (SIPT) suggest difficulties processing proprioceptive information, tactile information and with sensory-based motor planning and coordination.
- Standardized scores (COP-R) suggest difficulties processing proprioceptive information affecting postural control, motor planning, and proximal joint stability.
- Paul demonstrates co-occurring sensory problems more than cognitive factors interfering with motor planning and control.
- Paul has problems organizing, initiating, and completing simple action sequences with gross and fine motor skills, most notably handwriting.
- Handwriting, copying designs, and low scores on the fine motor integration tests of the BOT-2 may relate to visual motor planning difficulties to be further explored.
- Although cognitive factors may contribute to motor planning problems, Paul has little evidence of decreased cognition or ideation. Paul's language abilities and enjoyment of reading are two of his strengths.

The impact to participation:

- Paul's motor challenges impact his participation in daily activities at home and school with decreased performance in self-help skills, academics, and play.
- Paul's frustration with play at school and home is a result of his decreased skill level, as opposed to an emotional or sensory based regulation problem. Without intervention, these secondary psychosocial consequences can persist and increase as he ages with increasing demands.

The clinician recommends:

- Ongoing intervention by occupational therapy in the outpatient clinic. Also, evaluation results will be given to parents and teachers with recommendations for therapy services, sensory strategies, and environmental supports across contexts.
- Postural control can be further assessed, possibly using the Pediatric Clinical Test of Sensory Interaction for Balance (Lotfi et al., 2017), as part of a comprehensive PT evaluation.
- Evaluation results will be given to parents and teachers with recommendations for therapy services, sensory strategies, and environmental supports across contexts.

Having determined that motor planning problems impacting Paul's engagement and participation in everyday activities are influenced by sensory processing, the clinician chooses to use sensory integration treatment and task-specific motor learning approaches.

Step 3: Paul's Blended Intervention

Paul's clinician combines a sensory integration approach and elements of task specific motor learning with feedback from his motor performance as follows:

Box 6.4   Paul's Interventions

Paul's therapist uses the COPM to identify goals for Paul.

For dressing, a high parent priority for Paul, the OT educates the parents on modifications to the task and environment of dressing. Recommendations included: loose-fitting sweat pants and tee-shirts; using Velcro for shoes and other fastenings; and a toggle can be used on jacket zippers.

Based on the COPM, the clinician identifies Paul's desire to ride his bike without training wheels "more than anything." Also, Paul wishes to decrease the time it takes him to get dressed every morning. At school, he would like to play Legos and soccer with his friends during recess. For fun, he likes watching TV and playing video games. The parents prefer Paul to play outside rather than playing videogames.

- The clinician will provide opportunities for augmented sensory input (tactile, proprioception, visual, and vestibular) and challenges to facilitate adaptive responses while given verbal feedback about his motor performance. See Figure 6.2.

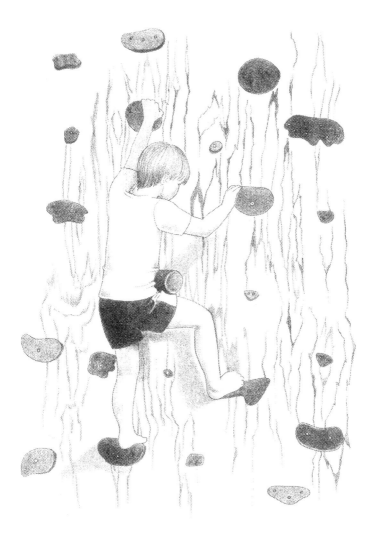

Figure 6.2 Child Using Visually Guided, Adaptive Movements and Receiving Verbal Feedback While Climbing to the Top

- During task specific activities, the clinician will use costumes to facilitate dressing. Ball skills will be addressed by throwing and catching different-sized, textured, and weighted balls. Verbal information will be provided to support his learning.
- Initially, task practice will focus on consistency of task parameters and demands to be successful. Over time, task, environment, and movement demands will vary with complexity as Paul becomes more proficient. See Figure 6.3.

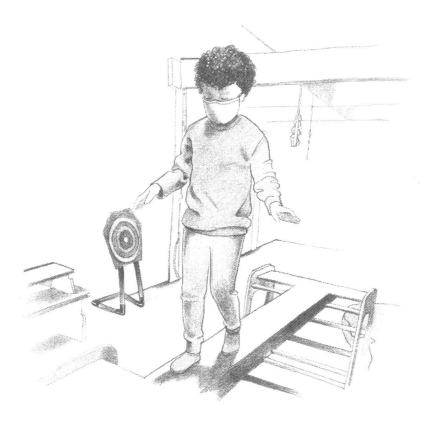

Figure 6.3 Child Creating a Path to Walk Slowly and Carefully to the Magic Castle

- The clinician will require Paul to motor plan, and problem solve arranging mats and other play equipment in the play environment. Different equipment will be used to facilitate negotiating the play environment, such as using a scooter board to move from place to place.

- Postural control and bilateral motor coordination while learning to ride a bike without training wheels will be addressed in sessions delivered in the community.
- Paul's clinician will educate his parents about SIT, learning how to structure tasks and adapt to his environment.
- To address his participation, learning, and performance in school activities, such as handwriting, Paul may benefit from OT in school providing environmental support and other strategies.

Conclusion

This chapter illustrates the complexity and heterogeneity of children with DCD or motor problems using Paul's case study. As presented within this chapter, research demonstrates that children with DCD and motor problems may have multiple challenges requiring a "motor" assessment and the consideration of various levels of the ICF-CY across contexts. Furthermore, as recent research examines and supports a high incidence of sensory processing problems in children classified as DCD, it is essential to evaluate sensory processing and its impact. A multilevel approach (a combination of process-oriented and task-oriented approaches) is recommended to address all ICF levels and promote participation. Clinicians can utilize this chapter to guide them in improving outcomes by using evidence-based practices and to blend effectively therapeutic approaches for each child with motor problems and those with DCD.

References

Adams, I. L. J., Steenbergen, B., Lust, J. M., & Smits-Engelsman, B. C. M. (2016). Motor imagery training for children with developmental coordination disorder-study protocol for randomized controlled trial. *BMC Neurology, 16*, Article 5. https://doi.org/10.1186/s12883-016-0530-6

Allen, S., & Casey, J. (2017). Developmental coordination disorders and sensory processing and integration: Incidence, associations and co-morbidities. *British Journal of Occupational Therapy, 80*(9), 549–557. https://doi.org/10.1177/0308022617709183

American Academy of Pediatrics. (2012). Sensory integration therapies for children with developmental and behavioral disorders. *Pediatrics, 129*(6), 1186–1189. http://pediatrics.aappublications.org/cgi/doi/10.1542/peds.2012-0876

American Psychiatric Association. (2013). *Diagnostic and statistical manual of mental disorders* (5th ed.). https://doi.org/10.1176/appi.books.9780890425596

Asunta, P., Viholaien, T., Ahonen, T., & Rintala, P. (2019). Psychometric properties of observational tools for identifying motor difficulties. *BMC Pediatrics, 19*, 322–335. https://doi.org/10.1186/s12887-019-1657-6

Ayres, A. J. (1963). The development of perceptual-motor abilities: A theoretical basis for treatment of dysfunction. *The American Journal of Occupational Therapy, 17*(6), 127–135.

Ayres, A. J. (1965). Patterns of perceptual-motor dysfunction in children: A factor analytic study. *Perceptual Motor Skills, 20*, 335–368.

Ayres, A. J. (1972). *Sensory integration and learning disorders*. Western Psychological Services.

Ayres, A. J. (1979). *Sensory integration and the child*. Western Psychological Services.

Ayres, A. J. (1985). *Developmental dyspraxia and adult onset apraxia*. Sensory Integration International.

Ayres, A. J. (1989). *Sensory integration and praxis tests manual*. Western Psychological Services.

Ayres, A. J. (2005). *Sensory integration and the child* (25th Anniversary ed.). Pediatric Therapy Network. (Original work published 1979).

Ayres, A. J., Mailloux, Z., & Wendler, C. L. W. (1987). Developmental apraxia: Is it a unitary function? *Occupational Journal of Research, 7*(2), 93–110.

Barnett, A. L., & Hill, E. L. (2019). *Understanding motor behavior in developmental coordination disorder*. Routledge.

Barnhart, R. C., Davenport, M. J., Epps, S. B., & Nordquist, V. M. (2003). Developmental coordination disorder. *Physical Therapy & Rehabilitation Journal, 83*(8), 722–731. https://doi.org/10.1093/ptj/83.8.722

Bieber, E., Smits-Engelsman, B. C. M., Sgandurra, G., Cioni, G., Feys, H., Guzzetta, A., & Klingels, K. (2016). Manual function outcome measures in children with developmental coordination disorder (DCD): Systematic review. *Research Developmental Disabilities, 55*, 114–131. doi:10.1016/j.ridd.2016.03.009

Blanche, E. I., Reinoso, G., & Blanche Kiefer, D. (2021). *Structured observations of sensory integration-motor (SOSI-M) & comprehensive observations of proprioception (COP-R)*. Administration Manual. Academic Therapy Publications (ATP).

Blank, R., Barnett, A. L., Cairney, J., Green, D., Kirby, A., Polatajko, H., Rosenblum, S., Smits-Engelsman, B., Sugden, D., Wilson, P., & Vincon, S. (2019). International clinical practice recommendations on the definition, diagnosis, assessment, intervention, and psychosocial aspects of developmental coordination disorder. *Developmental Medicine & Child Neurology, 61*, 242–285. https://doi.org/10.1111/dmcn.14132

Blank, R., Smits-Engelsman, B., Polatajko, H., & Wilson, P. (2012). European academy for childhood disability (EACD): Recommendations on the definition, diagnosis and intervention of developmental coordination disorder (long version). *Developmental Medicine & Child Neurology, 54*(1), 54–93. https://doi.org/10.1111/j.1469-8749.2011.04171.x

Bundy, A., & Lane, S. (2020). *Sensory integration and practice*. F. A. Davis.

Cabello, L. (2019). Diagnostic challenge and importance of the clinical approach of the developmental coordination disorder. *Archives of Argentina Pediatrics, 117*(3), 199–204. http://dx.doi.org/10.5546/aap.2019.eng.199

Cancer, A., Minoliti, R., Crepaldi, M., & Antonietti, A. (2020). Identifying developmental motor difficulties: A review of tests to assess motor coordination in children. *Journal of Functional Morphology and Kinesiology, 5*(1), 16–28. https://doi:10.3390/jfmk5010016

Cermak, S. A. (2011). Reflections on 25 years of dyspraxia research. In *Ayres dyspraxia monograph* (25th Anniversary ed.). Pediatric Therapy Network.

Dannemiller, L., Mueller, M., Leitner, A., Iverson, E., Kaplan, S. L. (2020). Physical therapy management of children with developmental coordination disorder: An evidence-based clinical practice guideline from the academy of pediatric physical therapy of the American physical therapy association. *Pediatric Physical Therapy, 32*(4), 278–213. doi:1097/PEP.0000000000000753

Delgado-Lobete, L., Pertega-Diaz, S., Santos-del-Riego, S., & Montes-Montes, R. (2020). Sensory processing patterns in developmental coordination disorder, attention deficit hyperactivity disorder and typical development. *Research in Developmental Disabilities, 100.* https://doi.org/10.1016/j.ridd.2020.103608

Elbasan, B., Kayihan, H., & Duzgun, I. (2012). Sensory integration and activities of daily living in children with developmental coordination disorder. *Italian Journal of Pediatrics, 38*(14). www.ijponline.net/38/1/14

Ferguson, G. D., Jelsma, J., Versfeld, P., & Smits-Engelsman, B. C. M. (2014). Using the ICF framework to explore the multiple interacting factors associated with developmental coordination disorder. *Current Developmental Disorders Reports, 1*, 86–10. doi:10.1007/s40474-014-0013-7

Fong, S. S. M., Ng, S. S. M., & Yiu, B. P. H. L. (2013). Slowed muscle force production and sensory organization deficits contribute to altered postural control strategies in children with developmental coordination disorder. *Research and Developmental Disabilities, 34*, 3040–3048. http://dx.doi.org/10.1016/j.ridd.2013.05.035

Gomez, A., & Sirigu, A. (2015). Developmental coordination disorder: Core sensorimotor deficits, neurobiology and etiology. *Neuropsychologia, 79*, 272–287. doi:10.1016/j.neuropsychologia.2015.09.032

Goyen, T.-A., Lui, K., & Hummel, J. (2011). Sensorimotor skills associated with motor dysfunction in children born extremely preterm. *Early Human Development, 87*(7), 489–93. doi:10.1016/j.earlhumdev.2011.04.002

Gubbay, S. S., Ellis, E., Walton, J. N., & Court, S. D. (1965). Clumsy children. A study of apraxic and agnosic defects in 21 children. *Brain: A Journal of Neurology, 88*(2), 295–312.

Harrowell, I., Hollen, L., Lingam, R., & Emond, A. (2018). The impact of developmental coordination disorder on educational achievement in secondary school. *Research in Developmental Disabilities, 72*, 13–22. http://dx.doi.org/10.1016/j.ridd2017.10.014

Heus, I., Weezenberg, D., Severijnen, S., Vlieland, T. V., & van der Holst, M. (2020). Measuring treatment outcomes in children with developmental coordination disorder; Responsiveness of six outcome measures. *Disability and Rehabilitation*, 1–12. https://doi.org/10.1080/09638288.2020.1785022

Kilroy, E., Cermak, S. A., & Aziz-Zadeh, L. (2019). A review of functional and structural neurobioiology of the action observation network in autism spectrum disorder and developmental coordination disorder. *Brain Sciences*, 9(4), 75. doi:10.3390/brainsci9040075

Kim, H. Y. (2020). Relationship between mastery motivation and sensory processing difficulties in South Korean children with developmental coordination disorder. *Occupational Therapy International, 2020*, Article 6485453. https://doi:10.1155/2020/6485453

Laszlo, J. I., & Bairstow, P. J. (1985). *Perceptual-motor behaviour: Developmental assessment in therapy*. Holt, Rinehart, and Winston.

Licari, M. K., Rigoli, D., & Piek, J. P. (2019). Biological and genetic factors in DCD. In A. Barnett & E. Hill (Eds.), *Understanding motor behavior in developmental coordination disorder*. Routledge.

Li, K.-Y., Su, W.-J., Fu, H.-W., & Pickett, K. A. (2015). Kinesthetic deficit in children with developmental coordination disorder. *Research in Developmental Disabilities, 38*, 125–133. https://doi.org/10.1016/j.ridd.2014.12.013

Lotfi, Y., Kahlaee, A. H., Sayadi, N., Afshari, P. J., & Bakhshi, E. (2017). Test-retest reliability of the pediatric clinical test of sensory interaction for balance in 4–6 years old children. *Auditory and Vestibular Research, 26*(4), 202–208. https://doaj.org/article/5fc66e241cc241ea90002f1e9ad83200

Macnab, J. J., Miller, L. T., & Polatajko, H. (2001). The search for subtypes of DCD: Is cluster analysis the answer? *Human Movement Science, 20*, 49–72. doi:10.1016/S0167-9457(01)00028-8

Mailloux, Z., Mulligan, S., Smith Roley, S., Blanche, E., Cermak, S., Coleman, S. G., Bodison, S., & Lane, C. J. (2011). Verification and clarification of patterns of sensory integrative dysfunction. *American Journal of Occupational Therapy, 65*(2), 143–151. doi:10.5014/ajot.2011.000752

Martini, R., Mandich, A., & Green, D. (2014). Implementing a modified cognitive orientation to daily occupational performance approach for use in a group format. *British Journal of Occupational Therapy, 77*(4), 214–219. https://doi.org/10.4276/030802214X13968769798917

Mikami, M., Hirota, T., Takahashi, M., Adachi, M., Saito, M., Koeda, S., Yoshida, K., Sakamoto, Y., Kato, S., Nakamura, K., & Yameda, J. (2020). Atypical sensory processing profiles and their association with motor problems in preschoolers with developmental coordination disorder. *Child Psychology and Human Development*. https://doi.org/10.1007/s10578-020-01013-5

Miyahara, M., Lagisz, M., Nakagawa, S., & Henderson, S. (2020). Intervention for children with developmental coordination disorder: How robust is our recent evidence? *Child: Care, Health and Development, 46*, 397–406. https://doi.org/10.1111/cch.12763

O' Dea, Á., & Connell, A. (2016). Performance difficulties, activity limitations and participation restrictions of adolescents with developmental coordination disorder (DCD). *British Journal of Occupational Therapy, 79*(9), 540–549. doi:10.1177/0308022616643100

Parham, L. D., Cohn, E. S., Spitzer, S., Koomar, J. A., Miller, L. J., Burke, J. P., Brett-Green, B., Mailloux, Z., May-Benson, T. A., Smith Roley, S., Schaaf, R. C., Schoen, S. A., & Summers, C. A. (2007). Fidelity in sensory integration intervention research. *American Journal of Occupational Therapy, 61*, 216–227. https://doi.org/10.5014/ajot.61.2.216

Polatajko, H. J., & Mandich, A. (2004). *Enabling occupation in children: The cognitive orientation to daily occupational performance (CO-OP) approach*. CAOT Publications ACE.

Preston, N., Magallón, S., Hill, L. J. B., Andrews, E., Ahern, S. M., & Mon-Williams, M. (2017). A systematic review of high quality randomized controlled trials investigating motor skill programmes for children with developmental coordination disorder. *Clinical Rehabilitation*, *31*(7), 857–870. https://doi.org/10.1177/0269215516661014

Purcell, C., Scott-Roberts, S., & Kirby, A. (2015). Implications of DSM-5 for recognizing adults with developmental coordination disorder (DCD). *British Journal of Occupational Therapy*, *78*, 295–302. https://doi.org/10.1177/0308022614565113

Schaaf, R. C., Dumont, R. L., Arbesman, M., & May-Benson, T. A. (2018). Efficacy of occupational therapy using ayres sensory integration®: A systematic review. *American Journal of Occupational Therapy*, *72*(1), 1–9. https://doi.org/10.5014/ajot.2018.028431

Smits-Engelsmen, B. C. M., Blank, R., van der Kay, A.-C., Mosterd-van der Meijs, R., Vlugt-van den Brand, E., Polatajko, H. J., & Wilson, P. H. (2013). Efficacy of interventions to improve motor performance in children with developmental coordination disorder: A combined systematic review and meta-analysis. *Developmental Medicine and Child Neurology*, *55*(3), 229–237. doi:10.1111/dmcn.12008

Smits-Engelsman, B. C. M., Vincon, S., Blank, R., Quadrado, V., Polatajko, H., & Wilson, P. (2018). Evaluating the evidence for motor-based interventions in developmental coordination disorder: A systematic review and meta-analysis. *Research in Developmental Disabilities*, *74*, 72–102. doi:10.1016/j.ridd.2018.01.002

Vaivre-Douret, L., Lalanne, C., & Golse, B. (2016). developmental coordination disorder, an umbrella term for motor impairments in children: Nature and co-morbid disorders. *Frontiers in Psychology*. https://doi.org/10.3389/fpsyg.2016.00502

Watling, R., & Hauer, S. (2015). Effectiveness of ayres sensory integration ® and sensory-based interventions for people with autism spectrum disorder: A systematic review. *American Journal of Occupational Therapy*, *69*(5), 1–11. https://doi.org/10.5014/ajot.2015.018051

Wilson, P. H., Ruddock, S., Smits-Engelsman, B., Polatajko, H., & Blank, R. (2013). Understanding performance deficits in developmental coordination disorder. *Developmental Medicine and Child Neurology*, *55*(3), 217–28. doi:10.1111/j.1469-8759.2012.04436.x

Yu, J. J., Burnett, A. F., & Sit, C. H. (2018). Motor skill interventions in children with developmental coordination disorder: A systematic review and meta-analysis. *Archives of Physical Medicine and Rehabilitation*, *99*(10), 2076–2099. https://doi.org/10.1016/j.apmr.2017.12.009

Zwicker, J. G., Yoon, S. W., MacKay, M., Petrie-Thomas, J., Rogers, M., & Synnes, A. R. (2013). Perinatal and neonatal predictors of developmental coordination disorder in very low birthweight children. *Archives of Disease in Childhood*, *98*, 118–122.

7 Combining Approaches
Children Under 3 Years

Mary Hallway and Kim Barthel

Objectives

1. To identify developmental issues in children with various diagnoses from birth–3 and how they impact participation.
2. To describe assessment tools used to evaluate areas of development in children birth–3.
3. To apply a clinical reasoning model to identify therapeutic intervention approaches and supporting evidence for their efficacy that can be integrated with the birth–3 populations.

Understanding early signs of developmental delay or disability and the interventions addressing them are among the first steps in becoming a proficient clinician in early intervention (EI). When children cannot perform developmental skills comparable to same-aged peers, the term *developmental delay* is used (Department of Developmental Services, 2013). The term *developmental disability* refers to an identifiable condition that involves physical, learning, language, and or behavioral impairments impacting participation in daily activities (Rice et al., 2014). Therefore, an essential part of the early identification process is differentiating between a delay and a disability.

Referral and Diagnostic Considerations

Parents, physicians, or high-risk infant follow-up clinics often are the first to identify developmental concerns and challenges occurring before, during, or after birth. Therefore, when a child is referred for intervention, the clinician needs to gather comprehensive information on the child's birth, medical and developmental history, diagnosis, and the parents' primary concerns.

Step 1: Gathering Information on the Child's Functional Problems and Diagnostic Considerations

When conducting the evaluation, factors to consider are the funding source, the context in which the evaluation is conducted, family

DOI: 10.4324/9781003050810-9

constraints, and the child's needs. As described in Chapter 2, the referral information helps identify the family's priorities and guides the choice of assessment tools to be used to detect early signs of developmental problems. The assessment process includes parent questionnaires, skilled observations, and standardized assessments. Table 7.4 identifies standardized tools to evaluate sensory, motor, developmental and attachment issues in EI, and the assessment table in Appendix A describes these tools in detail. The following sections focus on assessments most recognized in the literature of sensory processing, motor performance, cognitive and social-emotional development.

Sensory Assessment

Sensory processing impairments are present early in life in a variety of diagnoses, including prematurity, Down's syndrome, and cerebral palsy (CP) and have been linked to a later diagnosis of autism spectrum disorder (ASD) and dyspraxia (Baranek et al., 2006; Bro ring et al., 2017; Cabral de Paula Machado et al., 2017; Germani et al., 2014; Lönnberg et al., 2018; Niutanen et al., 2019; Will et al., 2019). Sensory processing disorders (SPD) in young children manifest in two areas; regulation/modulation of behavioral/emotional responses to sensory experiences and sensory-motor issues impacting motor performance (Blanche & Gunter, 2020; Niutanen et al., 2019; Ryckman et al., 2018) that impact

Table 7.1 Observations of Sensory Issues in Infants

	Sensory Systems		
Signs of SPD	*Tactile*	*Vestibular*	*Visual and Auditory*
Clinical signs of Hyperresponsiveness	Negative response to grooming and dressing activities Decreased molding into caretakers or pulls away or arches when held close Dislike of hands messy and will not finger feed self Difficulties with feeding and transitioning to textures Occasional toe walking	Distressed when swinging supported in an infant swing, lifted or moved in space, riding in a car, tipped backward while supported to be put down in the crib or to have hair rinsed	Distressed in response to household noises, i.e., vacuum cleaner, coffee grinder, leaf blower Agitated when in multisensory environments, i.e., grocery store, mall, family gatherings

(Continued)

Table 7.1 (Continued)

Signs of SPD	Sensory Systems		
	Tactile	Vestibular	Proprioception
Clinical Signs of Hypores-ponsiveness	Delayed or decreased response when touched Decreased awareness of food left in the mouth Seeks tactile input Delayed development of tool use, i.e., spoon, crayon	Seeks out movement activities, i.e., bouncing, swinging, rocking, jumping Slow response to movement	Overstuffs mouth Limits movement, stays in place Rough when handling toys, pushes firmly when releases objects Occasional toe walking

Source: Based on Blanche & Gunter, 2020; Dunn, 2014; Stallings-Sahler, 1998; Szklut, 2014; Tauman et al., 2017; Williamson & Anzalone, 2001)

social interaction, play, self-help development and participation in family life. Table 7.1 includes frequently observed signs of sensory issues in young children.

Motor Performance Assessment

Motor deficits are present in various diagnoses and often are the initial reason for referral and evident expression of a disorder (Novak et al., 2017). Early signs of atypical movement are commonly associated with a later diagnosis of CP and other developmental disabilities. However, other diagnoses and challenges such as ASD, SPD and developmental coordination disorder (DCD) exhibit atypical positions and subtle motor difficulties such as absent or brief crawling, preference for static positions such as supine, hesitancy navigating stairs, head lag in pull to sit and less mobile postural responses during reaching (Fallang & Hadders-Algra, 2005; Flanagan et al., 2012; Flanagan et al., 2019; May-Benson et al., 2009). Hence, it is crucial for clinicians to understand the range of typical motor development to identify subtle or apparent motor delays and abnormalities during the assessment as these may be critical indicators of a need for intervention.

One avenue to obtain information about movement in young children is through skilled movement analysis which requires understanding typical movement development as it serves as the foundation for identifying atypical movement strategies (Novak et al., 2017). Observations include analyzing the child's self-initiated movements and mobility preferences in different positions that may occur while administering

Table 7.2 Early Signs of Atypical Movement Development

Abnormal general movements (GM) at 2–4 months post-term; abnormal fidgety movements; limitations in variation and variability of motor behavior and the following related to CP classifications based on Novak et al., 2017:

Dyskinesia:
- Finger spreading and circular arm movements
- Twisting upper extremity (UE) and neck movements
- Difficulties with movement initiation, execution, and termination
- Initiation of movement impacts postures
- Hypotonia, increased muscle tone, and or fluctuating muscle tone

Hemiplegia:
- Asymmetry in UE movements and hand preference
- One direction motor transition, i.e., leading with the same leg when cruising

Quadriplegia:
- Head lag
- Increased bilateral finger flexion
- Poor reaching in supine
- Trunk flexion in supported sitting

Diplegia:
- UE function better compared to lower extremities (LE)
- Toe walking
- Difficulty with isolated movements at hips and knees

performance-based standardized assessments (Table 7.4) or during functional tasks and free play (Bierman et al., 2016). Table 7.2 includes early signs of atypical movement development seen in children who later may be diagnosed with CP.

Recent evidence suggests an interrelationship between deficits in early motor development and cognitive skills which will be covered in the next section (Heineman et al., 2018).

Assessment of Cognitive Development

Young children's cognitive development is influenced by sensory, motor, environmental, and parental factors and impacts social development, play, behavior and learning (Frolek Clark & Schlabach, 2013; Omizzolo et al., 2014). Evidence for impairments in cognition can coincide with sensory modulation problems and exists in some young children who experience a brain insult before age 3 (Adams et al., 2015; Anderson et al., 2010; Bro ring et al., 2017; Omizzolo et al., 2014). Environmental factors, parental depression, and negative parent-infant interactions can also adversely influence the development of cognition in children (Rhoades et al., 2011).

Standardized assessments containing a cognitive domain such as the Bayley-4 (Bayley & Aylward, 2019) can be used to assess cognitive development. Clinicians can also use play-based assessments to observe the child during self-directed activities in natural contexts to provide information on how they learn. However, inconsistent reliability and validity of play-based assessments make them useful as a supplement to standardized testing but should not be used alone (O'Grady & Dusing, 2015). Cognitive and language development are intertwined; both contributing to social-emotional development. Cognitive skills as measured by developmental assessments have also been found to improve in response to intervention (Blanche et al., 2016).

Assessing Engagement and Attachment

Parent-child engagement and attachment are two critical components of emotional development (Schore, 2003). The acquisition of behavioral/emotional self-regulation and the ability to establish secure attachments and positive relationships with others during early childhood form the foundation for developing social-emotional competence and overall well-being (National Scientific Council on the Developing Child, 2004). Adverse childhood experiences such as; prematurity, hospitalization, abuse, neglect, caregiver depression or mental illness, conditions of social risk and poverty, domestic violence, institutional care, and foster care are potential risk factors that potentially could impair the development of engagement and attachment. Children with sensory challenges are at risk for interruptions in attachment. Given that self-regulation limitations exist in young children with SPD, caregivers often experience challenges establishing attachment, soothing dysregulation, and managing exploratory behaviors. More than half of children with sensory challenges display insecure attachment features (Mubarak et al., 2017). Since engagement and attachment are relevant to the development of social-emotional competence in all children, assessment of this domain is of particular importance even when the therapist suspects ASD, trauma stress-related disorders (TSRD), or SPD as there is neurobiological overlap within these diagnoses (Phelps & Fogler, 2018). Table 7.3 identifies behaviors that need to

Table 7.3 Signs of Attachment Issues

- Dysregulated emotions
- Psycho-somatic experiences
- Dissociation, confusion, repetitive behaviors
- Oppositional, distrustful, compliant, aggressive behaviors
- Difficulties with language and learning
- Repeated relational trauma themes in the form of interpersonal enactments, in play and fantasy lives
- Anxiety
- Difficulty with attention span and impulse control

Source: Van der Kolk, 2017

be considered when evaluating attachment issues; however, some of these behaviors coexist in children with other diagnoses, i.e., SPD and ASD.

Co-regulation is a dynamic back and forth interaction between caregiver and child that influences each other's affective state and establishes a secure attachment foundation. When parents encounter difficulty interacting with their children, clinicians need to examine the interplay of all the contributing factors involved. Insecure attachment arises from caregiving that is out-of-sync with the child's attachment cues. For example, when a caregiver is consistently unavailable to modulate an infant's

Table 7.4 Assessments Used in EI

Area of Focus and Assessments	Comments
Sensory	
Sensory Profile-2 (SP-2), (Dunn, 2014)	SP-2 is useful in identifying sensory processing issues impacting behavioral and emotional responses.
Sensory Processing Measure-Preschool (SPM-P) (Miller Kuhaneck et al., 2010)	SPM helps identify issues in motor planning.
Sensory Experiences Questionnaire version 2.0 (SEQ-2.0) (available from the author) (Baranek, 1999; Baranek et al., 2006)	
The Test of Sensory Functions in Infants (TSFI) (DeGangi & Greenspan, 1989).	TSFI evaluates five areas of sensory reactivity and processing
Early identification of atypical quality of motor development	
The Prechtl Qualitative Assessment of General Movements (GMA) (Einspieler et al., 2004)	GMA use before five months corrected age.
Hammersmith Infant Neurological Examination (HINE) (Haataja et al., 1999)	GMA and HINE have high sensitivity for identifying infants at risk for CP. GMA has identified children later diagnosed with developmental coordination disorder (DCD) (Hadders-Algra et al., 2004; Novak et al., 2017).
The Test of Infant Motor Performance (TIMP) (Campbell et al., 2004, 2012)	TIMP: at eight weeks, infants with CP performed poorly on items requiring anti-gravity and balanced flexor/extensor muscle control but well on items requiring extension patterns (Barbosa et al., 2005)
Alberta Infant Motor Scale (AIMS) (Piper & Darrah, 1994)	
Toddler and Infant Motor Evaluation (TIME) (Miller & Roid, 1994) (out of publication).	TIMP, AIMS and TIME are useful for assessing the quality of movement.
Developmental	
Bailey-4 (Bayley & Aylward, 2019)	Bayley-4 includes subtests for many areas of development, i.e., motor, cognitive.
Peabody Developmental Motor Scale-2 (PDMS-2) (Folio & Fewell, 2000)	

(*Continued*)

Table 7.4 (Continued)

Area of Focus and Assessments	Comments
Attachment	
The CARE Index (Crittenden, 2010) Functional Emotional Assessment Scale (FEAS) (Greenspan et al., 2001) Cassidy Marvin Preschool Attachment Coding System (MAC) (Cassidy et al., 1992) Crittenden's Preschool Attachment Assessment (PAA) (Crittenden, 2006; Crittenden et al., 2007).	MAC and PAA can be scored during the Ainsworth extended method of the strange situation procedure (Deneault et al., 2020)

aroused state, the infant will learn to inhibit displaying their negative emotions by withdrawing or presenting as overly bright in their emotions. Ambivalent responses arise in infants when caregiver responses are unpredictable, resulting in an exaggerated expression of negative emotions and arousal (Crittenden & Landini, 2015).

Therapists working in EI are often required to clinically reason the impact of these many factors influencing engagement and attachment and ultimately social-emotional development. Assessment of these areas can occur through parent/caregiver interviews or standardized assessments (Table 7.4). The Developmental, Individual Difference, Relationship-Based (DIR®/FloortimeTM) model (Greenspan & Wieder, 2008) is a framework that helps clinicians conduct a comprehensive assessment using skilled observations (refer to Appendix B).

Blending Intervention Approaches Most Often Utilized with Young Children

The choice of appropriate interventions for young children is often complex, requiring consideration of many variables such as the child's age, diagnosis, areas of need, disciplines involved in the intervention process, frequency, and service delivery setting. The following section discusses the critical components for effective service delivery identified in EI:

1. Intervention must be family centered (Hutchon et al., 2019; Kingsley & Mailloux, 2013; van Wassenaer-Leemhuis et al., 2016).
2. Intervention requires multiple frames of reference to address the multi-system impairments impacting young children's development which changes over time (Hutchon et al., 2019; Park et al., 2014; Spittle & Treyvaud, 2016).
3. Intervention must consider contextual factors and promote enriched environments that support development (Hadders-Algra et al., 2017; Hutchon et al., 2019; Morgan et al., 2013; Spittle & Treyvaud, 2016).

Intervention Must be Family-Centered

Family-centered care recognizes the family as at the center of the child's life and decision making, and hence integration of care is guided by the family in partnership with the clinician. Caregiver participation is pivotal to successful EI outcomes (Hadders-Algra et al., 2017; Hutchon et al., 2019; Kingsley & Mailloux, 2013; van Wassenaer -Leemhuis et al., 2016). Standard delivery models utilized within family-centered care include child-focused, participation-based, and or routines-based. Child-focused care refers to clinician-administered interventions that address the child's impairments. Participation-based care refers to specific therapeutic techniques carried out by caregivers at home after being trained by clinicians; examples are teaching sensory strategies or therapeutic handling (Akhbari Ziegler & Hadders-Algra, 2020; Kemp & Turnbull, 2014). Interventions embedded within daily activities and routines are referred to as routine-based interventions. (Hughes-Scholes & Gavidia-Payne, 2016; McWilliam, 2016). This last model uses collaborative decision-making and caregiver coaching to empower families to foster their child's developmental needs and enhance their participation in daily routines (Kemp & Turn-bull, 2014; Akhbari Ziegler & Hadders-Algra, 2020). Evidence supports positive outcomes for participation-based and routine-based models of intervention; however, caregivers benefit more from the latter approach because they are actively involved in enhancing their child's self-efficacy (Hwang et al., 2013; Kemp & Turnbull, 2014). For in-depth information on caregiver coaching, refer to Rush and Sheldon (2011).

Diverse Frames of References to Support Intervention

Intervention requires multiple frames of reference to address the multi-system impairments impacting young children's development, which change across time. Blending approaches with infants focusing on parent-infant interaction, sensory processing, motor skill acquisition, and caregiver education will positively impact self-regulation, social engagement, communication, motor and cognitive development (Hadders et al., 2017; Jaegerman & Klein, 2010; Khurana et al., 2020; Park et al., 2014; Spittle et al., 2015). Approaches most often blended in EI include sensory integration treatments (SIT), relationship-based interventions (RBI), neurodevelopmental treatment (NDT) and motor training programs based on motor learning principles. Appendix B describes these approaches.

Sensory Integration Treatment (SIT)

SIT supports young children's development by emphasizing three complementary processes:

- Helping parents and caregivers understand the sensory contributions to their child's behavior.

- Providing individualized direct intervention designed to remediate identified sensory problems
- Using sensory enriched interventions
                    (Blanche & Gunter, 2020; Whitcomb et al., 2015)

Reframing behavior and helping parents understand their child's specific sensory needs and how they relate to behavior can foster the relationship between the child and caregiver. For example, an infant with tactile sensitivity may arch away from their parent while being held or comforted. Over time, the parent may interpret this action as emotional rejection by the child rather than tactile hyperresponsivity, setting the stage for an attachment disruption (Whitcomb et al., 2015). Suppose a toddler frequently seeks out movement by throwing themselves backward during daily routines. In that case, the parent may interpret this as the child resisting participating instead of a hyporesponsive to vestibular input, resulting in treating it as a behavior that needs extinguishing. Coaching the caregiver on the child's sensory preferences helps parents observe their child's sensory and regulatory needs and matching their response to their child's needs (Jaegermann & Klein, 2010; Jorge et al., 2013).

Blanche and Gunter (2020) describe two sensory intervention models in EI; the first directly addresses sensory processing impairments, and the second utilizes sensory enriched interventions. Direct intervention targets sensory processing impairments identified through the assessment process. Clinicians create affordances by using objects and the environment to address the child's sensory needs; for example, having a toddler who is hyperresponsive to touch push a weighted toy cart to provide increased proprioceptive input while carefully noting changes in the

Table 7.5 Evidence for Sensory Interventions

Sensory Interventions	Outcomes	Reference
Treatment based on SI principles for preterm infants addressed: tactile, oculomotor, and adaptive motor skills	Positive outcomes on TSFI	Pekçetin et al., 2016
Tactile and deep pressure via moderate touch pressure massage with preterm infants	Positive outcomes in weight gain, neurodevelopment and feeding tolerance	Özdermir et al., 2019; Seiiedi-Biarag & Mirghafourvand, 2020; Lu et al., 2020
Sensory strategies and enriched gym based on SIT in a group program for young children with sensory processing difficulties (See Chapter 15, Program 2)	Improved scores on Bayley-3 in gross motor, cognitive and language	Blanche et al., 2016

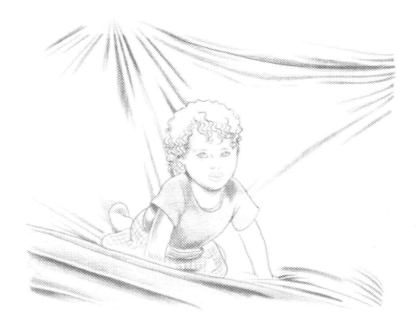

Figure 7.1 Sensory Enriched Interventions: Using lycra material to provide deep pressure and proprioception simultaneously facilitating self-initiated movements.

child's arousal and affective state. Therapists providing direct intervention with young children need to monitor their arousal and emotional state in response to sensory input and adjust accordingly. The evidence for using SIT to address sensory impairments in EI is limited; however, there is more significant evidence for the use of sensory enriched interventions (Blanche & Gunter, 2020). Table 7.5 outlines the evidence.

Relationship-Based Interventions

RBI is a primary and integral component of holistic blended approaches in EI. Evidence indicates that parental sensitivity and attunement directly impact infants' development of self-regulatory competencies and relationship development skills (Hambrick et al., 2019), which are foundational for social-emotional competence. Social-emotional competence is an integration of sensory, motor, cognitive and communication skills. Occupational therapists bring to EI a distinct blend of knowledge combining SIT, NDT, and RBI to address these foundational skills. For example, parents educated on reading their babies' stress signals (i.e., change in state, arousal level) can better respond in a manner that supports a child's nervous system homeostasis during activities that challenge the child's sensory or motor systems. (Hutchon et al., 2019; Van Hus et al.,

2013, 2016; van Wassenaer-Leemhuis et al., 2016). Relationship-based interventions are integrated into the clinician's skill set as components of the overall intervention. Two such relationship-based interventions are modified interactional guidance (MIG) and (DIR®/Floortime).

MIG is a parent coaching model that helps parents learn to tune into their children sensitively. Within the context of play, the therapist highlights moments of sensitivity within a videotaped play scheme, enhancing parent's skills through emphasis on the rehearsal of these attunement skills in everyday contexts. The focus of MIG is to develop secure attachment patterns between caregivers and children, emphasizing comfort and safety and environmental exploration. This intervention model was developed specifically to target attachment-related ruptures as contributions to a child's dysregulation and behavioral concerns (Madigan et al., 2006).

DIR®/Floortime can be used in EI to attend to multiple aspects of developmental skills simultaneously through play while promoting parent-child interactions (Stewart, 2008).

SIT and DIR have often been combined in EI as they both rely on the child's motivation to move in space freely and use sensory equipment. However, their focus is different and needs to be acknowledged when combining these two approaches (see Chapter 14).

Table 7.6 Evidence for Interventions using Therapeutic Handling Based on NDT Principles

Motor Intervention	Outcomes	Reference
Physical Therapy (PT) primarily using handling based on NDT principles	Equally effective when compared to a program based on motor learning principles	Hielkema et al., 2019
NDT principles used with preterm infants	Improved motor performance based on the TIMP	Lee, 2017
PT trained caregivers to provide therapeutic handling to increase postural control, head control, and midline orientation	Improved motor performance based on the TIMP, parent-infant attachment and the parent's sense of competency	Øberg et al., 2018; Ustad et al., 2016
Therapist provided motor interventions, including handling for high-risk preterm infants	Positive short-term outcomes in motor development	Khurana et al., 2020

Motor Interventions

A systematic review of EI's impact on motor development includes appraisals of NDT and motor training programs using principles from motor learning (Case-Smith et al., 2013; Hadders-Algra et al., 2017, Khurana et al., 2020; Morgan et al., 2016).

NEURODEVELOPMENTAL TREATMENT (NDT)

NDT is used with young children with a variety of diagnoses. Evidence for NDT with young children at risk for movement disorders, i.e., CP, has been inconclusive (Morgan et al., 2016; Spittle et al., 2015). However, Table 7.6 presents research supporting the use of therapeutic handling based on NDT principles.

Hadders-Algra et al. (2017) identify blending NDT therapeutic handling with principles from motor learning may be necessary for young children who present with more significant motor challenges; however, those who exhibit less challenge benefit most from intervention focused on self-initiated movements allowing for trial and error learning. These findings are consistent with NDT principles, emphasizing reducing the amount of therapeutic handling as the child effectively masters new motor skills.

NDT is combined with SIT in EI as understanding movement as an expression of sensory processing is pivotal with this population. While NDT emphasizes the acquisition of movement components necessary for participation, SIT contributes by focusing on sequencing these movements in motor planning. Understanding movement also assists the therapist in identifying motor planning issues during the first year of life (Flanagan et al., 2019)

MOTOR TRAINING PROGRAMS BASED ON MOTOR LEARNING THEORY (MTP)

MTP requires several ingredients that lead to successful outcomes in motor development in young children; focusing on task-specific goal-oriented activities, encouraging infant-initiated motor behavior and participation, and promoting trial and error to enhance learning (Hadders-Algra et al., 2017; Hielkema et al., 2019; Khurana et al., 2020; Morgan et al., 2016). These ingredients can be blended with SIT as child-initiated participation is inherent in SIT. Higher dosing and intervention provided early are critical findings to better motor outcomes in EI (Hadders-Algra et al., 2017) which are essential to consider when treating young children exhibiting atypical motor development.

Contextual Factors and Enriched Environments That Support Development

Contextual factors and enriched environments (EE) are at the forefront when clinicians treat young children, as EI is often provided in-home or in other natural environments where they participate (i.e., clinic, daycare, playground, community activities). Evidence supports intervention across multiple environments being most effective and that no one single environment is better than the other (Kingsley & Mailloux, 2013; Spittle & Treyvaud, 2016). The basis for selecting the most appropriate context for intervention depends on family values and preferences, government mandates, payor, the child's impairments, and intervention approach(es) utilized to address them.

Helping caregivers provide an EE is beneficial to developmental outcomes with young children (Hadders-Algra et al., 2017; Spittle & Treyvaud, 2016) and promotes learning in one or more areas of development (Hutchon et al., 2019; Morgan et al., 2013). Blending approaches can promote EE and optimize outcomes. Table 7.7 describes how approaches can create EE and ways clinicians can partner with caregivers in creating EE.

Table 7.7 Creating Enriched Environment Opportunities Through Caregiver Activities

EE Opportunities	Caregiver Activities	Research	Approaches
Creating an environment that stimulates social-emotional development within a parent-infant context	Teaching sensitivity and co-regulation by helping caregivers read their child's non-verbal cues and responding in a manner that supports the relationship, i.e., observing when a child is becoming overstimulated and modifying their tone of voice, affect and physical response	Hambrick et al., 2019; Morgan et al., 2013	MIG, DIR, SI
Enhancing motor development by providing opportunities for child-initiated exploration, play and modifying the physical environment	Presenting foods during snack time that facilitates a specific grasp Offering low furniture or objects available for pulling up to stand	Hadders-Algra et al., 2017; Hutchon et al., 2019; Morgan et al., 2013, 2016	NDT, MTP
Enhancing motor development by providing opportunities for practice within daily routines	Training in therapeutic handling to enhance optimal alignment during carrying, dressing, grooming, feeding, motor transitions and play	Hadders-Algra et al., 2017	NDT, MTP

(*Continued*)

EE Opportunities	Caregiver Activities	Research	Approaches
Adapting the child's physical and social environment relative to the sensory demands to suit the sensory needs of the child and enhance participation	Anticipating potentially disturbing events and preparing for transitions. Adapting the physical environment: Calm settings, minimal distractions and controlled sensory "flow" for children with sensory hyperresponsiveness Rich sensory environment, opportunities for active sensory-based exploration for children with sensory hyporesponsiveness	Williamson & Anzalone, 2001	SI

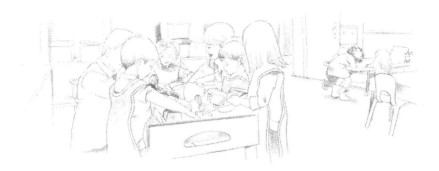

Figure 7.2 Enriched Environments: Adapting the Child's Physical and Social Environment by Including Sensory Rich Opportunities Such as This Tactile Table for Children Who are Hyporesponsive to Sensory input.

The following case study of James illustrates the EI process from assessment to intervention.

Box 7.1   James Case Study

James is a 15-month-old referred to OT by his physical therapist (PT) because of the following concerns; did not like to be placed on his back by his caregiver, especially during diaper changes; did not like to play with textured toys; cried during self-care activities, i.e., hair washing, bathing, and when handled by the PT and had difficulties being consoled. James' birth history was uncomplicated. James was diagnosed with torticollis at four months and received physical therapy for eight months.

OT evaluation occurred in a clinic setting and at James' home using the Toddler Sensory Profile-2 (SP-2), The Care Index, and the Bayley-4 assessments. SP-2 results suggested significant scores in tactile, vestibular, oral sensory processing, behavioral, sensitivity and avoiding. Furthermore, the mother reported the following behaviors to occur frequently:

- Tactile: Upset when hair brushed, nails clipped, resists cuddling, dislikes dressing/undressing and knees or feet on the carpet, avoids messy hands, touching grass or sand.
- Vestibular Processing: Upset when being lifted in and out of the tub, being tipped back or laid down, i.e., washing hair, changing diapers
- Oral Sensory Processing: food texture preferences, difficulties transitioning onto pureed and textured food.
- Behavioral: Irritable, upset in new settings

Care Index evaluation, parent's score exhibited low parental sensitivity with controlling behavior, perceiving James as demanding and challenging. CARE Index categorized James in the disorganized controlling category of attachment.

Bayley-4 subscores were as follows:

Gross and fine motor and adaptive behavior scale were below age level; parents identified difficulties with self-care items, i.e., irritability during dressing, hair washing.
Social-emotional, cognitive and language subtests standard scores were within the normal range.

Table 7.8 summarizes the assessment data and hypotheses using RAM.

Table 7.8 Summary of James' Data, Hypothesis, and Interpretation

First Phase: Data (Issues in participation, observations, other available information)	*Second Phase: Hypotheses Generation/ Interpretations*
Reason for referral: Did not like to be tipped backward on his back for diaper changes	Gravitational insecurity (GI) Poor postural control
Reason for referral and parent questionnaire: Cries during therapeutic handling by his PT and during self-care activities at home, i.e., grooming, dressing	Tactile hyperresponsiveness Poor self-regulation

(*Continued*)

First Phase: Data (Issues in participation, observations, other available information)	Second Phase: Hypotheses Generation/ Interpretations
Parent report: Difficulties being consoled with touch. Is easily frustrated, "easily angered" with new people, places, or changes in routine.	Tactile hyperresponsiveness Poor self-regulation Attachment difficulties
Parent questionnaire: Irritable when placed on a ball by PT, upset when being lifted in/ out of tub and head tilted back in space.	Vestibular hyperresponsivity /GI
Observations during testing: Trunk movements in sagittal and frontal planes during gross motor transitions, i.e., sit to quadruped and delays in age-appropriate transitions, i.e., pull to stand	Poor postural control Weak postural muscles (abdominal obliques) Limited range of motion in neck and trunk musculature due to torticollis Poor motor planning
Observation during testing: Immature grasp pattern	Weak intrinsic hand musculature Poor tactile discrimination
Skilled observations: Upset and fearful with movement, i.e., swinging supported, when sitting on the ball with support from mom	Vestibular hyperresponsivity /GI
Skilled observations: Does not like to transition onto moving equipment or sit with feet unsupported, i.e., on a high bench	Vestibular hyperresponsivity /GI
Home observation: Cried with face wiping, fussed during spoon-feeding purees, and cried when the puree dripped on his hand.	Tactile hyperresponsiveness Poor self-regulation
Home observation: James was overly focused upon his mom's emotional state, was sensitive to her vocal tone and facial expression, exhibiting stress responses relative to his mom's social cues.	Poor self-regulation Attachment Difficulties
Home observation: James' mom responded to James' irritability, dysregulation by either displaying frustration, anger, or disconnection from him. She became upset with him when he expressed discomfort, whether it was because of a "will not" or a "cannot." She expressed not feeling like a good mother because she could not help James feel better when he was upset.	At risk for Attachment Difficulties

(*Continued*)

Table 7.8 (Continued)

First Phase: Data (Issues in participation, observations, other available information)	Second Phase: Hypotheses Generation/ Interpretations

Third Phase: Counting Data points and Conclusion

Most often Observed Signs
Poor self-regulation (4)
Vestibular hyperresponsivity/Gravitational insecurity (GI) (4)
Tactile Hyper-responsive (3)
Difficulties with Attachment (3)

Areas needing further exploration to assess the impact on gross motor and fine motor skills:
Poor postural control (2)
Weak postural muscles (1)
Poor motor planning (1)
Weak intrinsic hand muscle (1)
Limited range of motion in neck and trunk musculature due to torticollis (1)

Box 7.2   Case Study Hypothesis Generation

Based on weighing the data points, James' assessment results supported the following conclusion: tactile and vestibular hyperresponsiveness and GI impacting arousal level, affect, self-regulation, play, attachment, feeding and participation during self-care activities. James' parent's low sensitivity score based on the CARE Index, difficulties understanding and addressing James' sensory hyperresponsivity and controlling behavior appeared to contribute to attachment difficulties.

Addressing sensory processing issues influencing arousal, affect, self-regulation, organization of behavior, and participation during self-care activities was a primary OT focus. Interventions blended SIT and MIG, including parent coaching on parent-child interaction within the context of the clinic and home as primary approaches. Integrating NDT and motor learning principles supported motor skills. Therapy sessions included setting up a sensory environment incorporating objects that would motivate James to engage in play-based activities and helping James' parent understand the relationship between James' sensory impairments and behaviors. Therapeutic use of self when his mother shared her feelings, vulnerability and supporting her readiness to explore community infant mental health resources. Following six months of OT, James was referred to a group program to practice his skills with peers and his mother received coaching with other caregivers. Table 7.9 describes the intervention process.

Table 7.9 James' Impairments, Treatment Activities Used and Interventions Blended

Areas Addressed	Treatment Activities	Interventions
Tactile Hyperrespon- siveness	Crawling between two large bolsters provided deep pressure and resistance to James' movement A vibrating toy against a rubber inner tube while James pats the tube with his hands until he initiated touching the vibrator Use of a neoprene compression vest and deep pressure hugs from his mother integrated into daily routines in preparation for and during tactile-based self-care activities.	SI
	Facilitated self-initiated gross movements, i.e., rolling, while on Lycra material suspended by therapist and parent partially supported on the floor Deep pressure touch was used as tolerated when the therapist facilitated active trunk movements in all planes during James' self-initiated movement in, out, on and off equipment.	SI, NDT, Motor learning principles
GI and Hyperrespon- sive to Vestibular	Sat supported in an infant swing on a bungy with LE on the supporting surface allowed James to initiate moving the swing by bouncing Sat supported on an inflated tire with feet on the floor and bounced Sat on a peanut ball and bounced while James' mother sat on the ball supporting him from behind	SI
Poor Self-Regulation	Helped parent understand and reframe James' "difficult" behaviors, i.e., arching, turning away and pushing mom away with his hands when touched, diminished emotional response and the need to slow down her interactional style with James.	MIG
	Coached parent on maternal sensitivity, teaching how to read James' behavioral cues when he becomes hyperresponsive to touch by providing opportunities for him to take a break or engaging in more integrating sensory input such as deep pressure or proprioceptive activities.	MIG & SI

(Continued)

Table 7.9 (Continued)

Areas Addressed	Treatment Activities	Interventions
Difficulties with Attachment	Coached parent on creating more physical space between them, slowing down her speech's pace, ensuring her body and face were in a position where he could look at her before she spoke to him with accompanying modulation of her emotional expressions. Videotape analysis and coaching helped James' parent observe herself as successful in her interaction with him and learned how to incorporate the sensory strategies into a modified engagement style through telehealth.	MIG & SI

Conclusion

Providing useful EI requires a holistic, integrated skill set of assessment and treatment strategies when addressing the complex and multi-faceted needs of young children and their families. This chapter introduced clinicians to the various frames of reference and approaches in an integrated, problem-solving manner, allowing them the opportunity to comprehend the clinical reasoning required when providing EI services.

References

Adams, J. N., Feldman, H. M., Huffman, L. C., & Loe, I. M. (2015). Sensory processing in preterm preschoolers and its association with executive function. *Early Human Development, 91*(3), 227–233. https://doi.org/10.1016/j.earlhumdev.2015.01.013

Akhbari Ziegler, S., & Hadders-Algra, M. (2020). Coaching approaches in early intervention and paediatric rehabilitation. *Developmental Medicine & Child Neurology, 62*(5), 569–574. https://doi.org/10.1111/dmcn.14493

Anderson, P. J., De Luca, C. R., Hutchinson, E., Roberts, G., & Doyle, L. W. (2010). Underestimation of developmental delay by the new Bayley-III scale. *Archives of Pediatrics & Adolescent Medicine, 164*(4), 352–356. https://doi.org/10.1001/archpediatrics.2010.20

Baranek, G. T. (1999). *Sensory experiences questionnaire (SEQ)*. University of North Carolina at Chapel Hill. Unpublished manuscript.

Baranek, G. T., David, F. J., Poe, M. D., Stone, W. L., & Watson, L. R. (2006). Sensory experiences Questionnaire: Discriminating sensory features in young children with autism, developmental delays, and typical development. *Journal of Child Psychology and Psychiatry, 47*(6), 591–601. https://doi.org/10.1111/j.1469-7610.2005.01546.x

Barbosa, V. M., Campbell, S. K., Smith, E., & Berbaum, M. (2005). Comparison of test of infant motor performance (TIMP) item responses among children with cerebral palsy, developmental delay, and typical development. *American Journal of Occupational Therapy, 59*(4), 446–456. https://doi.org/10.5014/ajot.59.4.446

Bayley, N., & Aylward, G. P. (2019). *Bayley scales of infant and toddler development screening test* (4th ed.). Technical Manual Pearson.

Bierman, J. C., Franjoine, M. R., & Hazzard, C. M. (Eds.). (2016). *Neuro-developmental treatment: A guide to NDT clinical practice.* Thieme.

Blanche, E. I., Chang, M. C., Gutiérrez, J., & Gunter, J. S. (2016). Effectiveness of a sensory enriched early intervention group program for children with developmental disabilities. *American Journal of Occupational Therapy, 70*(5), 7005220010p1–7005220010p8. https://doi.org/10.5014/ajot.2016.018481

Blanche, E. I., & Gunter, J. (2020). Sensory processing. In J. B. Benson (Ed.), *Encyclopedia of infant and early childhood development* (2nd ed., Vol. 2, pp. 116–124). Elsevier. https://doi.org/10.1016/b978-0-12-809324-5.23602-x

Bröring T., Oostrom, K. J., Lafeber, H. N., Jansma, E. P., & Oosterlaan, J. (2017). Sensory modulation in preterm children: Theoretical perspective and systematic review. *PLoS One, 12*(2), e0170828. https://doi.org/10.1371/journal.pone.0170828

Cabral de Paula Machado, A. C., de Oliveira, S. R., de Castro Magalhães, L., Marques de Miranda, D., & Bouzada, M. C. F. (2017). Sensory processing during childhood in preterm infants: A systematic review. *Revisita Paulista Pediatria, 35,* 92–101.

Campbell, S., Girolomi, G., Kolobe, T. H. A., Osten, E. T., & Lenke, M. C. (2004, 2012). *Test user's manual for the test of infant motor performance V.3 for the TIMP version 5.* S. K. Campbell. www.thetimp.com

Case-Smith, J., Clark, G. J. F., & Schlabach, T. L. (2013). Systematic review of interventions used in occupational therapy to promote motor performance for children ages birth–5 years. *American Journal of Occupational Therapy, 67*(4), 413–424. https://doi.org/10.5014/ajot.2013.005959

Cassidy, J., Marvin, R. S., & The MacArthur Working Group. (1992). *Attachment organization in preschool children: Procedures and coding manual.* Unpublished manuscript, University of Virginia, 125–131.

Crittenden, P. M. (2006). A dynamic-maturational model of attachment. *Australian and New Zealand Journal of Family Therapy, 27*(2), 105–115. https://doi.org/10.1002/j.1467-8438.2006.tb00704.x

Crittenden, P. M. (2010). *CARE-index. Infants. Coding manual.* Family Relations Institute.

Crittenden, P. M., Claussen, A., & Kozlowska, K. (2007). Choosing a valid assessment of attachment for clinical use: A comparative study. *Australian and New Zealand Journal of Family Therapy, 28*(2). https://doi.org/10.1375/anft.28.2.78

Crittenden, P. M., & Landini, A. (2015). Attachment relationships as semiotic scaffolding systems. *Biosemiotics, 8*(2), 257–273. https://doi.org/10.1007/s12304-014-9224-x

DeGangi, G. A., & Greenspan, S. I. (1989). *Test of sensory functions in infants.* Western Psychological Services.

Department of Developmental Services (DDS). (2013). *Compilation of early start statutes and regulations* (9th ed.). www.dds.ca.gov/EarlyStart

Deneault, A. A., Bureau, J. F., Yurkowski, K., & Moss, E. (2020). Validation of the preschool attachment rating scales with child-mother and child-father dyads. *Attachment & Human Development, 22*(5), 491–513. https://doi.org/10. 1080/14616734.2019.1589546

Dunn, W. (2014). *Sensory Profile™2.* Pearson.

Einspieler, C., Prechtl, H. F., Bos, A. F., Ferrari, F., & Cioni, G. (2004). Prechtl's method on the qualitative assessment of general movements in preterm, term and young infants. In *Clinics in developmental medicine* (p. 167). Mac Keith Press.

Fallang, B., & Hadders-Algra, M. (2005). Postural behavior in children born preterm. *Neural Plasticity, 12*(2–3), 175–182. https://doi.org/10.1155/ np.2005.175

Flanagan, J. E., Landa, R., Bhat, A., & Bauman, M. (2012). Head lag in infants at risk for autism: A preliminary study. *American Journal of Occupational Therapy, 66*(5), 577–585. https://doi.org/10.5014/ajot.2012.004192

Flanagan, J. E., Schoen, S., & Miller, L. J. (2019). Early identification of sensory processing difficulties in high-risk infants. *American Journal of Occupational Therapy, 73*(2), 7302205130p1–7302205130p9. https://doi.org/10.5014/ ajot.2018.028449

Folio, M. R., & Fewell, R. R. (2000). *Peabody developmental motor scales. Examiners manual.* Pro-ED.

Frolek Clark, G., & Schlabach, T. (2013). Systematic review of occupational therapy interventions to improve cognitive development in children ages birth–5 years. *American Journal of Occupational Therapy, 67*(4), 425–430. https:// doi.org/10.5014/ajot.2013.006163

Germani, T., Zwaigenbaum, L., Bryson, S., Brian, J., Smith, I., Roberts, W., & Vaillancourt, T. (2014). Brief report: Assessment of early sensory processing in infants at high-risk of autism spectrum disorder. *Journal of Autism and Developmental Disorders, 44*(12), 3264–3270. https://doi.org/10.1007/ s10803-014-2175-x

Greenspan, S. I., DeGangi, G., & Wieder, S. (2001). *The functional emotional assessment scale (FEAS): For infancy & early childhood.* Interdisciplinary Council on Development & Learning Disorders.

Greenspan, S., & Wieder, S. (2008). DIR®/Floortime™ model. *The International Council on Developmental and Learning Disorders.* https://doi.org/10.1093/ med/9780195371826.003.0068

Haataja, L., Mercuri, E., Regev, R., Cowan, F., Rutherford, M., Dubowitz, V., Dubowitz, L. (1999). Optimality score for the neurologic examination of the infant at 12 and 18 months of age. *Journal of Pediatrics, 135*(2 Pt 1), 153–161. https://doi.org/10.1016/s0022-3476(99)70016-8

Hadders-Algra, M., Boxum, A. G., Hielkema, T., & Hamer, E. G. (2017). Effect of early intervention in infants at very high risk of cerebral palsy: A systematic review. *Developmental Medicine & Child Neurology, 59*(3), 246–258. https://doi. org/10.1111/dmcn.13331

Hadders-Algra, M., Mavinkurve-Groothuis, A., Groen, S., Stremmelaar, E., Martijn, A., & Butcher, P. (2004). Quality of general movements and the development of minor neurological dysfunction at toddler and school age. *Clinical Rehabilitation, 18*(3), 287–299. https://doi.org/10.1191/0269215504cr730oa

Hambrick, E. P., Brawner, T. W., Perry, B. D., Brandt, K., Hofmeister, C., & Collins, J. O. (2019). Beyond the ACE score: Examining relationships between timing of developmental adversity, relational health and developmental outcomes in children. *Archives of Psychiatric Nursing, 33*(3), 238–247. https://doi.org/10.1016/j.apnu.2018.11.001

Heineman, K., Schendelaar, P., Van den Heuvel, E., & Hadders-Algra, M. (2018). Motor development in infancy is related to cognitive function at 4 years of age. *Developmental Medicine & Child Neurology, 60*(11), 1149–1155. https://doi.org/10.1111/dmcn.13761

Hielkema, T., Boxum, A. G., Hamer, E. G., La Bastide-Van Gemert, S., Dirks, T., Reinders Messelink, H. A., & Hadders-Algra, M. (2019). LEARN2MOVE 0–2 years, a randomized early intervention trial infants at very high risk of cerebral palsy: Family outcome and infant's functional outcome. *Disability and Rehabilitation*, 1–9. https://doi.org/10.1080/09638288.2019.1610509

Hughes-Scholes, C. H., & Gavidia-Payne, S. (2016). Development of a routines-based early childhood intervention model. *Educar em Revista*, (59), 141–154. https://doi.org/10.1590/0104-4060.44616

Hutchon, B., Gibbs, D., Harniess, P., Jary, S., Crossley, S. L., Moffat, J. V., & Basu, A. P. (2019). Early intervention programmes for infants at high risk of atypical neurodevelopmental outcome. *Developmental Medicine & Child Neurology, 61*(12), 1362–1367. https://doi.org/10.1111/dmcn.14187

Hwang, A. W., Chao, M. Y., & Liu, S. W. (2013). A randomized controlled trial of routines based early intervention for children with or at risk for developmental delay. *Research in Developmental Disabilities, 34*(10), 3112–3123. https://doi.org/10.1016/j.ridd.2013.06.037

Jaegermann, N., & Klein, P. S. (2010). Enhancing mothers' interactions with toddlers who have sensory-processing disorders. *Infant Mental Health Journal: Official Publication of the World Association for Infant Mental Health, 31*(3), 291–311. https://doi.org/10.1002/imhj.20257

Jorge, J., de Witt, P. A., & Franzsen, D. (2013). The effect of a two-week sensory diet on fussy infants with regulatory sensory processing disorder. *South African Journal of Occupational Therapy, 43*(3), 28–34. https://doi.org/10.1080/j006v16n04_01

Kemp, P., & Turnbull, A. P. (2014). Coaching with parents in early intervention: An interdisciplinary research synthesis. *Infants & Young Children, 27*(4), 305–324. https://doi.org/10.1097/iyc.0000000000000018

Khurana, S., Kane, A. E., Brown, S. E., Tarver, T., & Dusing, S. C. (2020). Effect of neonatal therapy on the motor, cognitive, and behavioral development of infants born preterm: A systematic review. *Developmental Medicine & Child Neurology, 62*(6), 684–692. https://doi.org/10.1111/dmcn.14485

Kingsley, K., & Mailloux, Z. (2013). Evidence for the effectiveness of different service delivery models in early intervention services. *American Journal of Occupational Therapy, 67*(4), 431–436. https://doi.org/10.5014/ajot.2013.006171

Lee, E. (2017). Effect of neuro-development treatment on motor development in preterm infants. *Journal of Physical Therapy Science, 29*(6), 1095–1097. https://doi.org/10.1589/jpts.29.1095

Lönnberg, P., Niutanen, U., Parham, L. D., Wolford, E., Andersson, S., Metsäranta, M., & Lano, A. (2018). Sensory-motor performance in seven-year-old children born extremely preterm. *Early Human Development, 120*, 10–16. https://doi.org/10.1016/j.earlhumdev.2018.03.012

Lu, L., Lan, S., Hsieh, Y., Lin, L., Chen, J., & Lan, S. (2020). Massage therapy for weight gain in preterm neonates: A systematic review and meta-analysis of randomized controlled trials. *Complementary Therapies in Clinical Practice, 39,* 101168. https://doi.org/10.1016/j.ctcp.2020.101168

Madigan, S., Hawkins, E., Goldberg, S., & Benoit, D. (2006). Reduction of disrupted caregiver behavior using modified interaction guidance. *Infant Mental Health Journal: Official Publication of the World Association for Infant Mental Health, 27*(5), 509–527. https://doi.org/10.1002/imhj.20102

May-Benson, T., Koomar, J. A., & Teasdale, A. (2009). Incidence of pre-, peri-, and post-natal birth and developmental problems of children with sensory processing disorder and children with autism spectrum disorder. *Frontiers In Integrative Neuroscience, 3.* https://doi.org/10.3389/neuro.07.031.2009

McWilliam, R. (2016). Birth to three: Early intervention. *Handbook of Early Childhood Special Education,* 75–88. https://doi.org/10.1007/978-3-319-28492-7_5

Miller-Kuhaneck, H., Ecker, C. E., Parham, L. D., Henry, D. A., & Glennon, T. J. (2010). *Sensory processing measure-preschool (SPM-P): Manual.* Western Psychological Services.

Miller, L. J., & Roid, G. H. (1994). *The TIME Toddler and Infant Motor Evaluation: A standardized assessment.* Therapy Skill Builders.

Morgan, C., Darrah, J., Gordon, A., Harbourne, R., Spittle, A., Johnson, R., & Fetters, L. (2016). Effectiveness of motor interventions in infants with cerebral palsy: A systematic review. *Developmental Medicine & Child Neurology, 58*(9), 900–909. https://doi.org/10.1111/dmcn.13105

Morgan, C., Novak, I., & Badawi, N. (2013). Enriched environments and motor outcomes in cerebral palsy: Systematic review and meta-analysis. *Pediatrics, 132*(3), e735–e746. https://doi.org/10.1542/peds.2012-3985

Mubarak, A., Cyr, C., St-André, M., Paquette, D., Emond-Nakamura, M., Boisjoly, L., & Stikarovska, I. (2017). Child attachment and sensory regulation in psychiatric clinic referred preschoolers. *Clinical Child Psychology and Psychiatry, 22*(4), 572–587. https://doi.org/10.1177/1359104516667997

National Scientific Council on the Developing Child. (2004). *Children's emotional development is built into the architecture of their brains* (Working Paper No. 2). www.developingchild.net

Niutanen, U., Harra, T., Lano, A., & Metsäranta, M. (2019). Systematic review of sensory processing in preterm children reveals abnormal sensory modulation, somatosensory processing and sensory-based motor processing. *Acta Paediatrica, 109*(1), 45–55. https://doi.org/10.1111/apa.14953

Novak, I., Morgan, C., Adde, L., Blackman, J., Boyd, R. N., Brunstrom-Hernandez, J., & De Vries, L. S. (2017). Early, accurate diagnosis and early intervention in cerebral palsy: Advances in diagnosis and treatment. *JAMA Pediatrics, 171*(9), 897–907. https://doi.org/10.1001/jamapediatrics.2017.1689

Øberg, G., Ustad, T., Jørgensen, L., Kaaresen, P., Labori, C., & Girolami, G. (2018). Parents' perceptions of administering a motor intervention with their preterm infant in the NICU. *European Journal of Physiotherapy, 21*(3), 134–141. https://doi.org/10.1080/21679169.2018.1503718

O'Grady, M. G., & Dusing, S. C. (2015). Reliability and validity of play-based assessments of motor and cognitive skills for infants and young children: A systematic review. *Physical Therapy, 95*(1), 25–38. https://doi.org/10.2522/ptj.20140111

Omizzolo, C., Scratch, S. E., Stargatt, R., Kidokoro, H., Thompson, D. K., Lee, K. J., Cheong, J., Neil, J., Inder, T. E., Doyle, L. W., & Anderson, P. J. (2014).

Neonatal brain abnormalities and memory and learning outcomes at 7 years in children born very preterm. *Memory, 22*(6), 605–615.

Özdermir, S., & Yildiz, S. (2019). The effects of massage on the weight gain of preterm infants: A systematic review. *Journal of Traditional Medical Complementary Therapies, 2*(1), 33–41. https://doi.org/10.5336/jtracom.2018-62885

Park, H. Y., Maitra, K., Achon, J., Loyola, E., & Rincón, M. (2014). Effects of early intervention on mental or neuromusculoskeletal and movement-related functions in children born low birthweight or preterm: A meta-analysis. *American Journal of Occupational Therapy, 68*(3), 268–276. https://doi.org/10.5014/ajot.2014.010371

Pekçetin, S., Akı, E., Üstünyurt, Z., & Kayıhan, H. (2016). The efficiency of sensory integration interventions in preterm infants. *Perceptual and Motor Skills, 123*(2), 411–423. https://doi.org/10.1177/0031512516662895

Phelps, R. A., & Fogler, J. M. (2018). Tangled roots and ramifications: The early histories of autism spectrum disorder and reactive attachment disorder. In *Trauma, Autism, and Neurodevelopmental Disorders* (pp. 5–18). Springer. https://doi.org/10.1007/978-3-030-00503-0_2

Piper, M. C., & Darrah, J. (1994). *Motor assessment of the developing infant.* W.B. Saunders Company.

Rhoades, B., Greenberg, M., Lanza, S., & Blair, C. (2011). Demographic and familial predictors of early executive function development: Contribution of a person-centered perspective. *Journal of Experimental Child Psychology, 108*(3), 638–662. https://doi.org/10.1016/j.jecp.2010.08.004

Rice, C., Van Naarden Braun, K., Kogan, M. D., Smith, C., Kavanagh, L., & Strickland, B., & Blumberg, S. J. (2014, September 12). *Screening for developmental delays among young children-national survey of children's health, United States, 2007.* Center for Disease Control and Prevention. www.cdc.gov/mmwr/preview/mmwrhtml/su6302a5.htm

Rush, D. D., & Sheldon, M. L. (2011). *The early childhood coaching handbook.* Paul H. Brookes.

Ryckman, J., Hilton, C., Rogers, C., & Pineda, R. (2018). Sensory processing disorder in preterm infants during early childhood and relationships to early neurobehavior. *Early Human Development, 113*, 18–22. https://doi.org/10.1016/j.earlhumdev.2017.07.012

Schore, A. N. (2003). Development of the right brain and its role in early emotional life. In *Emotional development in psychoanalysis, attachment theory, and neuroscience: Creating connections* (pp. 23–54). https://doi.org/10.4324/9780203420362_part_1

Seiiedi-Biarag, L., & Mirghafourvand, M. (2020). The effect of massage on feeding intolerance in preterm infants: A systematic review and meta-analysis study. *Italian Journal of Pediatrics, 46*, 1–10. https://doi.org/10.1186/s13052-020-0818-4

Spittle, A., Orton, J., Anderson, P. J., Boyd, R., & Doyle, L. W. (2015). Early developmental intervention programmes provided post hospital discharge to prevent motor and cognitive impairment in preterm infants. *Cochrane Database of Systematic Reviews, 11.* https://doi.org/10.1002/14651858.cd005495.pub4

Spittle, A., & Treyvaud, K. (2016, December). The role of early developmental intervention to influence neurobehavioral outcomes of children born preterm. In *Seminars in perinatology* (Vol.40, No. 8, pp. 542–548). WB Saunders. https://doi.org/10.1053/j.semperi.2016.09.006

Stallings-Sahler, S. (1998). Sensory integration: Assessment and intervention with infants and young children. In J. Case-Smith (Ed.), *Pediatric occupational therapy and early intervention* (pp. 223–254). Butterworth-Heinemann.

Stewart, K. B. (2008). Outcomes of relationship-based early intervention. *Journal of Occupational Therapy, Schools, & Early Intervention, 1*(3–4), 199–205. https://doi.org/10.1080/19411240802589395

Szklut, S. (2014). Early identification and intervention of sensory issues in the birth to 3 year population. *OT Practice, 19*, 19.

Tauman, R., Avni, H., Drori-Asayag, A., Nehama, H., Greenfeld, M., & Leitner, Y. (2017). Sensory profile in infants and toddlers with behavioral insomnia and/or feeding disorders. *Sleep Medicine, 32*, 83–86. https://doi.org/10.1016/j.sleep.2016.12.009

Ustad, T., Evensen, K. A. I., Campbell, S. K., Girolami, G. L., Helbostad, J., Jørgensen, L., & Øberg, G. K. (2016). Early parent-administered physical therapy for preterm infants: A randomized controlled trial. *Pediatrics, 138*(2), e20160271. https://doi.org/10.1542/peds.2016-0271

Van der Kolk, B. A. (2017). Developmental trauma disorder: Toward a rational diagnosis for children with complex trauma histories. *Psychiatric Annals, 35*(5), 401–408. https://doi.org/10.3928/00485713-20050501-06

Van Hus, J. W. P., Jeukens-Visser, M., Koldewijn, K., Geldof, C. J., Kok, J. H., Nollet, F., & Van Wassenaer-Leemhuis, A. G. (2013). Sustained developmental effects of the infant behavioral assessment and intervention program in very low birth weight infants at 5.5 years corrected age. *The Journal of Pediatrics, 162*(6), 1112–1119. https://doi.org/10.1016/j.jpeds.2012.11.078

Van Hus, J. W. P., Jeukens-Visser, M., Koldewijn, K., Holman, R., Kok, J. H., Nollet, F., & Van Wassenaer-Leemhuis, A. G. (2016). Early intervention leads to long-term developmental improvements in very preterm infants, especially infants with bronchopulmonary dysplasia. *Acta Paediatrica, 105*(7), 773–781. https://doi.org/10.1111/apa.13387

van Wassenaer-Leemhuis, A. G., Jeukens-Visser, M., van Hus, J. W., Meijssen, D., Wolf, M. J., Kok, J. H., & Koldewijn, K. (2016). Rethinking preventive post-discharge intervention programmes for very preterm infants and their parents. *Developmental Medicine & Child Neurology, 58*, 67–73. https://doi.org/10.1111/dmcn.13049

Whitcomb, D. A., Carrasco, R. C., Neuman, A., & Kloos, H. (2015). Correlational research to examine the relation between attachment and sensory modulation in young children. *American Journal of Occupational Therapy, 69*(4), 6904220020p1–6904220020p8. https://doi.org/10.5014/ajot.2015.015503

Will, E. A., Daunhauer, L. A., Fidler, D. J., Raitano Lee, N., Rosenberg, C. R., & Hepburn, S. L. (2019). Sensory processing and maladaptive behavior: Profiles within the down syndrome phenotype. *Physical & Occupational Therapy in Pediatrics, 39*(5), 461–476. https://doi.org/10.1080/01942638.2019.1575320

Williamson, G. G., & Anzalone, M. E. (2001). *Sensory integration and self-regulation in infants and toddlers: Helping very young children interact with their environment.* Zero to Three: National Center for Infants, Toddlers and Families, 2000 M Street, NW, Suite 200, Washington, DC 20036–3307.

Part 3

Contexts & Community Programs

8 Incorporating Nature in the Context of Sensory Integration Treatment

Gustavo Reinoso, Laura Kula, and Erna Imperatore Blanche

The importance of studying the interaction between the person and the environment is emphasized in several theoretical and intervention models (Kaplan, 1983; Law, 1991; Law et al., 1996) as well as in the International Classification of Functioning, Disability and Health (ICF) (WHO, 2001). The analysis of the interaction often highlights increasing participation through adaptations made to the built environment or indoor spaces, but seldom addresses the importance of nature and its impact on health. This is striking because children's opportunities for free outdoor play have declined at the same time that children's physical health, mental health, psychological resilience, and sense of personal control also declined (Lanza, 2012). The purpose of this chapter is to 1) provide a short review of the literature about the effects of environments on health and wellness; 2) emphasize the importance and the affordances of nature as well as considerations to embed nature-based space elements into designed built spaces; and 3) address the need to incorporate, and infuse health producing affordances of nature in the interventions process in all environments.

Defining Environments and Their Effects on Health

Built environments are defined as spaces that are deliberately constructed, including outdoor spaces altered by human activity (The Committee on Environmental Health, 2009). Natural environments, on the other hand, are defined in a variety of ways depending upon their interpretation. In the early intervention literature, the definition of natural environment is "any setting that is part of the everyday routine of the child and family where incidental learning happens" (Dunst et al., 2006, p. 4). This definition of natural environment guides early intervention practices, and by this definition, homes and day-care centers are considered "natural" regardless of the physical space where they occur. **This definition of "natural environment" is not the one that will be utilized in this chapter.** For other disciplines (e.g., urban planning) natural environment is a term considered to be synonymous with outdoor spaces and

DOI: 10.4324/9781003050810-11

contact with nature or aspects of nature, an area that has been found to impact health and well-being (Bowler et al., 2010; Fjortoft & Sageie, 2000; Wheeler et al., 2012). This definition is the one utilized in this chapter, that is, natural environments refer to access to nature in outside environments, or aspects of outside environments. Natural environments are also subdivided into green and blue spaces. Green spaces include trees and vegetation, while blue spaces refer to water such as ponds, lakes, rivers, and oceans (Gascon et al., 2015, p. 4355). The evidence for the effects of outdoor green environments on children's health and well-being is increasing. Bowler et al. (2010) emphasized the importance of focusing on the spatial and social impact of activities performed in outdoor versus inside environments such as the experiential difference of walking in a park versus walking on a treadmill in a gym. In pediatrics, it would be important to consider the difference between playing in an indoor gym compared to an outdoor play structure. Given that different definitions of outdoor spaces include both the natural and built environments, research is difficult to synthesize and even more challenging to include in an intervention environment at a practical level (Taylor & Hochuli, 2017). Gathering information about a child's daily access to outdoor spaces, natural or built, green or blue, should be valuable in the evaluation process. In this chapter, we emphasize the importance of incorporating green outdoor spaces, built or natural, or adding natural elements into the clinical environment. We will use the term green space to describe research and interventions done in outdoor spaces where there is contact with vegetation.

The studies addressing green spaces cover a vast area, but are primarily outside the profession of occupational therapy (OT). In this section of the chapter we will discuss the effects of green spaces on health, and in particular, the effect of green spaces in urban areas as most children live in cities where access to parks and gardens is limited.

Bowler et al. (2010) reviewed twenty-five studies focusing on the impact of natural environments, or outdoor spaces, on individuals' well-being and concluded that natural environments have a direct and positive impact on well-being. Specifically, improvements can be measured in brain and cognitive development (Dadvand et al., 2015), children's attention (Dadvand et al., 2017), overall health (Giusti et al., 2017), and overall well-being (Krekel et al., 2016). Other literature reviews specific to the impact of green space on health describe long term effects on the physiological signs of stress, overall reported health, better health outcomes (Twohig-Bennett & Jones, 2018), improved mental health (Callaghan et al., 2020), and improved cognitive functions (de Keijzer et al., 2016; de Keijzer, 2018). However, the majority of these reviews also indicate that the heterogeneity and poor quality of many studies limits drawing definitive conclusions. Furthermore, a comprehensive summary provided by Barakat and colleagues (2019), described nature as healing for children with Autism Spectrum Disorder (ASD). They described the impact of nature on cognitive skills, creativity, attention, stress level, language, and social and emotional development. These authors thoroughly described the need to incorporate nature in the intervention process. Their recommendations on sensory gardens are included later in this chapter (Barakat et al., 2019).

When monitoring green space in urban areas, Van Herzele and Wiedermann (2003) identified several concepts to consider. These include the perceptions a person has of inside and outside city green spaces, the safety of those green spaces, and proximity and ease of access to them. It is clear that green spaces in urban environments are needed as their presence is correlated with well-being, while the presence of abandoned areas correlates with decreased life satisfaction (Krekel et al., 2016). Overall access to green spaces in urban environments may decrease children's life stress, including the psychological effects of stressful life events (Wells & Evans, 2003). The presence of green spaces may also impact daily routines as there are more opportunities for going outdoors and engaging in outdoor physical activity (de Vries et al., 2003).

The impact of sensory overload, mainly auditory, has also been studied in relation to different environments. For example, the effects of acute and chronic exposure to noise in urban environments decreases speech perception and listening comprehension in children (Szalma & Hancock, 2011). The presence of excessive noise in the environment may also affect non-auditory performance domains such as short-term memory, attention, pre-reading, reading and writing skills (Klatte et al., 2010). Most studies in this area have targeted specific environments such as schools, living in proximity to airports or road traffic noise (Clark, 2015; Hygge, 2003; Stansfeld et al., 2005). However, access or proximity to green space can have a mitigating effect on the negative impacts of noise levels. A study by Gidlöf-Gunnarsson and Öhrström (2007) indicated that increased availability to nearby green area and increasing time spent outside is important for well-being and daily behavior. These factors coincide with findings of reducing long-term noise annoyances and stress-related psychosocial symptoms. The authors proposed that future designs of urban green space locations should be easily accessible, provide lower noise levels from traffic and relief from environmental stress, and should include opportunities for relaxation and noise-free sections.

The Importance of Incorporating Outdoor Spaces in the Interventions Process

The ICF: Children and Youth Version (ICF-CY) identifies health to include the original definition describing health as "a state of complete physical, mental and social well-being and not merely the absence of disease or infirmity" (WHO, 2001, 2013). The ICF model also identifies environments as an area of intervention, and although occupational therapists incorporate this concept of health and environments in practice; most descriptions of environments are about the effects of built environments. More specifically, much has been written about built environments' exposure of sensory information that often exceeds children's coping abilities (Cermak et al., 2015). Less is written about green spaces and how to include these concepts, or elements of them in the intervention process. Based on the literature reviewed, the following concepts need to be incorporated in the evaluation and treatment process:

1. Incorporate questions about access to green spaces, including proximity, perception of the value of green spaces and safety issues.
2. Analyze the living and academic built environment giving special attention to their sensory aspects (visual, auditory, olfactory, etc.).
3. Address access at an individual level to green spaces as part of leisure occupations, daily routines, and daily habits. Addressing access at the system level is beyond the scope of this chapter.

Incorporate Questions About Access to Green Spaces Including Proximity, Perception of the Value of Green Spaces, and Safety Issues

Features that enable children to explore and experience aspects of the natural environment are important elements when occupational therapy practitioners (OTPs) design interventions. More research is needed on how to incorporate green spaces in children's lives. However, it is important to start by increasing attention to the impact of green spaces on participation. During the evaluation, the therapist may consider incorporating questions about children's living spaces, neighborhood safety, and percentage of time spent indoors versus outdoors. Access to natural environments is especially important for children with sensory processing disorders living in urban environments. Existing evaluations of the environment such as the Participation and Sensory Environment Questionnaire (PSEQ) can be used to analyze the impact of the sensory environment on participation as well as the type of sensory response exhibited by the child (Pfeiffer et al., 2017). Subsequently, carefully designed recommendations can be made across environments for inclusion of these sensory experiences.

Addressing the Sensory Aspects of the Built Environments

When intervening in the built environment, elements from nature and what is known about the effects of sensory input can be included in its design. Environmental modifications can include tailored lighting, sound reduction, spatial organization, and other multisensory considerations. For example, a recent study by Cermak and colleagues used ideas from Snozelen to make multisensory changes in the dental environment and thus decrease stress during teeth cleaning for children with ASD (Cermak et al., 2015; Shapiro et al., 2007). The environment used in Snozelen may not be inspired directly from research on nature, but offers elements found in nature: decreased auditory and visual overload, increased uniformity (decrease abrupt sensory changes), and exploration opportunities. Ideas emanating from Snozelen have been successful in decreasing stress in adults and children with disabilities, and are examples of adjustments that can be made in indoor spaces (Lotan & Gold, 2009). In the same way that the dental environment was modified, other environments such as grocery stores, classrooms, and many others need to be attended to and modified. Table 8.1 provides examples of modifications that can be incorporated into built environments, as well as their possible effects on sensory processing.

Address Access to Green Spaces as Part of Leisure Occupations, Daily Routines, and Daily Habits

The need for increased participation in green spaces, either in neighborhood gardens, schools, parks or farms is widely supported in the literature (Bell et al., 2008; Gill, 2014). However, with few exceptions, extending occupational therapy services into green spaces and natural environments is undervalued perhaps due to issues around logistics and cost. The existing programs addressing participation in green spaces include farms, sensory gardens, and nature.

Working in farms with children can be somewhat more difficult for interveners working in urban environments, however using a farm with animals may be a solution for summer camps and weekend recreational activities. Hickman and Harkness (2002) use animals and farms to address sensory modulation difficulties in children with a variety of disorders. Caring for farm animals can offer practitioners an avenue for providing the just right challenge while participating in a green space. Another program developed by Protopapadaki (2019) uses principles of sensory integration treatment in farms where children are encouraged to engage in specialized farm activities to provide the necessary sensory experiences while working on skills such as attention and motor planning. Occupational therapy practices may benefit from more fully exploring such outdoor delivery models. For example, Figueroa (2020) provides clinical services outdoors and describes nature based occupational therapy services, including camps and playgroups.

At a global level, recommendations emphasizing the importance of the child's relationship to nature include the work of Giusti et al. (2017). These authors created a framework to understand the qualities of situations that help children connect to nature by interviewing professionals with expertise in outdoor focused pedagogical approaches. They focused on the qualities of what constitutes a significant nature

Table 8.1 Examples of Environmental Modifications, Potential Effects on Sensory Processing, and Recommendations Based on Current Literature

Environmental aspect	Effects on sensory processing and integration	Recommendations
Presence of multiple objects, multiple wall paintings, mirrors, and moving parts	Decreased attention, decreased processing speed, and overload on central visual connections.	Organize the environment (e.g., put things away, highlight what is relevant by decreasing competing bright stimuli), include at least one singular-colored wall in the treatment environment.
Indoor/outdoor noise (i.e., traffic, shopping centers)	Decreased language development and listening skills, attention, over-responsivity, regulatory issues.	Specially designed walls and windows, carpeted floor, adaptations to chair legs and tables.
Artificial Lighting	Hyperresponsiveness, regulation issues, and decreased attention.	Use spaces with windows that allow fresh air and natural light.
Multiple colored mats and busy floor patterns	Decreased attention, poor visual perceptual and spatial skills, over-orientation to detail.	Singular color mats (e.g., avoid multiple color squares in intervention and clinical settings), clear contrast between floors/mats and walls, furniture, doors, and windows.
Lack of restorative quiet spaces	Decreased opportunities for self-regulation.	Create places where a child can remove self from visual, auditory, and other sensory experiences (tents, enclosed spaces in playgrounds, nature gardens).
Lack of access to nature and green spaces in outside and inside environments	Decreased opportunities for the positive benefits of nature.	Create protected time where children freely engage with nature. Include trees, plants, water fountains in inside spaces and outside playgrounds.

situation, describing crucial elements such as the engagement of the senses, involvement of mentors, self-restoration, involvement of animals, and physical activity, among others. See Figure 8.1.

Other approaches existing in the literature include those focusing on sensory gardens. Hussein (2012, 2020) offers several ideas in the construction of sensory gardens, including attending to the choice of plant compositions and the sensory experiences derived from

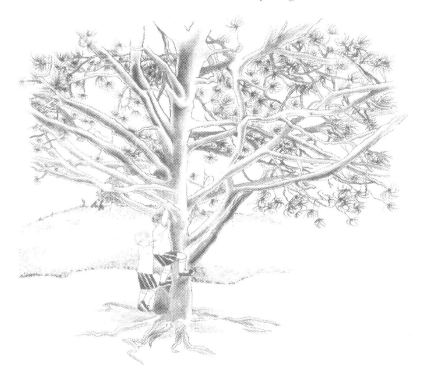

Figure 8.1 Climbing Trees Provides the Opportunity for Challenging Motor Planning and Enhance Proprioceptive Feedback

interacting with them. For example, colors, texture, and scents are important considerations during the construction of a sensory garden (Chiumento et al., 2018; Hussein, 2012, 2020). Furthermore, Barakat et al. (2019) established specific guidelines for designing sensory gardens that address hyporesponsiveness and hyperresponsiveness in children with ASD. They suggest using a savannah type landscape, similar plant sizes, pastel colors, monochromatic schemes, and small spaces for children who are hyperresponsive. For children who are hyporesponsive, they recommend using vivid colors, coarse textured plants, contrast, changes in topography, and large open spaces. Sensory gardens may be easier to incorporate in the therapeutic process. Occupational therapy clinics should consider having access to outdoor green spaces, even if they are smaller, for children to explore and play. Using plants to call attention to specific textures and scents, planting vegetables, and playing with water are simple activities that can be incorporated into any therapeutic routine in a built clinical environment.

Table 8.2 Addressing Sensory Systems in the Natural and Built Environments

Sensory systems	Natural Environment	Built Environment
Tactile	Gardening; collecting leaves, herbs, or flowers; building or arranging pebbles and rocks, crawling through grasses or sand, playing in the snow.	Roof-top soil bed; potted plants, ikebana's, green walls, indoor gardening beds, hydroponic pod towers, vertical vegetable gardens, sand boxes.
Vestibular	Swinging, gyroscopic-shaped playground equipment, vortex spin, rotating play climbers, Merry Go Round, seesaw spinner, trapeze, etc. Rolling down the hill, swinging on a tree branch, jumping/diving into a pool/pond.	Playground and classroom equipment that allows movement experiences (e.g., rocking chairs, balls, swings).
Proprioception	Climbing/planting tree, building/climbing fences, and landscape structures, climbing boulders or trees, hanging from trees, wading through water or snow.	Playground equipment that allows climbing, jumping, pushing, lifting, and carrying. Pushing of sand or wet sand in a sand table, carrying of watering cans full of water.
Visual	Natural sunlight, outdoor garden or green environment with contrasting colors or expansive green areas.	Decrease and/or cover fluorescent lighting, open windows and curtains, light colored walls, sunlight reaching light colored walls, orientation of windows (balancing light and heat), roof natural lighting construction (diffused light), smaller lamps.
Auditory	Nature sounds (wind, water, birds, moving trees).	Sound dampening walls, sound reducing paintings and acoustic panels, wearable sound canceling devices, utilize sound monitor equipment that offers visual feedback to classrooms. Incorporate sounds of nature such as small fountains, wind and wind chimes.

(*Continued*)

Sensory systems	Natural Environment	Built Environment
Olfactory	Planting herbs, trees, and flowers (e.g., jasmine, lavender, magnolias, mint), watering plants, cutting grass.	Potted plants, ikebanas, greenery walls, indoor gardening beds, hydroponic pod towers for herbs, essential oils, aroma humidifiers.

Focusing on the environment also requires attending to family routines and habits. Increasing access to green spaces and recreational areas can help increase physical activity (Babey et al., 2005) and compensate for depleted attention (Berto, 2005). Children are continually using their attention capacity in what is called *directed but also rapidly switching attention*. During these chunks of time, children attend to and rapidly shift attention between homework, surfing the internet, texting, playing video games, watching online videos, and watching TV, among many other competing tasks. This shifting of attentional units exhausts finite attentional resources and prevents concentrated, quality engagement. Some research now suggests that this type of attention, once depleted, is restored by actively engaging in green spaces such as taking a walk in nature (Berto, 2005). Building on the idea of movement breaks, including "nature breaks" where children engage with green spaces in the context of their daily routine, can be incorporated and measured as an intervention resource. Nature breaks can restore cognitive capacities to optimum levels (Berto, 2005; Faber Taylor et al., 2002; Harting et al., 2003; Kaplan, 1995; Tennessen & Cimprich, 1995). Table 8.2 provides examples of the use of specific sensory experiences in both the natural and built environment.

Conclusions

Blending therapeutic interventions offers attractive solutions for children with a variety of abilities and their families by considering their sensory needs as well as potential barriers in and across several environments. A step-by-step approach to tackling these problems should be undertaken, including the consideration of present and future realities, while taking into consideration the opportunities in natural environments or green spaces. The tables included should not be taken as recipes, but rather as examples of how space could be best utilized to meet children's needs across and specific to different contexts. The present and future profiles of children and the wishes of the families should also be carefully considered in combination with the basic human need for function and participation. The ultimate goal of blending SI with

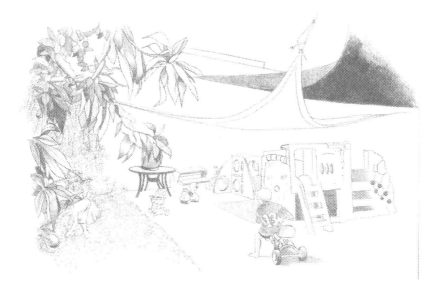

Figure 8.2 An Outside Treatment Environment Created in an Urban Context Designed to Treat Children During the Pandemic

other therapeutic interventions is to offer an environment that facilitates well-being, life satisfaction, the highest level of function and participation, and considers the current and future needs of child, family, and the community.

Interestingly, as the authors of this chapter explored information about natural environments, it was difficult to find data under the domain of occupational therapy due to the context of natural environments reflecting only on children's everyday built environments. Understanding the impact of environmental contexts on daily occupations and their relationship with health and well-being need to be further reviewed. Providing occupations in natural environments or built environments containing elements of green space encourages opportunities to register and modulate sensory processing experiences effectively, while also allowing simple adaptive responses to help organize behavior and learning.

Play is children's primary occupation and occupational therapists' main intervention. Children's play is intrinsically motivating and is a transaction between the child and the environment (Hollenbeck, 2017). The contribution of outdoor or green spaces (or the incorporation of elements of them) to health and well-being gives occupational therapists an additional realistic and beneficial tool during the intervention process.

References

Barakat, H. A. E. R., Bakr, A., & El-Sayad, Z. (2019). Nature as a healer for autistic children. *Alexandria Engineering Journal, 58*(1), 353–366.

Babey, S. H., Brown, E. R., & Hastert, T. A. (2005). *Access to safe parks helps increase physical activity among teenagers. Health policy research brief.* UCLA Center for Health Policy Research, UC. https://escholarship.org/uc/item/42x5z4jn

Bell, S., Hamilton, V., Montarzino, A., Rothnie, H., Travlou, P., & Alves, S. (2008). *Greenspace scotland research report, greenspace and quality of life: A critical literature review.* The Research Centre for Inclusive Access to Outdoor Environments Edinburg College of Art and Heriot-Watt University.

Berto, R. (2005). Exposure to restorative environments helps restore attentional capacity. *Journal of Experimental Psychology, 25,* 249–259.

Bowler, D. E., Buyung-Ali, L. M., Knight, T. M., & Pullin, A. S. (2010). A systematic review of evidence for the added benefits to health of exposure to natural environments. *BMC Public Health, 10,* 456. https://doi.org/10.1186/1471-2458-10-456

Callaghan, A., McCombe, G., Harrold, A., McMeel, C., Mills, G., Moore-Cherry, N., & Cullen, W. (2020). The impact of green spaces on mental health in urban settings: A scoping review. *Journal of Mental Health,* 1–15. https://doi.org/10.1080/09638237.2020.1755027

Cermak, S. A., Stein Duker, L. I., Williams, M. E., Dawson, M. E., Lane, C. J., & Polido, J. C. (2015). Sensory adapted dental environments to enhance oral care for children with autism spectrum disorders: A randomized controlled pilot study. *Journal of Autism and Developmental Disorders, 45*(9), 2876–2888. https://doi.org/10.1007/s10803-015-2450-5

Chiumento, A., Mukherjee, I., Chandna, J., Dutton, C., Rahman, A., & Bristow, K. (2018). A haven of green space: Learning from a pilot pre-post evaluation of a school-based social and therapeutic horticulture intervention with children. *BMC Public Health, 18*(1), 836. https://doi.org/10.1186/s12889-018-5661-9

Clark, C. (2015). *Aircraft noise effects on health: Report prepared for the UK airport commission* (Report Number 150427). Queen Mary University of London.

Committee on Environment Health. (2009). The built environment: Designing communities to promote physical activity in children. *Pediatrics, 123*(6), 1591–1598. https://doi.org/10.1542/peds.2009-0750

Dadvand, P., Nieuwenhuijsen, M. J., Esnaola, M., Forns, J., Basagana, X., Alvarez-Pedrerol, M., Rivas, I., Lopez-Vicente, M., De Castro Pascual, M., Su, J., Jerrett, M., Querol, X., & Sunyer, J. (2015). Green spaces and cognitive development in primary schoolchildren. *Proceedings of the National Academy of Sciences of the U S A, 112*(26), 7937–7942. doi:10.1073/pnas.1503402112

Dadvand, P., Tischer, C., Estarlich, M., Llop, S., Dalmau-Bueno, A., Lopez-Vicente, M., . . . Sunyer, J. (2017). Lifelong residential exposure to green space and attention: A population-based prospective study. *Environ Health Perspect, 125*(9), 97016. doi:10.1289/ehp694.

de Keijzer, C., Gascon, M., Nieuwenhuijsen, M. J., & Dadvand, P. (2016). Long-term green space exposure and cognition across the life course: A systematic review. *Current Environmental Health Reports, 3*(4), 468–477, PMID: 27730509, 10.1007/s40572-016-0116-x.

de Keijzer, C., Tonne, C., Basagaña, X., Valentín, A., Singh-Manoux, A., Alonso, J., Antó, J. M., Nieuwenhuijsen, M. J., Sunyer, J., & Dadvand, P. (2018). Residential surrounding greenness and cognitive decline: A 10-year follow-up of the whitehall II cohort. *Environmental Health Perspectives, 126*(7), 77003. https://doi.org/10.1289/EHP2875.

de Vries, S., Verheij, R. A., Groenewegen, P. P., & Spreeuwenberg, P. (2003). Natural environments – healthy environments? An exploratory analysis of the relationship between greenspace and health. *Environment and Planning A: Economy and Space, 35*(10), 1717–1731. https://doi.org/10.1068/a35111

Dunst, C. J., Bruder, M. B., Trivette, C. M., & Hamby, D. (2006). Everyday activity settings, natural learning environments and early intervention practices. *Journal of Policy and Practice in Intellectual Disabilities, 3*(1), 3–10.

Faber Taylor, A. F., Kuo, F. E., & Sullivan, W. C. (2002). Views of nature and self-discipline: Evidence from inner city children. *Journal of Environmental Psychology, 22*, 49–63.

Figueroa, L. (2020, November 14). *Outdoor kids. Everything you need to know to dress your child for outdoor play in wet or cold weather.* www.outdoorkidsot.com/blog/wet-weather-clothing

Fjortoft, I., & Sageie, J. (2000). The natural environment as a playground for children. *Landscape and Urban Planning, 48*(1), 83–97. doi:10.1016/S0169-2046(00)00045-1

Gascon, M., Triguero-Mas, M., Martínez, D., Dadvand, P., Forns, J., Plasència, A., & Nieuwenhuijsen, M. J. (2015). Mental health benefits of long-term exposure to residential green and blue spaces: A systematic review. *International Journal of Environmental Research and Public Health, 12*(4), 4354–4379. https://doi.org/10.3390/ijerph120404354

Gidlöf-Gunnarsson, A., & Öhrström, E. (2007). Noise and well-being in urban residential environments: The potential role of perceived availability to nearby green areas. *Landscape and Urban Planning, 83*, 115–126. doi:10.1016/j.landurbplan.2007.03.003

Gill, T. (2014). The benefits of children's engagement with nature: A systematic literature review. *Children Youth and Environments, 24*(2), 10–34.

Giusti, M., Svane, U., Raymond, C. M., & Beery, T. H. (2017). A framework to assess where and how children connect to nature. *Front Psychol, 8*, 2283. doi:10.3389/fpsyg.2017.02283

Harting, T., Evans, G. W., Jammer, L. D., Davis, D. S., & Garlin, T. (2003). Tracking restoration in natural and urban field settings. *Journal of Environmental Psychology, 23*, 109–123.

Hickman, L., & Harkness, L. (2002). Environment as a milieu for intervention: The farm. In A. C. Bundy, S. J. Lane, & E. A. Murray (Eds.), *Sensory integration: Theory and practice* (pp. 364–367). F.A. Davis.

Hollenbeck, J., Wagenfeld, A., Kaldenberg, J., & Honaker, D. (Eds.). (2017). *Foundations of pediatric practice for the occupation therapy assistant* (2nd ed., pp. 203–226). Slack. Inc.

Hussein, H. (2012). Affordances of sensory garden towards learning and self-development of special schooled children. *International Journal of Psychological Studies, 4*(1), 135.

Hussein, H. (2020). Design of sensory gardens for children with disabilities in the context of the United Kingdom. In *Place, pedagogy and play* (pp. 63–76). Routledge.

Hygge, S. (2003). Classroom experiments on the effects of different noise sources and sound levels on long-term recall and recognition in children. *Applied Cognitive Psychology, 17*, 895–914. doi:10.1002/acp.926

Kaplan, S. (1983). A model of person-environment compatibility. *Environment and Behaviour, 15*, 311–332.

Kaplan, S. (1995). The restorative benefits of nature: Toward an integrative framework. *Journal of Environmental Psychology, 15*, 169–182.

Klatte, M., Lachmann, T., Schlittmeier, S., & Hellbrück, J. (2010). The irrelevant sound effect in short-term memory: Is there developmental change? *European Journal of Cognitive Psychology, 22*, 1168–1191. doi:10.1080/095414409 03378250

Krekel, C., Kolbe, J., & Wustemann, H. (2016). The greener, the happier? The effect of urban land use on residential well-being. *Ecological Economics, 121*, 117–127. https://doi.org/10.1016/j.ecolecon.2015.11.005.

Lanza, M. (2012). *Playborhood: Turn your neighborhood into a place for play.* Free Play Press, ISBN: 9780984929818.

Law, M. (1991). The environment: A focus for occupational therapy. *Canadian Journal of Occupational Therapy, 58*, 171–179.

Law, M., Cooper, B., Strong, S., Stewart, D., Rigby, P., & Letts, L. (1996). The person-environment-occupation model: A transactive approach to occupational performance. *Canadian Journal of Occupational Therapy, 63*(1), 9–23. https://doi.org/10.1177/000841749606300103.

Lotan, M., & Gold, C. (2009). Meta-analysis of the effectiveness of individual intervention in the controlled multisensory environment (Snoezelen) for individuals with intellectual disability. *Journal of Intellectual & Developmental Disability, 34*(3), 207–215. https://doi.org/10.1080/13668250903080106

Pfeiffer, B., Coster, W., Tucker, C., & Piller, A. (2017). Development and content validity of the participation and sensory environment questionnaire. *Occupational Therapy in Mental Health.* Advanced online publication. http://dx.doi.org/10.1080/0164212X.2017.1383221.

Protopapadaki, M. (2019, June 20, 22). *Sensory integration in a green care farm.* The 6th European Sensory Integration Congress (ESIC). Thessaloniki, Greece.

Shapiro, M., Melmed, R. N., Sgan-Cohen, H. D., Eli, I., & Parush, S. (2007). Behavioural and physiological effect of dental environment sensory adaptation on children's dental anxiety. *European Journal of Oral Sciences, 115*(6), 479–483. https://doi.org/10.1111/j.1600-0722.2007.00490.x

Stansfeld, S. A., Berglund, B., Clark, C., Lopez-Barrio, I., Fischer, P., Öhrström, E., Haines, M. M., Head, J., Hygge, S., van Kamp, I., & Berry, B. F. (2005). Aircraft and road traffic noise and children's cognition and health: A cross-national study. *The Lancet, 365*(9475) 1942–1949.

Szalma, J. L., & Hancock, P. A. (2011). Noise effects on human performance: A meta-analytic synthesis. *Psychological Bulletin, 137*, 682–707. doi:10.1037/a0023987

Taylor, L., & Hochuli, D. F. (2017). Defining green space: Multiple uses across multiple disciplines. *Landscape and Urban Planning, 158*, 25–38. https://doi.org/10.1016/j.landurbplan.2016.09.024.

Tennessen, C. M., & Cimprich, B. (1995). Views to nature: Effects on attention. *Journal of Environmental Psychology, 15*, 77–85.

Twohig-Bennett, C., & Jones, A. (2018). The health benefits of the great outdoors: A systematic review and meta-analysis of greenspace exposure and health outcomes. *Environmental Research, 166,* 628–637. https://doi.org/10.1016/j.envres.2018.06.030.

Van Herzele, A., & Wiedermann, T. (2003). A monitoring tool for accessible and attractive green spaces. *Landscape and Urban Planning, 63,* 109–126.

Wells, N. M., & Evans, G. W. (2003). Nearby nature: A buffer of life stress among rural children. *Environment and Behavior, 35*(3), 311330. https://doi.org/10.1177/0013916503035003001.

Wheeler, B. W., White, M., Stahl-Timmins, W., & Depledge, M. H. (2012). Does living by the coast improve health and wellbeing? *Health Place, 18*(5), 1198–201. doi:10.1016/j.healthplace.2012.06.015.

World Health Organization. (2001). *International classification of functioning, disability and health: ICF.* World Health Organization. https://apps.who.int/iris/handle/10665/42407

World Health Organization. (2013). *World health report 2013: Research for universal health coverage.* World Health Organization.

9 School-Based Practice

Supporting Participation and Self-Determination

Lisa A. Test and Bryant Edwards

Results from the Occupational Therapy Compensation and Workforce study indicate that 18.8 percent of occupational therapists and 15.4 percent of occupational therapy assistants work in school settings as their primary area of employment (American Occupational Therapy Association [AOTA], 2020a). Of school-based practitioners, 85 percent reported utilizing a sensory integration approach, 9.3 percent indicated they did not, and another 5.6 percent indicated "other," which was described as either not knowing enough about sensory integration approaches or not feeling they apply enough to consider them (AOTA, 2010). The center point of the intervention may vary based upon each student, the student's therapeutic history, and the expected progress. Services are aimed at remediating deficits in participation skills; adapting and modifying environments or occupations; or providing consultations for the teacher and classroom staff in use of strategies within the school day. Intervening in schools requires knowledge of curriculum, educational standards, and age-appropriate school activities in which the students engage. At the conclusion of this chapter, readers will be able to utilize clinical reasoning to assess, determine needs, and plan intervention in the school setting; articulate various delivery models within the school setting; and understand how to systematically apply different treatment approaches to support student success. This chapter first presents information for how best to proceed through the school-based evaluation and intervention processes, and then utilizes four unique case examples to highlight key elements of this process.

Within the school setting, occupational therapy (OT) is recommended when a student needs the specialized services of OT in order to access and make progress within their educational program. The educational program consists of the academic, curriculum-based education, as well as social education that includes access to typically developing peers, engaging in social activities, and establishing and maintaining relationships (Law, 2002; United States Department of Education [USDE], 2004a, 2004b).

DOI: 10.4324/9781003050810-12

As previously discussed in the Reasoning in Action Model, this systematic process of assessment requires the practitioner to select appropriate methods of gathering information and to identify difficulties with functional participation. The therapist is then able to synthesize data from the assessment with current evidence that guides the selection of intervention approaches. In the school-based setting, the therapist evaluates the dynamic relationship between a student's skills, the curriculum demands and the student's expected participation. The questions guiding the therapist's choices are:

- What are the gaps in the student's performance?
- Do these gaps require an occupational therapist to intervene?
- Is using strategies to adapt the environment enough?
- Or should the student receive individualized services in order to promote optimal student learning and participation in educational activities?

Assessment and Hypothesis Generation

A school-based assessment utilizes similar methods as other practice settings including record reviews, student, and parent interviews, standardized evaluations, and skilled observation of the student's performance in various school contexts. The focus of the assessment is on identifying participation restrictions and activity limitations that limit students' access to their educational program. By identifying the students' strengths and educational supports, the practitioner is able to collaborate with the team to foster self-determination. Assessment requires knowledge of the curriculum, review of educational records, teacher and student interview, observation of the student in context (classroom, hallways, playground, cafeteria, etc.) and use of standardized measures. This allows the therapist to determine gaps, barriers and strengths to occupational performance and participation. The therapist synthesizes the data and collaborates with the team to establish goals. If services are warranted, the practitioner recommends a plan of care. The plan of care might incorporate some or all of the delivery methods identified Table 9.2. It may also be influenced by funding sources and the practitioner's role.

The therapist considers several factors when choosing assessment tools and/or intervention approaches in the school environment. Figure 9.1 illustrates factors guiding the therapist's clinical reasoning for assessment and intervention planning based on ICF-CY (World Health Organization, 2007), Educational Framework for Child Success (Torlakson, 2012), American Occupational Therapy Association (AOTA) Practice Framework (AOTA, 2020b), and the Individuals with Disabilities Education Improvement Act of 2004 (USDE, 2004b). The student is at the center of equally important factors to consider.

To develop goals, the practitioner must consider contextual and personal features; family's and school personnel's goals; the student's available supports and strengths; and the student's interests. Contextual Factors include the temporal, physical, social, cultural, and virtual environments where a student interacts. Contextual factors are important to consider during goal setting as they may be modified to improve the student's participation and performance or to assist with remediation of underlying skill deficits. Personal attributes are features of an individual, which includes habits, interests, and values. Strengths are the positive contextual factors, body structures and functions, and personal attributes that support expected and/or actual performance and participation.

The student's interests and motivations must also be ascertained to create meaningful and occupation-based treatment sessions tapping into the student's intrinsic motivation as much as possible. While establishing goals, it is key to attend to the evidence and frames of reference most appropriate for addressing these goals. The plan of care drives toward the established goals, and individual treatment sessions can continually be informed using this systematic approach of infusing best evidence.

Case Example 1: Isaac

In the following case, the clinical reasoning process utilized by a therapist within the assessment process is explored.

Isaac, a 4 ½-year-old boy, was referred for an OT assessment to determine his need for school-based services to access his educational program. He lives with his parents, maternal grandmother, and two sisters. His mother expressed concerns with his ability to follow directions, especially multiple-step commands. She said he demonstrates "unsafe' behaviors such as jumping off the sofa and pulling on objects. She reported he can complete work at home in a structured, one-to-one setting; but requires consistent prompting in larger, busier environments (classroom, community classes, etc.) to follow along with his peers. Isaac previously received OT in a school setting and in the home from an early intervention program. However, the family has moved, and he is no longer receiving OT. He is now in a private, faith-based preschool three days per week in a classroom with ten students and two teachers. Because of smaller class size, the teachers can prompt Isaac to remain on task or redirect him when he is off task. His mother's greatest concern as he transitions to Kindergarten, is if he can thrive in a full day, public school program.

During the interview, his current preschool teachers also expressed concerns Isaac may have difficulty focusing in a Kindergarten classroom setting. When the occupational therapist assessed Isaac, he was able to participate in many of the classroom activities at smaller centers with minimal prompting and general supervision by the teachers. However, during clinical observations of group activities, Isaac struggled, was often off-task, and required consistent verbal, visual and physical cues to remain engaged. During circle time, he was often observed leaning against peers, the table, and other surfaces.

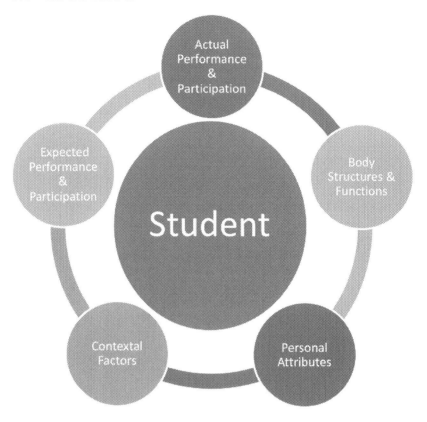

Figure 9.1 Student in Context

The therapist's initial hypothesis, based upon skilled observations, was that Isaac may have difficulties with sensory processing, as well as with motor skills. Therefore, standardized measures were selected to gather additional data. As suspected, Isaac presented with delayed fine motor and visual motor skills as based on observations and upon standardized scores of the Peabody Developmental Motor Scales, 2nd Edition (PDMS-2) and the Bruininks-Oseretsky Test of Motor Proficiency, 2nd Edition (BOT-2). He displayed average bilateral motor abilities during functional activities. Isaac appeared to have difficulty modulating sensory information as well as establishing and maintaining an optimal level of arousal in order to attend to and participate in meaningful activities and appropriately motor plan new movements. During the assessment, Isaac was in constant movement, running quickly from one area to the next, and requiring verbal prompting to maintain a seated position. Isaac's observed sensory processing difficulties (hyporesponsive to vestibular and proprioception information) were described by teachers and his parents and supported by the data from both the School and Home Forms of the Sensory Processing Measure and the Clinical Observations of Proprioception (COP).

Table 9.1 Clinical Reasoning of Isaac's Participation and Performance

Expected Performance (School-Based Goals):
1. Establish and maintain grasp on tools such as paint brush, crayons
2. Copy body and hand positions during movement-based classroom instruction
3. Remain seated during class instruction and participate in tabletop activities for 15 minutes

Contextual Factors	• Preschool classroom with natural light. • Door to outside play yard. • Two rectangular tables, carpeted area, couch, imaginative play area, sink area, and calendar area at front of the classroom. • Two classroom teachers, ten students. • Morning program, starting at 8 a.m. and ending at 11:45 a.m., five days per week. Each day follows the same routine. • Isaac and his family belong to a strong faith-based community. The preschool is part of the religious community in which the family lives. • Isaac lives with his two older sisters, father, mother, and maternal grandmother. • Isaac has supervised access to a computer tablet at home.
Personal Attributes	• Isaac enjoys playing sports. He has been exposed to a variety of sports, including T-ball and soccer.
Participation and Performance	• At home in constant movement, loves to jump on the bed, impacting ability to sit and attend for more than 5 minutes. • Within the classroom setting, he struggles to maintain an upright posture while sitting on the carpet. • Leans against the wall or his peers or shifts positions from seated to prone or side lying position. • Unable to copy body and arm movements during circle time movement activities. • Loose grasp on crayons; marks are light.
Body Structures and Function	• Low muscle tone • Strength within average range • Struggles to maintain an upright posture while sitting on the carpet

Table 9.1 illustrates some factors the therapist integrated into their clinical reasoning with respect to Isaac's participation and performance.

Intervention

Designing a meaningful data-driven intervention is based upon assessment results, literature review, knowledge of diagnosis, frames of references, and the therapist's clinical experience, which guide the therapist to select the appropriate frames of reference for intervention. Therapists

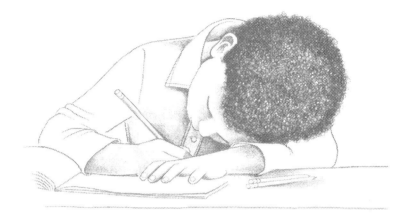

Figure 9.2 Isaac Was Often Observed Leaning on the Table During Classroom-Based Activities

also should tap into the student's interest, to develop an intervention that addresses the priorities identified.

The literature (Berry & Ryan, 2002; Nelson et al., 2009) indicates many occupational therapists use principles of Sensory Integration in combination with other frames of reference in their daily treatment planning (Reynolds et al., 2017). However, practitioners do not necessarily link the selected frames of reference with a solid, underlying rationale on how to combine them (Case-Smith, 2002). Furthermore, various delivery models are utilized in a school setting including individualized interventions within and outside the classroom; group interventions; and consultations with teachers or others. These methods require an understanding of sensory processing within the context of the educational environment. The complexity of practice requires therapists to be cognizant of the theoretical basis of the strategies being utilized. The American Occupational Therapy Association has underscored the relationship of sensory integration to learning (AOTA, 2015; Ayres, 2005). For example, a school-based occupational therapist may suggest an alternative seating arrangement informed by principles of Sensory Integration or a neurodevelopmental treatment frame of reference. These interventions may be employed in isolation or combined to achieve desired educational outcomes and increased student participation in the school setting. To effectively monitor student progress, practitioners must systematically implement school-based therapeutic strategies with a clear understanding of their theoretical basis.

Given the high percentages of occupational therapists working in schools identifying sensory integration in combination with other frames of reference as their preferred intervention practices (AOTA, 2010), there is a need for blending the application of multiple frames of reference in intervention planning.

There are several intervention delivery models used in schools. Table 9.2 presents the context in which the services are delivered and the focus of each model.

Table 9.2 Delivery Models Informed by Principles of Sensory Integration

Delivery MODEL	Context	Foci
Strategies, Tier 1 & Tier 2	Practitioner provides general and/or targeted strategies/ education to support all students or a select group of students	Strategies to support self-regulation Strategies to support executive function Opportunities for flexible seating/learning spaces (Cahill & Bazyk, 2020)
Direct, Push-in	Practitioner embeds services in the context of the classroom and/ or educational environment	Skill development Classroom intervention (whole or part) e.g., movement informed by SI followed by academic task, aligned with curriculum (Clark et al., 2019; Davies et al., 2019)
Direct, Pullout (therapy room)	Practitioner sees student in therapy room with specialized equipment or play yard with the use of playground equipment (able to provide opportunities for sensory input and control the rate and intensity)	Addressing underlying sensory based impairments and skills to promote engagement and organization of behavior (Smith, 2019)
Direct, Social Skills	Practitioner provides intervention in small group format	Social skills development using play based sensorimotor approach (Challita et al., 2019)
Virtual	Practitioner provides synchronous intervention	Synchronous services are provided through various technologies such as videoconferencing, mobile videoconferencing (face time), audio-only telephone calls, and real-time chat rooms to provide instant and engaging services (Cason et al., 2018)

(Continued)

Table 9.2 (Continued)

Delivery MODEL	Context	Foci
Indirect, Consultation/ Modification	Practitioner embeds data-driven sensory strategies	Sensory diet Adaptive equipment, e.g., ball chair or alternate seating (Bodison & Parham, 2018)
Parent Education/ Home Assignments	Practitioner consults with parents	Asynchronous strategies (e.g., may include pre-recorded videos, data files, digital photographs, virtual reality technologies, and electronic communications such as text messages or e-mail correspondences) for use in home and in community (AOTA, 2017)

Choosing any of the service delivery models identified in Table 9.2 requires taking into account the student's needs, the context of intervention delivery and the interaction between the two. Tier 1 and Tier 2 strategies are based upon a variety of models of practice and frames of reference, including principles of sensory integration, and provide general strategies to support student engagement and participation (Bazyk et al., 2009; Ohl et al., 2013; Reid et al., 2006). Programs 1 and 3 in Chapter 15 provide examples of programs related to student participation.

Within a Tier 1 or Tier 2 model, the practitioner provides strategies based upon their perspective and understanding of the relationship between the student, the environment, and the desired occupation. Within Tier 1, all students receive high quality instruction. The practitioner might collaborate with the teacher to look at the environment such as seating and lighting and suggest general strategies to be applied to the whole class. Within Tier 2, the intervention and strategies are targeted to a group of students. Using this delivery model, the teacher and therapist may collaborate to create activities embedded within classroom routine that incorporate various sensory experiences along with activities informed by motor learning theory (e.g., massed practice) or a biomechanical frame of reference (use of slant boards, improved ergonomic positioning, etc.). Student progress should be systematically appraised to ensure outcomes are being achieved.

As previously noted, pediatric occupational therapists employ a variety of intervention approaches. While sensory integration is one of the most often used frames of reference, developmental and behavioral approaches are commonly utilized, especially for children with autism

(Monz et al., 2019). Since autism is one of the primary diagnoses seen by school-based therapists, those therapists are often combining sensory integration with other approaches. Appendix B summarizes approaches and frames of reference to consider within school-based practice.

A school-based therapist often must balance between addressing contextual factors including the cultural, temporal, virtual, physical, and social environments, personal attributes including motivation and interests, body structure and function, and performance skills. If the physical environment presents barriers to occupational participation or performance, modifications and adaptations to the environment or the materials may be an appropriate form of intervention for improving participation. For example, allowing a student with a mobility challenge to have increased time to transition from one class to another may be a sufficient adaptation for that student to navigate the school environment. If personal attributes, such as habits and routines, are impacting performance patterns or participation, modifications, or adaptations such as a visual schedule to help organize the day may improve occupational participation or school performance. The occupational therapist can work on remediating underlying impairments through direct intervention or modifying the activities or the environments to improve performance and participation. Once therapists have identified the areas of difficulty impacting successful and meaningful participation, distinct frames of reference can be selected.

Case Example 1: Isaac (Continued)

To support Isaac in the educational setting, the practitioner addressed goals related to safe playground participation, on-task behaviors, and pre-writing performance. To improve motor planning skills and sensory modulation skills related to engagement in play and pre-writing activities, the therapist recommended a service delivery model incorporating both pull-out and push-in approaches. The therapist's hypothesis, (hyporesponsiveness to proprioceptive and vestibular information) led the practitioner to recommend a pull-out approach to access necessary suspended equipment. The intervention was informed by a Sensory Integration frame of reference, in this case, in the playground and therapy room. The push-in approach within the overall educational setting incorporated sensory integration, motor learning, visual-motor and biomechanical frames of reference. Using a dynamic clinical reasoning process, the therapist synthesized data related to Isaac's identified occupational performance deficits, his therapeutic history, current research, and his overall therapeutic potential to determine the recommended plan of care. The plan involved facilitated sensory opportunities on the playground and in the therapy room (climbing, swinging, and jumping) to provide Isaac the ability to better achieve an optimal state of arousal for engagement and participation in classroom activities. In addition, sensory strategies (such as movement breaks and increased opportunities for proprioceptive input) were also incorporated within his classroom setting. The therapist broke down the parts of the songs with arm and body movements in order for Isaac to learn the sequence. With repetition, Isaac was able to sequence the movements. After he had achieved optimal levels of arousal, the therapist embedded a variety of visual-motor activities (drawing, cutting, etc.) using different media (markers, crayons, chalk, clay, etc.) within the classroom and pull-out sessions. The therapist chose to utilize both a remedial approach (facilitated sensory opportunities, visual-motor activities) and a compensatory approach (sensory strategies) to help Isaac achieve his goals.

In the following example, a practitioner supports student participation informed by sensory integration using a consultative model. The focus is on a systematic and ongoing approach to the assessment process and the subsequent appraisal of outcomes. This approach guides the therapist in making necessary adjustments to the intervention plan, resulting in a blended approach.

Case Example 2: Francesca

Francesca, a 2nd grade student with a medical diagnosis of Attention Deficit Hyperactivity Disorder (ADHD) and a special education eligibility of Specific Learning Disability (SLD), was fully included within the general education setting, and received support from a special education teacher who collaborated with the general education teacher and Francesca's one-to-one aide. Francesca's developmental abilities were slightly below average, but overall, she possessed all requisite skills to be successful within the classroom setting given adequate accommodations; however, she had difficulty maintaining attention within the larger general education setting. The therapist collaborated with team members to develop Francesca's goal, which was to remain seated and on-task during teacher-led instruction, as measured by remaining in her seat for up to 20 minutes and answering questions or following teacher-led instructions.

The therapist's intervention plan was informed by a comprehensive assessment that determined Francesca's participation was best addressed in a least-restrictive environment through modifications within the classroom setting. Francesca's teacher and her mother were primarily concerned that Francesca struggled to remain attentive during classroom instruction, and she often distracted other students. The assessment included relevant teacher and parent interviews; use of the Sensory Processing Measure (SPM) and Miller Function and Participation Scales (MFUN); structured clinical observations and observation across contexts. Assessment indicated proprioceptive and vestibular hyporesponsiveness as it related to postural control and the ability to maintain attention as well as general lower adaptive functioning.

The OT considered Francesca's actual performance and participation in addition to her personal attributes, body structure and functions and contextual factors. The current evidence was reviewed to determine the best complementary approaches to improve her goal attainment. The identification of all of the factors influencing Francesca's performance, as well as relevant evidence related to her diagnosis, led the practitioner to determine the best approach included a combination of sensory integrative theory, biomechanical and cognitive-behavioral theory approaches (Uyanik et al., 2003).

The educational team initially implemented the use of an air cushion to provide proprioceptive opportunities throughout her day to improve attention to task, as well as a behavior chart to reward Francesca when she achieved certain objective milestones. A review of literature has indicated in-seat behavior and executive function for some children may improve with the use of an air cushion (Pfeiffer et al., 2008; Schilling et al., 2004; Umeda & Deitz, 2011). A data sheet was used by the aide over several weeks to track the amount of time Francesca was able to remain seated; the number of times Francesca responded to teacher-led questions, as well as the number of opportunities provided in the classroom.

After the first week, it was evident the air cushion was not effective, so the intervention plan was revised, but continued to combine both a sensory integrative, biomechanical, and cognitive-behavioral approach. The therapist then implemented use of a cushioned footstool placing Francesca in more efficient postural alignment, while also providing an opportunity for increased proprioceptive feedback through her lower extremities. The data showed this was more effective, but not yet sufficient. The general education teacher reported anecdotally that she felt that the footstool was beneficial. Although the use of sensory strategies was informed by data from the assessment, Francesca's response to those interventions was not fully yielding desired results. The therapist hypothesized the greater underlying challenge was behavioral in nature.

The practitioner decided to place motivating "Princess" stickers on the seat and the backrest of Francesca's chair to employ visual supports and cognitive strategies, so she would have a visual reminder to facilitate improved postural positioning. The data showed this approach combined with the footrest was effective, and coupled with the behavioral chart, provided Francesca the motivation and the means to successfully participate in her classroom for extended periods of time. Over the course of the next several months, Francesca eventually met her goal of attentively remaining seated for 20 minutes and participating in, and completing, teacher-led activities.

In the earlier example, the therapist determined the best and least-restrictive approach to supporting Francesca's successful participation involved combining both sensory integrative, biomechanical, and cognitive-behavior approaches, while also modifying the environment and the task. The systematic data collection allowed the therapist to determine the effectiveness of the intervention and adjust accordingly. Francesca's case is a prime example of the dynamic process of intervention planning and balancing the multiple areas of concern. While keeping Francesca at the center of focus with the desired goal, the OT combined frames of reference based upon knowledge of Francesca's diagnosis (ADHD) and relevant evidence along with personally motivating factors.

As with Francesca, it is paramount to maintain each student at the center of focus, and to individualize plans to best meet each student's need. Handwriting concerns are a frequent reason for OT referral and can result in different therapeutic approaches depending on the assessment data and the context of the intervention.

Case Example 3: Susie

Susie was benefitting from general strategies to support fine and visual motor development, however continued to fall behind her peers. She was referred for a school OT assessment secondary to continued difficulty with handwriting despite instructional support. Susie had significant difficulty copying designs as instructed by the practitioner. The therapist administered the Sensory Integration and Praxis Tests, the Beery-Buktenica Developmental Test of Visual-Motor Integration, 6th Edition (VMI) (Beery & Beery, 2010) and conducted skilled clinical observations as part of the comprehensive assessment. Based on a systematic analysis of the evaluation data, Susie received clinic-based OT to address underlying sensory integration deficits. She received a combination of pull-out OT in the clinic one time a week and push-in OT in the classroom on a monthly basis. Strategies were embedded into the instruction such as proper positioning to

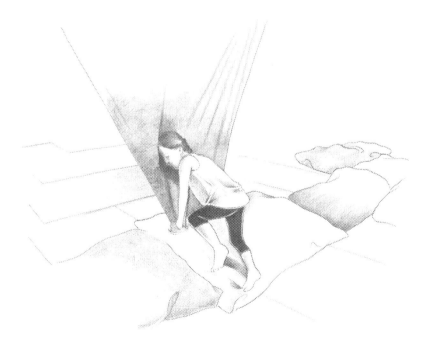

Figure 9.3 Susie Received Pull-Out, Clinic-Based Occupational Therapy Along With Push-In OT in the Classroom to Address Underlying Sensory Processing Deficits

promote optimal stability for distal control; mazes and connect the dots to facilitate improved visual motor and motor planning skills, and age-appropriate crossword puzzles to provide increased opportunities to practice writing letters within visual boundaries. Within a year, Susie began to figure out how to use her body and her organization in time and space improved and was provided increased opportunities to practice writing in a playful manner that promoted success. This positively affected her handwriting as well as other skill areas such as tying her shoes.

This last case example demonstrates how a common reason for referral (in this case, handwriting concerns), can be addressed using principles of Sensory Integration along with other therapeutic approaches when the assessment data warrants those approaches.

This chapter illustrates utilization of a systematic approach to assessment and intervention planning to provide tailored, data-informed OT within the educational setting. With particular focus on combining sensory integration theory with other treatment approaches, tangible case examples of the spectrum of service delivery models, as well as contrasting approaches to similar reasons for referral have been provided to reinforce the systematic approach to assessment and intervention. Working within the school setting requires knowledge of curricular expectations, therapeutic potential, and best practices informed by current evidence. This chapter highlights how practitioners can structure their clinical reasoning to integrate all of these data points in determining the most effective approach to address student outcomes and expected occupational performance, and foster self-determination.

References

American Occupational Therapy Association. (2010). 2010 Occupational therapy compensation and workforce study. AOTA, Incorporated.

American Occupational Therapy Association. (2015). Occupational therapy for children and youth using sensory integration theory and methods in school-based practice. American Journal of Occupational Therapy, 69(Suppl. 3), 6913410040p1–6913410040p20. https://doi.org/10.5014/ajot.2015.696s04

American Occupational Therapy Association. (2017). Guidelines for occupational therapy services in early intervention and schools. American Journal of Occupational Therapy, 71(Suppl. 2), 7112410010. https://doi.org/10.5014/ajot.2017.716s01

American Occupational Therapy Association. (2020a). 2015 Salary and workforce survey. AOTA.

American Occupational Therapy Association. (2020b). Occupational therapy practice framework: Domain and process. American Journal of Occupational Therapy, 74(7412410010). https://doi.org/10.5014/ajot.2020.74s2001

Ayres, A. J. (2005). Sensory integration and the child: Understanding hidden sensory challenges. Western Psychological Services.

Bazyk, S., Michaud, P., Goodman, G., Papp, P., Hawkins, E., & Welch, M. A. (2009). Integrating occupational therapy services in a kindergarten curriculum:

A look at the outcomes. American Journal of Occupational Therapy, 63(2), 160–171. https://doi.org/10.5014/ajot.63.2.160

Beery, K. E., & Beery, N. A. (2010). Beery VMI administration, scoring, and teaching manual (6th ed.). NCS Pearson Inc.

Berry, J., & Ryan, S. (2002). Frames of reference: Their use in paediatric occupational therapy. British Journal of Occupational Therapy, 65(9), 420–427. https://doi.org/10.1177/030802260206500905

Bodison, S. C., & Parham, L. D. (2017). Specific sensory techniques and sensory environmental modifications for children and youth with sensory integration difficulties: A systematic review. American Journal of Occupational Therapy, 72, 1–11. https://doi.org/10.5014/ajot.2018.029413

Cahill, S. M., & Bazyk, S. (2020). School-based occupational therapy. Case-Smith's Occupational Therapy for Children and Adolescents, 627–658.

Case-Smith, J. (2002). Effectiveness of school-based occupational therapy intervention on handwriting. American Journal of Occupational Therapy, 56, 17–25. https://doi.org/10.5014/ajot.56.1.17

Cason, J., Hartmann, K., Jacobs, K., & Richmond, T. (2018). Telehealth in occupational therapy. The American Journal of Occupational Therapy, 72, 1–18. https://doi.org/10.5014/ajot.2018.72s219

Challita, J., Chapparo, C., Hinitt, J., & Heard, R. (2019). Effective occupational therapy intervention with children demonstrating reduced social competence during playground interactions. British Journal of Occupational Therapy, 82(7), 433–442. https://doi.org/10.1177/0308022619832467

Clark, G. F., Watling, R., Parham, L. D., & Schaaf, R. (2019). Occupational therapy interventions for children and youth with challenges in sensory integration and sensory processing: A school-based practice case example. American Journal of Occupational Therapy, 73(3), 7303390010p1–7303390010p8. https://doi.org/10.5014/ajot.2019.733001

Davies, A., Shure, J., Jones, L., LaRossa, K., & Watling, R. (2019). The evidence for sensory-based interventions (SBIs) for a school setting. American Journal of Occupational Therapy, 73(4_Supplement_1), 7311520385p1–7311520385p1. https://doi.org/10.5014/ajot.2019.73s1-po2025

Law, M. (2002). Participation in the occupations of everyday life, 2002 distinguished scholar lecture. American Journal of Occupational Therapy, 56, 640–649. https://doi.org/10.5014/ajot.56.6.640

Monz, B. U., Houghton, R., Law, K., & Loss, G. (2019). Treatment patterns in children with autism in the United States. Autism Research, 12(3), 517–526. https://doi.org/10.1002/aur.2070

Nelson, A., Copley, J., Flanigan, K., & Underwood, K. (2009). Occupational therapists prefer combining multiple intervention approaches for children with learning difficulties. Australian Occupational Therapy Journal, 56(1), 51–62. https://doi.org/10.1111/j.1440-1630.2007.00712.x

Ohl, A. M., Graze, H., Weber, K., Kenny, S., Salvatore, C., & Wagreich, S. (2013). Effectiveness of a 10-week Tier-1 response to intervention program in improving fine motor and visual – Motor skills in general education kindergarten students. American Journal of Occupational Therapy, 67(5), 507–514. https://doi.org/10.5014/ajot.2013.008110

Pfeiffer, B., Henry, A., Miller, S., & Witherell, S. (2008). Effectiveness of disc'O'sit cushions on attention to task in second-grade students with attention difficulties. American Journal of Occupational Therapy, 62, 274–281. https://doi.org/10.5014/ajot.62.3.274

Reid, D., Chiu, T., Sinclair, G., Wehrmann, S., & Naseer, Z. (2006). Outcomes of an occupational therapy school-based consultation service for students with fine motor difficulties. Canadian Journal of Occupational Therapy, 73(4), 215–224. https://doi.org/10.1177/000841740607300406

Reynolds, S., Glennon, T. J., Ausderau, K., Bendixen, R. M., Kuhaneck, H. M., Pfeiffer, B., Watling, R., Wilkinson, K., & Bodison, S. C. (2017). Using a multifaceted approach to working with children who have differences in sensory processing and integration. American Journal of Occupational Therapy, 71(2), 7102360010p1–7102360010p10. https://doi.org/10.5014/ajot.2017.019281

Schilling, D. L., & Schwartz, I. S. (2004). Alternative seating for young children with autism spectrum disorder: Effects on classroom behavior. Journal of Autism and Developmental Disorders, 34(4), 423–432. https://doi.org/10.1023/b:jadd.0000037418.48587.f4

Smith, M. C. (2019). Sensory integration: Theory and practice. FA Davis.

Torlakson, T. (2012). Guidelines for occupational therapy and physical therapy in California public schools. California Department of Education.

Umeda, C., & Deitz, J. (2011). Effects of therapy cushions on classroom behaviors of children with autism spectrum disorder. American Journal of Occupational Therapy, 65(2), 152–159. https://doi.org/10.5014/ajot.2011.000760

United States Department of Education. (2004a). Building the legacy: IDEA 2004. http://idea.ed.gov/explore/home

United States Department of Education. (2004b). Individuals with Disabilities Education Improvement Act of 2004.

Uyanik, M., Bumin, G., & Kayihan, M. (2003). Comparison of different therapy approaches in children with Down syndrome. Pediatrics International, 45, 68–73. https://doi.org/10.1046/j.1442-200x.2003.01670.x

World Health Organization. (2007). International classification of functioning, disability, and health: Children & youth version: ICF-CY. World Health Organization.

10 Incorporating Sensory Integration Approaches in Pediatric Mental Health

Shelby Surfas and Bryant Edwards

Occupational therapy practice has historically traced its professional roots in mental health since the moral treatment movement (Peloquin, 1989). Early on, professionals saw the value in empowering people with mental health needs through participation in meaningful activities, which yielded positive, humanizing results for many. Peloquin (1989) argued that the profession of occupational therapy, unlike the moral treatment movement, must continually evolve within changing contexts, redefining the value of occupation and articulating the power of interventions aimed at promoting participation. Since that time, the occupational therapy profession has evolved, shaped by increased knowledge, evidence, and sociopolitical systems. The increased knowledge about how sensory processing relates to mental health diagnoses is one of those areas in which knowledge has evolved. Hence, interveners need to be cognizant of the relationship between these two variables when working with children with sensory processing disorder (SPD) as well as when working in mental health settings.

Hayley's Story

'I've always been hiding in plain sight. In high school I excelled in language arts, yet barely passed my science and math classes. I enjoyed the camaraderie through tennis and fencing; yet was always klutzy. As a young adult, I struggled navigating the subway system, university campus, and my student worker schedule and duties. I found myself unable to socialize or concentrate, spending consecutive days in my dorm room, avoiding everything. I quickly fell behind, collected debt, and dropped out before the first semester ended. I would re-enroll only to find myself dropping back out again and again. My depression was treated through medications and psychotherapy. Years later, as a young adult, I was diagnosed with dyspraxia and sensory processing difficulties. This was my "ah ha moment" to my own narrative.'

DOI: 10.4324/9781003050810-13

> *It's not that I am stupid or incompetent or clumsy. Little things became crystal clear. I can't get enough of "mud runs," "water parks," or "bouncy houses," yet, must always grip the subway handles so tightly to prevent falling. I will always panic at the sight of a combination lock, parallel parking spot, or chopsticks, yet may perform a heartfelt monologue with ease. The internal turmoil is devastating, while on the outside people have no idea. I simultaneously fear and hope that they will see me.*

The focus of this chapter will be to:

- Highlight the value in systematically combining sensory integration approaches when intervening with children in mental health settings; and
- Illustrate how mental health approaches can be enfolded into the care of children identified with sensory processing needs.

Relationship Between Sensory Processing and Mental Health

Although there is research supporting the correlation between mental health and sensory processing (Bailliard & Whigham, 2017; DeSantis et al., 2011; Kagan, 2018), clinicians are just beginning to ask how and why this relationship exists. In adults, symptoms of anxiety and depression have been significantly correlated with sensory overresponsiveness and have been found to show lower rates of perceived social supports (Kinnealey et al., 2011). Sensory processing has also been linked to depression (Champagne & Koomar, 2011; Serafini, 2016), anxiety (Crucianelli et al., 2016; Hazen et al., 2008; Koomar, 1996; Lane et al., 2012), complex trauma, and insecure attachment (Fraser et al., 2017; Linkugel et al., 2020; Pat-Horenczyk & Yochman, 2020; Walbam, 2019), requiring interventions that address the sensory processing issues as well as emotional stability, reactivity, and self-awareness. Existing evidence also supports combining sensory processing approaches with mental health approaches (Bailliard & Whigham, 2017; Barnes et al., 2008; Champagne & Koomar, 2011; Fraser et al., 2017; Dowdy et al., 2020; May-Benson & Teasdale, 2019).

The interest in the interconnectivity of sensory processing and its impact on mental health is growing (Kannenberg, 2016; Lynch et al., 2017; Scanlan & Novak, 2015). Within the adult literature, sensory-motor approaches have been described as interventions to support those with mental health needs in more effectively self-regulating their emotions and arousal levels (Sutton et al., 2013). Scanlan and Novak (2015) further posited that "the available research appears to suggest that adopting sensory approaches to care may be effective in supporting reduced distress and reduced behavioral disturbances in consumers." As occupational therapists (OTs) working with children with mental health diagnoses, evaluations should include an appraisal of sensory processing abilities to determine if sensory approaches can facilitate improved participation in meaningful activities across changing contexts.

Hayley's story exemplifies the link between sensory processing and mental health. At first, many children with sensory processing challenges like Hayley may successfully fit into the social demands of the environment. Yet, deep underneath, their confidence suffers, with a disabling impact on mental health over time. Although qualitative measures of participation may appear to indicate that the child is successful, the depletion of emotional resources accumulates over time. In her words:

> *'Fifteen years later, I still have trouble with the occupations of day to day life, but I have figured out how to adapt, cope and compensate. If dyspraxia and sensory processing can be caught early and treated instead of ignored, maybe other people won't have to go to hell and back like I have.'*

Hayley's case is clear; without therapy, she struggled but was able to perform until her reserves were depleted. The ramifications negatively impacted her own mental health over time, as she became depressed and withdrew, socially isolating herself. Simultaneously, society did not offer the supports necessary for Hayley to thrive, reinforcing the isolation.

Serving Children With Mental Health Needs

Children across settings can present with mental health needs, be it within the hospital setting, the school setting, or community clinics. To best frame things, the initial focus here is on children specifically referred for occupational therapy due to the impact of a mental health diagnosis. Subsequently, the chapter will explore the consideration of the long-term narrative of mental health issues and well-being in children with sensory processing diagnoses and will conclude with case examples highlighting both.

For children and youth referred for mental health interventions to address symptoms associated with diagnoses of mental illness, severe behavior disorders, and autism spectrum disorders, the evidence suggests that focusing on social skill development, as well as on play, leisure, and recreation, is most effective (Arbesman et al., 2013). In their systematic review on addressing mental health in children and youth, Arbesman et al. (2013), analyzed and categorized the most effective treatment approaches for individualized interventions, prevention and reduction of mental health disorders, and promotion of overall mental health for populations and groups. The themes that emerged through this systematic review demonstrate the evolution of the profession to address mental health issues across the continuum from general strategies to intensive interventions (Arbesman et al., 2013). Common approaches within occupational therapy working with individuals with mental health needs include cognitive-behavioral approaches, interpersonal therapy (Markowitz & Weissman, 2004), and ecological models, all while balancing an occupation-based delivery of those services (Ashby et al., 2017; Sarsak, 2018). These lenses guide the therapist to evaluate function through

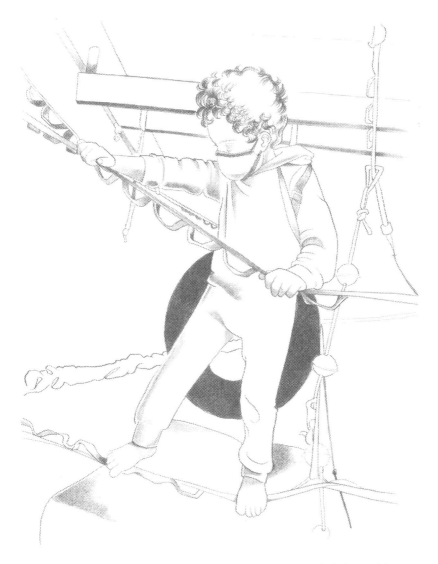

Figure 10.1 Addressing praxis challenges using an approach informed by sensory integration boosts confidence and competence in typical activities, and may decrease withdrawal and isolation behaviors.

psychosocial lenses and apply these approaches through occupation- or activity-driven services. However, broadening the therapeutic perspective to consider how sensory processing influences a child's self-regulation, their ability to adapt to changing environments, or their ability to perform meaningful activities effectively provides another framework through which to strengthen that child's resilience and social supports. Depending on the setting, funding sources, and therapists' knowledgebase and skill set, practitioners can and should reflect on how best to assess for and utilize sensory integration principles within their delivery of care. If need be, therapists should refer for more intense provision of sensory integration therapy. Conversely, therapists working primarily to address sensory processing needs should reflect on underlying mental health needs, addressing what is within their scope and skill set, and referring to other appropriate services as needed.

Some children with mental health diagnoses may have hidden sensory processing difficulties. Also, those children with sensory processing impairments may have unrecognized emotional symptoms. Children with underlying sensory processing impairments spend tremendous resources developing emotional coping abilities (Bar-Shalita & Cermak, 2016). Ayres (1972) stated that emotional experiences in the first five years of life are intertwined with sensory motor experiences. Assessment, therefore, requires skilled interpretation by the therapist, simultaneously weaving together and teasing apart standardized data and clinical impressions.

When evaluating a child's participation, as well as qualitative performance, therapists may first interpret the visible and reported behaviors through a sensory processing perspective. With Hayley, her initial outreach for support was related to the mental health challenges she was facing with social isolation and depression – collateral damage from underlying issues with dyspraxia that left her feeling inadequate, incompetent, and overwhelmed. Her situation differs slightly in that a sensory integrative approach earlier in life might have *prevented* later mental health challenges or may have *promoted* her own competence and resilience in dealing with adversity in life. Using Hayley as an example, we might note that because of underlying impairments with sensory processing, she struggled with effective performance in activities in which she was interested, like tennis or fencing. This struggle exacerbated feelings of fear and incompetence and eventually led Hayley to withdraw from those social occupations. Simultaneously, we may also need to consider that, perhaps, Hayley's mental health and psychosocial needs are not caused by her dyspraxia, and that a pure sensory-based approach will not help to remediate those challenges. So, it is imperative that OTs explore complementary perspectives to support children, like Hayley, in their mental health development in order to promote optimal participation.

Promoting Mental Health for Children With Sensory Processing Difficulties

While Hayley initially searched for support because of the impact of withdrawal and depression, it is important to consider that she could have been referred for occupational therapy services in her childhood to address concerns with incoordination, clumsiness, and performance of age-appropriate occupations. In that case, the therapist might have identified difficulties with sensory integration that adversely impacted Hayley's ability to plan movements effectively, and to participate in occupations of her choice such as tennis or fencing. The therapist might have focused entirely on addressing the underlying motor planning difficulties, utilizing a sensory integrative approach, perhaps enfolding elements of motor acquisition. Clinicians working with young children could have an even more profound impact if they also incorporated approaches shown to be effective in supporting mental health development. In this chapter, this process of considering multiple perspectives is described as the process of "zooming out."

When therapists zoom out by considering multiple perspectives related to sensory processing, motor performance and mental health, it allows for the development of various interpretations opening various opportunities to incorporate different approaches into practice to best meet the needs of the child. Considering and combining approaches that target safe and secure social development with sensory processing approaches allows the therapist to facilitate optimal participation and performance in meaningful activities. In order to most appropriately and effectively achieve this, therapists must conduct a thorough and systematic evaluation of performance and participation.

Evaluation Process

While holding the previous discussion in mind, clinicians also need to "zoom in" during the clinical evaluation. Zooming in informed by the zoomed-out view requires therapists to systematically consider the specific elements linked to sensory integration theory and overlapping with mental health perspectives. This process will then drive intervention approaches in a systematic manner. The following will present the three steps of the Reasoning in Action Model (RAM) as a process, then will walk the reader through this process across case examples.

Step 1: Choosing the Best Method to Gather Information

The first step in every evaluation is considering the participation issues that bring the child for an evaluation or intervention. The participation issues, diagnosis and other pertinent information help the clinician choose the assessments to use to uncover the child's occupational barriers and challenges. Observations and interviews are pivotal in pediatric mental health practice. When possible, additional information, such as questionnaires related to daily patterns, such as sleep will be helpful (Foitzik, 2018). The AOTA Occupational Profile Template (AOTA, 2020) may provide organization for the therapist to examine the environmental context, performance patterns and client factors supporting or inhibiting participation in meaningful occupation. Beginning the evaluation with an occupational-based tool, such as the Short Child Occupational Profile (SCOPE) (O'Brien et al., 2019), reinforces the centrality of occupation for the therapist, client, family, and funding source. Questionnaires for the caregiver, teacher, as well as self-reports for the child may reveal patterns of performance that vary across physical and social contexts, and allow the therapist the opportunity to gain both a sense of the child's actual and perceived success and the perceived success and performance of the child by themselves and others. These may include the Behavior Assessment System for Children (BASC) (Burback, 2020) and/or sensory-based questionnaires. Performance based assessments, such as the Miller Function and Participation Scales (M-FUN), provide the clinician an opportunity to watch how the child may approach, interact, enjoy, and find satisfaction in a variety of structured and standardized activities. The therapist is also encouraged to screen for adverse childhood experiences and adverse community environments (the "pair of ACES") (Ellis & Dietz, 2017; Ellis, 2018). For example, adverse childhood experiences may include neglect, abuse or family separation, while adverse community experiences include poverty, violence and community disruption (such as a global pandemic and systemic racism). Clinicians should consider employing healing centered engagement principles (Ginwright, 2018), as this pair of ACES may interfere with the child's opportunity for occupational experiences that support typical development (Lynch et al., 2017).

The evaluation process is a critical "diagnostic" step as interveners must be expert interviewers, observers, and decoders. Considering strategies, such as warm up activities and sentence starters, to move the discomfort of information gathering, into a rich and enjoyable experience of revealing the child's personhood and narrative as an occupational being (Morrison & Smith, 2013; Teachman & Gibson, 2013). The interview process provides a direction; evidence based standardized assessments and skilled observations provide the details necessary to more precisely 'diagnose' the origin of a challenge.

Step 2: Identifying the Difficulties, and Step 3: Choosing the Intervention Methods and Strategies

Most children referred for services present challenges in occupational participation that relate to a variety of interwoven elements of social, emotional, physical, developmental and environmental factors. The next and most challenging step is for the therapist to consider how sensory processing may influence the child's underlying factors (i.e., attention, confidence, playfulness, self-regulation, motivation, coordination, endurance) and how they influence the child's participation. Children diagnosed with anxiety disorder often show increased fear with new, unpredictable, and imposed sensory experiences. This is anxiety inducing for any child; however, a child with heightened levels of sensory responsiveness and limited proficiency for self-regulation or inconsistent access to caregivers to support in co-regulation will form maladaptive coping strategies (Weaver & Darragh, 2015).

Once the social, emotional, physical, developmental, and environmental factors are identified, the intervention unfolds. In the next two cases, these concepts are applied by analyzing common behaviors occurring during occupational performance problem areas. In each of the cases, at least two interpretations for the child's behavior are considered, one is sensory based, the other relates to common pediatric mental health issues.

Case Example 1

Resisting Tooth Brushing and Nail Clipping: Anxiety or Tactile Hyperresponsiveness?

Children who present patterns of limited engagement in typical activities, such as mealtimes, may be labeled as having a generalized anxiety disorder or obsessive compulsive disorder, yet in a subset of these cases, a sensory sensitivity or hyperresponsiveness is the primary cause for the onset of these psychiatric symptoms (Hazen et al., 2008; Zucker et al., 2015). Discernment of the degree to which the child's sensory sensitivities, the caregivers' interactive style, and the environment influence the participation issue is critical. Self-care occupations, such as toothbrushing, nail clipping, applying sunblock, dressing and hair washing are highly dependent on the child and caregiver emotional attunement, and the child's past experiences reinforcing occupational performance coaching with caregivers (Kraversky, 2019; Ruttle et al., 2011). Occupational performance coaching is an approach in which therapists guide and coach parents and caregivers in the achievement of goals for themselves and their child. Furthermore, research suggests that parent – child tactile interaction is crucial for social comfort and as a foundation for social engagement throughout life (Kennedy et al., 2004; Kingsley, 2020).

Crystal, a 3-year-old child, is referred for occupational therapy from the developmental psychologist who has been working with the family due to concerns that the child has generalized anxiety. Of note, the child often resists or tantrums when engaging in hygiene activities, such as face washing, toothbrushing and nail trimming. The therapist first begins by gathering information through family interview, skilled observation in the home environment, and use of an occupation-based assessment, the SCOPE. Results of the assessment information is organized in Table 10.1, with subsequent identification of difficulties and determination of approaches to take within treatment in Table 10.2.

Table 10.1 Case 1: Information Gathered, Interpretation, and Conclusion

Information Gathered from Step 1	Interpretation	Conclusion (Step 2: Identification of Difficulties)
Child tolerates nail-clipping, yet when the caregiver negatively comments on child's hygiene, indicating disappointment with dirty nails, the child's level of resistance and sensitivity is heightened.	Anxiety Parent-child Interaction Sensory Hyper-responsiveness	Child shows inconsistent reactivity with sensory stimulus, with dramatic changes in sensitivity and reactivity as a child's social-emotional well-being fluctuates.
Child has never tolerated nail clipping with anyone besides her grandfather. Her grandfather first engages his granddaughter in rough play, then allows her to drive the pacing of the clipping based on her reactivity, while holding her with consistent pressure, and maintaining the familiar routine.		Child shows consistent fear reactivity with sensory stimulus, with only slight or no changes in sensitivity as child's social-emotional well-being fluctuates.

Table 10.2 Case 1: Intervention Methods and Strategies

Step 3: Choose the Intervention Methods and Strategies
Hypothesis: Tactile hyperresponsiveness
Intervention Approaches Utilized: Sensory Integration Strategies and Occupational Performance Coaching

Coach caregiver to enter into activity with a calm, relaxed, and realistic expectation of their child prior to each occupational interaction. If caregiver is feeling anxious, coach them to narrate and model for the child strategies they use to help calm themselves down before proceeding.
Allow opportunities for playful control (Whitebread, 2018).
Increase proprioceptive feedback.
Encourage play where child is allowed clear boundaries for safety and drives their own opportunities for confronting challenging situations (Whitebread, 2018).
Consider role playing, pretend play, and virtual activities to promote habituation.

Intentional obstruction paired with increased time and space.
Intentional avoidance to enhance empowerment and internal locus of control.
Inclusion of caregiver into the activity as a graded goal.

Case Example 2

Accident Prone: Hyporesponsiveness to Vestibular and Proprioceptive Sensory Input or Neglect?

Occupations which require effective memory of discrimination of pain sensations, to prevent physical harm, include dressing appropriately for extreme weather, safe handling of dangerous objects (knives, fire, pets, hammer, chemicals, etc.), and cautiousness when trying new physical activities (pumping a swing, walking on a balance beam, crossing the street, shaving, etc.). As we grow and begin to take risks, we look to our caregivers to provide us with feedback regarding safety as well as our own muscle and sensory memory to determine whether or not to try something. While emotionally balanced children with healthy attachments will take risks beyond those that their caregivers are comfortable with, children with trauma experiences will often take risks for the sake of the risk rather than the pleasure of the experience (Howard et al., 2020). Furthermore, patterns noted in children with trauma exposure include both extreme drive toward and extreme avoidance of activities that may lead to danger. The child with externalizing tendencies may show decreased fear; the child with internalizing tendencies may show excessive fear. Watters et al. (2020), found positive indicators of resilience as a mitigating factor in teen and caregiver internalizing measures. Further, abuse is related to an overall increase in internalizing symptoms such as depression, anxiety, withdrawn behaviors, and somatic complaints. Having an awareness of healing centered engagement approaches, wherein the practitioner promotes a healing approach, incorporating holistic elements including culture, spirituality, civic engagement, and community healing. This approach focuses on facilitating well-being at the individual and systems level (Ginwright, 2018).

Taino, a 6-year-old child, was referred for occupational therapy due to concerns with sensory processing by his developmental pediatrician. Specifically, the child appeared to be seeking out high risk sensory and social experiences, putting himself at increased danger for serious injury. The therapist began the evaluation by interviewing the child on his interests, interviewing the family, performing skilled observations walking from the family's home to an outdoor park setting, and through administering a parent-based questionnaire (SPM) and a performance-based assessment (M-FUN). Results of the assessment information is organized in Table 10.3, with subsequent identification of difficulties and determination of approaches to take within treatment in Table 10.4.

Table 10.3 Case 2: Information Gathered, Interpretation, and Conclusion

Information Gathered from Step 1	Interpretation	Conclusion (Step 2: Identification of Difficulties)
Child is accident prone, thrives in conditions which provide intense sensory feedback with few motor demands, and is lethargic/low arousal when required to stay in sedentary and familiar daily routines.	Anxiety Parent-child Interaction Sensory Hyper-responsiveness	Hypo-responsiveness which prompts the child to engage in unsafe activities due to lack of sensory feedback, thus may look to others to help them stay aware of their surrounding and determine safety.
Child is easy going with changes in environment (weather, bugs, dirt, fireworks, motorcycle, surprises, flavors).		
Child observed climbing on top of a structure and jumping down when others are watching; choosing to walk in the street instead of sidewalk when traffic is moving quickly; and places themselves in danger for peer attention.		Trauma as he often engages in unsafe activities due to disconnection from emotions or feelings, thus, may seek out and engage in activities that others may discourage to help them feel something at all.
Child was able to use a dinner knife to cut a piece of fruit; exert force to open/close a door that is jammed; tell a pet not to approach them.		

Table 10.4 Case 2: Intervention Methods and Strategies

Step 3: Choose the Intervention Methods and Strategies
Hypothesis: Developmental Complex Trauma
Intervention Approaches Utilized: Sensory strategies and Healing Centered Engagement
Facilitate strong, safe, and positive social emotional attachment experiences with caregiver during co-occupations.
Increase support for caregiver and child connection, intentional de-emphasis on therapist and child relationship.
Define and organize occupations with family: those as safe, allowable, encouraged, and those that are dangerous, scary, and not allowed.
Avoid situations which require a high level of adult cueing and increase situations which allow for a high level of child driven play within an emotionally safe environment.
Explore culturally grounded environments that promote feelings of wellness, well-being and belonging.
Sensory-motor explorative play is highly encouraged, with limited rules or expectations beyond safety (emotional and physical). Opportunity for repetitious movement and routines throughout a predictable schedule.

Conclusion

This chapter is the start to acknowledging the awareness of current gaps in our evaluative process as it relates to the interconnectivity between mental health and sensory processing, which is currently focused on discrete elements of one's emotional and sensory differences, rather than the learned adaptations and patterns of resilience. While still at its infancy, we must learn to distinguish the patterns and common symptoms rooted in mental health, sensory processing, and the most effective intervention to promote resilience and growth in the whole child.

As we have seen with Haley, the literature indicates one's resilience is formed by a complex feedback interaction over time; facilitating coping mechanisms that allow the person to function in the world (Cosbey et al., 2012; Dean et al., 2018; Dunn et al., 2016; Kinnealey, 2011). In these coping mechanisms, we use the experiences and resources available to us. Therefore, it is important that during the evaluation and the intervention process, these coping mechanisms need to be identified in relationship to the underlying root of the problem. Clinicians must take a broad view and consider the various and dynamic roots underlying any challenge a child faces, so that they can plan appropriate interventions to facilitate resilience and well-being.

References

American Occupational Therapy Association. (2020). Occupational therapy practice framework: Domain and process (4th ed). *American Journal of Occupational Therapy*, *74*(Suppl. 2), 7412410010. https://doi.org/10.5014/ ajot2020. 74S2001

Arbesman, M., Bazyk, S., & Nochajski, S. M. (2013). Systematic review of occupational therapy and mental health promotion, prevention, and intervention for children and youth. *American Journal of Occupational Therapy*, *67*(6), e120–e130.

Ashby, S., Gray, M., Ryan, S., & James, C. (2017). An exploratory study into the application of psychological theories and therapies in Australian mental health occupational therapy practice: Challenges to occupation-based practice. *Australian Occupational Therapy Journal*, *64*(1), 24–32.

Ayres, A. J. (1972). *Sensory integration and learning disorders*. Western Psychological Services.

Bailliard, A. L., & Whigham, S. C. (2017). Centennial topics – Linking neuroscience, function, and intervention: A scoping review of sensory processing and mental illness. *American Journal of Occupational Therapy*, *71*, 7105100040. http://doi.org/10.5014/ajot.2017.024497

Barnes, K. J., Vogel, K. A., Beck, A. J., Schoenfeld, H. B., &. Owen, S. V. (2008). Self-regulation strategies of children with emotional disturbance. *Physical & Occupational Therapy in Pediatrics*, *28*(4), 369–387. doi:10.1080/01942630802307127

Bar-Shalita, T., & Cermak, S. A. (2016). Atypical sensory modulation and psychological distress in the general population. *American Journal of Occupational Therapy*, *70*(4), 7004250010p1–7004250010p9. https://doi.org/10.5014/ajot.2016.018648.

Burback, S. (2020). *Construct validity of the behavior assessment system for children-teacher rating scales (BASC-3 TRS): Comparisons with the adjustment scales for children and adolescents (ASCA). (4783)*, Masters Thesis, Eastern Illinois University. https://thekeep.eiu.edu/theses/4783

Champagne, T., & Koomar, J. (2011). Expanding the focus: Addressing sensory discrimination concerns in mental health. *Mental Health Special Interest Section Quarterly, 34*(1), 1–4.

Cosbey, J., Johnston, S. S., Dunn, M. L., & Bauman, M. (2012). Playground behaviors of children with and without sensory processing disorders. *OTJR: Occupation, Participation and Health, 32*(2), 39–47.

Crucianelli, L., Cardi, V., Treasure, J., Jenkinson, P., & Fotopoulou, A. (2016). The perception of affective touch in Anorexia Nervosa. *Psychiatry Research, 239*. doi:10.1016/j.psychres.2016.01.078

Dean, E. E., Little, L., Tomchek, S., & Dunn, W. (2018). Sensory processing in the general population: Adaptability, resiliency, and challenging behavior. *American Journal of Occupational Therapy, 72*(1), 7201195060p1–7201195060p8.

DeSantis, A., Harkins, D., Tronick, E., Kaplan, E., & Beeghly, M. (2011). Exploring an integrative model of infant behavior: What is the relationship among temperament, sensory processing, and neurobehavioral measures? *Infant Behavior and Development, 34*(2), 280–292. doi:10.1016/j.infbeh.2011.01.003

Dowdy, R., Estes, J., Linkugel, M., & Dvornak, M. (2020). Trauma, sensory processing, and the impact of occupational therapy on youth behavior in juvenile corrections. *Occupational Therapy in Mental Health, 36*(4), 373–393.

Dunn, W., Little, L., Dean, E., Robertson, S., & Evans, B. (2016). The state of the science on sensory factors and their impact on daily life for children: A scoping review. *OTJR: Occupation, Participation and Health, 36*(2_suppl), 3S-26S.

Ellis, W. (2018, November). Community resilience: A framework for equity. In *APHA's 2018 annual meeting & expo (Nov. 10-Nov. 14)*. American Public Health Association.

Ellis, W., & Dietz, W. (2017). A new framework for addressing adverse childhood and community experiences: The building community resilience (BCR) model. *Academic Pediatrics, 17*(7S), S86–S93.

Foitzik, K., & Brown, T. (2018). Relationship between sensory processing and sleep in typically developing children. *American Journal of Occupational Therapy, 72*, 7201195040. https://doi.org/10.ajot.2018.027524

Fraser, K., MacKenzie, D., & Versnel, J. (2017). Complex trauma in children and youth: A scoping review of sensory-based interventions. *Occupational Therapy in Mental Health, 33*(3), 199–216.

Ginwright, S. (2018). The future of healing: Shifting from trauma informed care to healing centered engagement. *Occasional Paper, 25.*

Hazen, E. P., Reichert, E. L., Piacentini, J. C., Miguel, E. C., Do Rosario, M. C., Pauls, D., & Geller, D. A. (2008). Case series: Sensory intolerance as a primary symptom of pediatric OCD. *Annals of Clinical Psychiatry, 20*(4), 199–203.

Howard, A. R. H., Lynch, A. K., Call, C. D., & Cross, D. R. (2020). Sensory processing in children with a history of maltreatment: An occupational therapy perspective. *Vulnerable Children and Youth Studies, 15*(1), 60–67. doi:10.1080/17450128.2019.1687963

Kagan, J. (2018). Perspectives on two temperamental biases. *Philosophical Transactions of the Royal Society B, 373*, 20170158. http://dx.doi.org/10.1098/rstb.2017.0158

Kannenberg, K. (2016). Occupational therapy services in the promotion of mental health and well-being. *The American Journal of Occupational Therapy, 70*, 1–15.

Kennedy, A. E., Rubin, K. H., D. Hastings, P., & Maisel, B. (2004). Longitudinal relations between child vagal tone and parenting behavior: 2 to 4 years. *Developmental Psychobiology, 45*(1), 10–21.

Kingsley, K., Sagester, G., & Weaver, L. L. (2020). Interventions supporting mental health and positive behavior in children ages birth–5 yr: A systematic review. *American Journal of Occupational Therapy*, 74(2), 7402180050p1–7402180050p29.

Kinnealey, M., Koenig, K. P., & Smith, S. (2011). Relationships between sensory modulation and social supports and health-related quality of life. *American Journal of Occupational Therapy*, 65(3), 320–327. http://doi.org/10.5014/ajot.2011.001370

Koomar, J. A. (1996). *Vestibular dysfunction is associated with anxiety rather than behavioral inhibition or shyness* (Order No. 9530623). ProQuest Dissertations & Theses Global. (304242818).

Kraversky, D. G. (2019). Occupational performance coaching as an ultimate facilitator. *OT Practice*, 24(11), CE1–7. www.aota.org/~/media/Corporate/Files/Publications/CE-Articles/CE_Article_November_2019.pdf

Lane, S. J., Reynolds, S., & Dumenci, L. (2012). Sensory overresponsivity and anxiety in typically developing children and children with autism and attention deficit hyperactivity disorder: Cause or coexistence? *The American Journal of Occupational Therapy*, 66, 595–603. http://dx.doi.org/10.5014/ajot.2012.004523

Linkugel, M., Dvornak, M., Estes, J., Snodgrass, R., Klein, K., & Williams, A. (2020). Trauma, Sensory processing, and the impact of OT on youth in juvenile corrections. *American Journal of Occupational Therapy*, 74(4_Supplement_1), 7411515432p1–7411515432p1.

Lynch, A., Ashcraft, R., & March Tekell, L. (2017). Understanding children who have experienced early adversity: Implications for practitioners practicing sensory integration. *SIS Quarterly Practice Connections*, 2(3), 5–7.

Markowitz, J. C., & Weissman, M. M. (2004). Interpersonal psychotherapy: Principles and applications. *World Psychiatry*, 3(3), 136.

May-Benson, T., & Teasdale, A. (2019). Validation of a sensory-based trauma-informed intervention program using qualitative video analysis. *American Journal of Occupational Therapy*, 73(4_Supplement_1), 7311520393p1–7311520393p1.

Morrison, T. L., & Smith, J. D. (2013). Working alliance development in occupational therapy: A cross-case analysis. *Australian Occupational Therapy Journal*, 60, 326–333. https://doi.org/10.1111/1440-1630.12053

O'Brien, J., Hoffman, J., & Moreau, E. (2019). Measuring OT intervention outcomes using the short child occupational profile (SCOPE). *American Journal of Occupational Therapy*, 73(4_Supplement_1), 7311515347p1–7311515347p1.

Pat-Horenczyk, R., & Yochman, A. (2020). Sensory modulation in children exposed to continuous traumatic stress. *American Journal of Occupational Therapy*, 74(4_Supplement_1), 7411505189p1–7411505189p1.

Peloquin, S. M. (1989). Moral treatment: Contexts considered. *American Journal of Occupational Therapy*, 43(8), 537–544.

Ruttle, P. L., Serbin, L. A., Stack, D. M., Schwartzman, A. E., & Shirtcliff, E. A. (2011). Adrenocortical attunement in mother – Child dyads: Importance of situational and behavioral characteristics. *Biological Psychology*, 88(1), 104–111.

Sarsak, H. I. (2018). Overview: Occupational therapy for psychiatric disorders. *Journal of Psychology and Clinical Psychiatry*, 9(5), 518–521.

Scanlan, J. N., & Novak, T. (2015). Sensory approaches in mental health: A scoping review. *Australian Occupational Therapy Journal*, 62(5), 277–285.

Serafini, G., Gonda, X., Canepa, G., Pompili, M., Rihmer, Z., Amore, M., & Engel-Yeger, B. (2016). Extreme sensory processing patterns show a complex association with depression, and impulsivity, alexithymia, and hopelessness. *Journal of Affective Disorders*, 210, 249–257. https://doi.org/10.1016/j.jad.2016.12.019

Sutton, D., Wilson, M., Van Kessel, K., & Vanderpyl, J. (2013). Optimizing arousal to manage aggression: A pilot study of sensory modulation. *International Journal of Mental Health Nursing, 22*(6), 500–511.

Teachman, G., & Gibson, B. E. (2013). Children and youth with disabilities: Innovative methods for single qualitative interviews. *Qualitative Health Research, 23*(2), 264–274.

Walbam, K. M. (2019). Integrating connection: A mixed-methods exploration of sensory processing and attachment. *Infants & Young Children, 32*(1), 43–59.

Watters, E. R., & Wojciak, A. S. (2020). Childhood abuse and internalizing symptoms: Exploring mediating & moderating role of attachment, competency, and self-regulation. *Children and Youth Services Review, 117,* 105305.

Weaver, L. L., & Darragh, A. R. (2015). Systematic review of yoga interventions for anxiety reduction among children and adolescents. *American Journal of Occupational Therapy, 69*(6), 6906180070p1–6906180070p9.

Whitebread, D. (2018). Play: The new renaissance. *International Journal of Play, 7*(3), 237–243. http://doi.org/10.1080/21594937.2018.1532952

Zucker, N., Copeland, W., Franz, L., Carpenter, K., Keeling, L., Angold, A., & Egger, H. (2015). Psychological and psychosocial impairment in preschoolers with selective eating. *Pediatrics, 136*(3), e582–e590. http://doi.org. 10.1542/peds.2014-2386

11 Provision of Occupational Therapy in the Pediatric Hospital Setting

Bryant Edwards and Kimberly Grenawitzke

Occupational therapy practice within an acute, pediatric hospital presents challenging opportunities for provision of care while meeting the needs of the patients and their families. As in all pediatric care, therapists are working with the child with consideration of the diagnosis, the child's interests, the goals of the family, and family culture and routines. Additional layers of complexity include the onset of the diagnosis and the patient and family's coping, the prognosis of the diagnosis, the severity of the impairments related to the diagnosis, and collaboration and communication as part of the interdisciplinary team.

A report outlining trends for acute hospital admissions from 2012 revealed that the top three diagnostic categories were related to the respiratory system, digestive system, and the nervous system. Musculoskeletal and connective tissue systems were the fifth highest reason for admission (Witt et al., 2015). When looking at admissions to pediatric hospitals, pneumonia/acute bronchitis/asthma, appendicitis, and epilepsy/seizures were among the most common conditions for which children are hospitalized (Witt et al., 2015). For any of these diagnoses, occupational therapy is often involved in care, regardless of medical acuity.

It is important to distinguish between the acute hospital setting (acute) and the acute or inpatient rehabilitation (rehab) setting, as this chapter will focus only on the acute setting. Within the acute setting, the goal of therapy is to facilitate a safe discharge to the next level of care. Oftentimes, this means that the patient is discharged home or to the community, to inpatient rehab, or to a sub-acute facility. Due to the complexity of the patient population served in the hospital setting, multiple frames of reference are considered when delivering occupational therapy services.

The successful acute care occupational therapist (OT) is one who uses clinical reasoning in the determination of evaluation, setting goals and intervention approaches within the rapidly-changing hospital setting. Pragmatic reasoning takes into account various factors that may influence therapy, including space, reimbursement, resources, available equipment, and time (Schell & Cervero, 1993). In the acute setting, therapists must

DOI: 10.4324/9781003050810-14

consider the influence of the client's length of stay, the timing of services in coordination with the rest of the team, appropriateness of specific interventions in-regards to medical acuity, and available space and materials. Acute care stays are typically short, with a focus on medically stabilizing a patient and facilitating the transition to the next level of care. Although a biomedical frame of reference tends to dominate acute inpatient occupational therapy practice, sensory-based and developmental interventions and environmental sensory considerations can and do integrate in practice models in the pediatric acute setting (Edwards, 2020). This chapter highlights ways in which occupational therapists in the acute hospital setting can utilize the sensory environment, sensory experiences, and sensory-based approaches in combination with other treatment approaches to support improved occupational performance and participation for pediatric clients.

Case Study

Karina, a 15-year-old female with acute myeloid leukemia, was admitted to the hospital to initiate chemotherapy treatment, and potentially undergo a life-saving bone marrow transplant. As the clinician begins reviewing Karina's chart, she quickly notices not only the medical complexity of this patient's case, but that she has been progressively getting sicker since admission to the hospital. Just after the therapy order was placed, a rapid response team code was called due to medical de-compensation, and the child was transferred to the pediatric intensive care unit (PICU). Due to swift decline in respiratory function and alertness, Karina was intubated and started on multiple medications to keep her calm and sedated, as well as support her heart function while she underwent strong chemotherapy treatments to get her cancer under control.

The clinician begins by confirming with the medical team that Karina is appropriate to be seen for therapy, noting her change in status and transfer to the Pediatric Intensive Care Unit (PICU). The nurse practitioner managing Karina's care recommends that the OT initiates a bed level evaluation and maintains close communication with the medical team regarding progressing her mobility and activity levels. The therapist begins her evaluation by checking in with the bedside nurse regarding how Karina has been doing since her transfer to the PICU, and how her family is coping. The nurse explains that Karina's family speaks very little English, and despite having medical interpreters present at the time of admission and transfer to the PICU, the family is struggling to understand what is happening with Karina. They are strongly guided by their faith and are praying that God will help Karina recover from her illness. The nurse also explains that her family feels that Karina is under the influence of a bad omen, and they are waiting for their priest from their hometown in Guatemala to arrive to bless Karina and protect her during her treatment. They have requested that no additional medical interventions be done until Karina is blessed by their priest. The nurse shares the therapist could see Karina for a bed-level evaluation nonetheless.

Acute care pediatric occupational therapists should consider the diagnosis and the functional impairments caused by the diagnosis, and also the impact that hospitalization, stress, and varied amounts of medical trauma have on the patient and their family. In Karina's case, although a "bottom up" approach may be utilized initially in which the therapist focuses on addressing component deficits, the occupational therapist's goals are always individualized, wide reaching, and focused on future occupational participation. In acute care occupational therapy, it is common in the PICU to begin with a biomechanical frame of reference, evaluating range of motion, strength, alertness/orientation, as well as a cognitive frame of reference to assess one's ability to follow commands. This is typically the therapy approach due to medical acuity, limited patient engagement, and an environment that is inappropriate for use of typical therapy tools and equipment, making it difficult to consider a more occupation-based approach. It is also important to consider the impact this assessment may have on the family who is confused, experiencing stress, and feeling overwhelmed and lost. In the example of Karina, in order to respect the family's wish to "avoid" any additional medical interventions prior to their priest arriving, the therapist must decide how to approach initiating the assessment, as well as how to communicate their findings with the family. This determination must consider the current diagnosis and state of the patient, the family's needs and wishes, while focusing on the bigger picture. The clinician must ask, "What can I do now to support her occupational engagement later?"

The therapist, accompanied by a qualified interpreter, began by introducing themselves and discussing their role as an occupational therapist. The clinician reassured the family that their role was to help keep Karina comfortable while she was being treated medically, with the goal of helping her return to her favorite daily activities. The therapist then took a complete occupational history of Karina from her parents, asking what they were doing with or for Karina regarding activities of daily living (ADLs), social interactions (talking with her, holding her hand, reading to her, etc.), and any leisure activities (listening to music, watching tv, etc.). Through this history, the clinician gleaned valuable information from Karina's parents about her life prior to diagnosis. Karina was an excellent student and excelled in art and history classes. She had a younger brother, who she proudly cared for after school when her parents were at work. She was active in her religious youth group and sang in the choir. Her parents proudly spoke of Karina and her accomplishments. Although she was independent in all ADLs prior to becoming ill, Karina's parents revealed that since being admitted to the hospital, they helped her with some ADLs, including brushing her hair, and washing her face and limbs. Her parents were very concerned that she was not yet able to eat, and asked "When can she eat again?" many times during the session, as they felt oral feeding would improve her chances of recovery.

The clinician first approached the observational aspect of the assessment by working through the parents, asking if they would demonstrate how they performed those activities. The therapist offered to help by retrieving the necessary materials, assisting as needed. By doing so, the therapist gained the trust of the family by respecting their routines and roles as caregivers. The clinician observed that Karina's parents easily moved Karina's arms in a variety of planes during the washing activity with no obvious restrictions in range. The clinician asked for permission to move Karina's arms, and the family was agreeable. The therapist continued the assessment in this manner; alternating between empowering the family to demonstrate how they cared for Karina and then allowing the therapist to do a more skilled, hands-on assessment.

Ultimately, the clinician identified that Karina was completely dependent for all occupations, presented with global flaccidity, but was responsive to certain stimuli including auditory and tactile (cold). The therapist maintained an awareness of the cultural aspects of Karina's care that would need to be considered, as well as the longer narrative of Karina's story. The clinician synthesized these considerations with their clinical observations to help determine the therapeutic plan of care, which focused on combining a biomechanical approach of providing bedside exercises to maintain Karina's joint integrity and range of motion along with a sensory-based approach to promote enhanced responsivity, orientation, and awareness, eventually supporting motor function and performance skills. The literature regarding the efficacy of sensory strategies in the pediatric brain injury population is mixed, but due to Karina's significant impairments, the therapist chose to incorporate sensory strategies and then assess for clinical effectiveness in this specific situation (Chang et al., 2016; Padilla & Domina, 2016). Because of the lack of clear supporting literature consistently available in acute pediatrics, the acute care occupational therapist must apply the best available literature and carefully assess efficacy of these interventions.

For the next week, the therapist followed Karina two times for gentle range of motion, to train caregivers in performing ADLs, and to monitor Karina's alertness. The therapist also fabricated resting hand splints to maintain functional positioning. When the therapist would visit Karina, they would assess her response to tactile stimuli, verbal/auditory stimuli, kinesthetic stimulation (PROM), and gustatory stimulation. If Karina showed any type of response to a stimulus, the clinician would document it. At this point in her recovery an approach heavy in sensory-based treatment strategies was appropriate to initiate Karina's brain injury rehabilitation (Lancioni et al., 2010). A coma stimulation program was initiated with familiar tactile and olfactory inputs from Karina's life, including a stuffed animal from home with a small amount of her grandmother's perfume sprayed on it (Megha et al., 2013; Padilla & Domina, 2016). The OT also began an oral hygiene program to protect against aspiration pneumonia while Karina was intubated, as well as provide alerting stimulation (Hua et al., 2016). With support from the nurse, the therapist taught Karina's parents how to perform oral hygiene carefully and effectively with the endo-tracheal tube in place. The clinician communicated regularly with the attending physicians to ensure the oral hygiene program was effective in reducing dental caries and pneumonia risk. Karina accepted the prescribed treatment regimen without changes in her vital signs or notable agitation, but minimal change in her responsiveness was observed, despite many of her sedatives being lifted by the medical team. Although the coma stimulation program did not yield consistent and sustained improvement of alertness and orientation, Karina's passive range of motion was maintained through stretching and exercises, and Karina's family reportedly felt more comfortable and empowered to handle Karina and her care. Additionally, Karina never presented with aspiration pneumonia during her early ICU stay, which is a well-known complication of prolonged intubation. Karina's priest was able to visit and bless her prior to initiation of high dose chemotherapy. Based upon Karina's response to the intervention plan, the OT decided to continue to promote the family performing passive range of motion and oral hygiene, while the therapist routinely assessed for higher levels of alertness to determine when to advance care. Because the family wanted to continue to incorporate tactile (stuffed animal), olfactory and auditory (familiar music) stimulation, and the OT and medical team determined there were no adverse responses to it, the therapist encouraged the family to continue in order to promote their continued involvement in care.

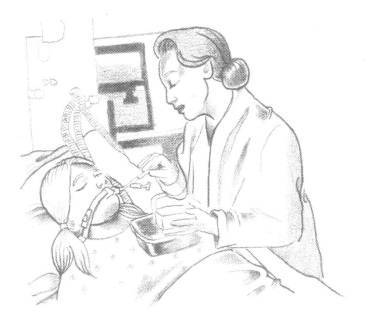

Figure 11.1 The Occupational Therapist Provided Tactile and Gustatory Experiences Through an Oral Hygiene Program That also Served to Reduce the Risk of Infections

About two weeks after her transfer to the PICU and one week of chemotherapy, Karina suffered a massive hemorrhagic stroke in the right Middle Cerebral Artery territory. Although this was discussed as a potential complication of her chemotherapy, Karina's family was shocked, surprised, and devastated. Although she declined neurologically, the medical team was able to wean the ventilator, and eventually extubate Karina to nasal canula.

As a significant change in Karina's functional status was expected, the OT completed a re-evaluation, focusing more on her neurologic presentation. Her family had stepped out of the room when the OT arrived. The OT found that Karina was awake, but with only reflexive responses to stimulation. She was hypo-reflexive at this time. She blinked as a response to threat, and had clonus in her left ankle and wrist, as well as increased tone in her finger, wrist, and elbow flexors. Her left shoulder was beginning to show signs of subluxation. She also was presenting with increased tone in her neck, pulling her head into right rotation and left head tilt. Karina appeared uncomfortable and potentially in pain. The therapist immediately notified the nurse of her high FLACC score (evidence-based pain scale for non-verbal patients), who was able to administer an as needed (PRN) medication to help her relax (Merkel et al., 2002). In addition to increased tone, Karina was noted with open mouth posture and drooling, and would intermittently moan during passive range of motion and stretching. Knowing that Karina was left-handed immediately focused the OT's attention to caring for her hemiplegic upper extremity that was beginning to show signs of spasticity.

The therapist initiated a shoulder subluxation and tone management program including positioning strategies, as well as use of a custom resting hand splint to maintain and improve range of motion of the left hand. Although the literature supports neuromuscular electrical stimulation (NMES) as a treatment approach with strong evidence to support shoulder subluxation management, the clinician employed procedural reasoning to understand Karina and her underlying health condition and what approaches and procedures were appropriate (Fleming, 1991). As a patient with cancer, NMES may be contraindicated, so the OT decided to take the aforementioned approach, which is moderately supported in the literature (Cole & Cox, 2019). Karina's oral hygiene program was continued, as prevention of aspiration pneumonia remained an important medical goal (Huang et al., 2016). In addition, the therapist wanted to focus on controlling and adapting the sensory environment (Lombardi et al., 2002). Although initially the therapist attempted to use sensory stimulation to increase arousal and alertness, with Karina's change in neurologic status due to the stroke, the OT wanted to ensure that the sensory environment promoted brain recovery without overstimulation. Therefore, the therapist educated Karina's nursing team about brain injury and the need for low sensation visual and auditory environments for healing (Meyer et al., 2010). Karina's television was always turned off, only one provider spoke in the room at a time, the lights were kept low, and all actions were slowly described verbally as they were taking place. Karina's family was also educated about protecting her healing brain (Dang et al., 2017). The goal was to provide education to her caregivers to ensure that all sensory stimulation was appropriately graded, as it was when done during therapy sessions by the therapist.

In addition, the OT increased Karina's frequency of therapy to daily, and began co-treating with physical therapy (PT) for neuromotor re-education and early activity and mobilization. Evidence shows that earlier involvement in therapy typically yielded greater progress (Cameron et al., 2015; Wieczorek et al., 2016). Therapy focused on utilizing neurodevelopmental treatment (NDT) strategies to practice rolling, transitioning to sit, and increasing tolerance of sitting at the edge of the bed in order to participate in meaningful ADLs. Through both her modulated sensory stimulation program and this early activity and mobilization program, Karina began to show more alertness, answering questions by nodding her head "yes" and "no" and following very simple motor commands. As mentioned previously, there is some level of expected improvement in function due to brain healing that is likely not related to direct therapy interventions but supported by a tailored sensory environment (Lombardi et al., 2002), so the clinician was diligent about continually assessing Karina's progress. The OT facilitated rote, repetitive, familiar sensory-motor activities with Karina like oral hygiene and face washing with hand over hand assistance. These activities were chosen based on the occupational therapist's strong understanding of motor learning theory, while utilizing olfactory and gustatory experiences within treatment approaches. Motor learning theory stipulates that consistent, repetitive practice of motor activities across a wide variety of circumstances builds the strongest skill in that area (Adolph, 2008).

As Karina's alertness improved, the medical team requested a dysphagia evaluation. Until this point, Karina was receiving all nutrition and hydration through a naso-gastric tube, or a temporary feeding tube, that was placed in her nose and delivered formula and fluids directly to her stomach. Knowing the prevalence of dysphagia for children who have experienced a brain injury, and as specialists in the mechanics of feeding, eating, and swallowing, as well as the psychosocial aspects of eating and mealtime, the acute care OT was uniquely suited to evaluate and manage Karina's feeding and swallowing needs (AOTA, 2017; Mendell & Arvedson, 2016).

The therapist began her evaluation by completing thorough oral and dental hygiene. Although the nursing staff maintained an oral care program, as oral feeding was being considered, it was crucial to ensure a clean mouth prior to initiating a dysphagia evaluation. In addition, oral hygiene provided another opportunity to initiate hand over hand engagement in a familiar occupation (tactile and proprioceptive input to the UE), as well as tactile, gustatory, and olfactory stimulation to the intra and extra oral space. Through completing oral hygiene, the OT was able to evaluate Karina's secretion management with and without additional sensory stimulation (poor at baseline, but significantly improved with tactile, gustatory, olfactory stimulation of oral hygiene), as well as her ability to coordinate oral musculature to spit. Karina presented with a left sided facial droop, poor lip closure on the left side, loss of fluid from the left lateral sulcus and inability to adequately seal her lips to swallow. Despite these deficits, Karina's alertness, engagement, and interest in eating, combined with her ability to manage secretions, indicated safe readiness to explore feeding in therapy.

To provide additional sensory stimulation as well as evaluate Karina's ability to swallow small volumes, the OT attempted trials of ice chips. Ice chips provide a cold, crunchy stimulus, as well as a volume-controlled trial of plain water. Literature supports the use of "free water" protocols as a way to improve hydration in critically ill patients despite dysphagia and aspiration risk. The literature shows that the risk of developing pulmonary complications from intake of water when the mouth is thoroughly cleaned through oral and dental hygiene is low – as there is less risk of bacteria laden saliva to be aspirated (Bernard et al., 2016). Through use of hand over hand assist, Karina demonstrated the ability to self-feed. She engaged in an immature munching pattern, driven by her right-sided musculature, but the sensory input from the cold, resistive ice chips improved her left-sided motor control. She demonstrated the ability to transition the bolus posteriorly and trigger a swallow, but the trigger appeared delayed. Although no immediate cough was noted, her breathing appeared slightly congested after this trial. It was determined that Karina would continue small trials of ice chips only *after* impeccable oral and dental hygiene was completed 2–3 times per day, and that occupational therapy would continue to assess her ability to transition to a less restrictive diet.

As her alertness improved and her medical status evolved, Karina was very motivated by food; specifically, the scents of familiar, family foods, and she often was very successful with self-feeding activities, like spoon feeding strawberry ice cream. The OT continued to evaluate her abilities to manage a wide variety of consistencies focused specifically on family foods. The therapist continued to work with Karina on improving the timing and strength of her swallow, utilizing compensatory techniques as well as remediation exercises like the Massako maneuver and Shaker exercise (Loret, 2015; Lundine et al., 2015; McCullough & Kim, 2013).

As her acceptance to hands-on intervention was improving, the OT issued a Giv-Mohr sling to support her left upper extremity and shoulder during transfers (Cole & Cox, 2019). A Giv-Mohr sling maintains the hemiplegic upper extremity down at the patient's side, the elbow in slight flexion, the wrist in functional extension, and provides proprioceptive/tactile input through the hand support of the sling, and has been shown to reduce vertical subluxation without overcorrecting (Dieruf et al., 2005). While her nurses and family were educated on safe commode and chair transfers towards her stronger side, therapy focused on transfers to her hemiplegic side, working on actively using her left upper extremity (LUE) as an assist during weight bearing tasks, increasing proprioceptive input to her LUE as well as more frequently incorporating the LUE into functional tasks (Jyotikant, 2016).

With significant progress, the therapist decided to re-evaluate Karina's occupational engagement, initiating a more "top down" approach, shifting from preparatory activities to actual occupations. This involved a focus on assessing Karina's needs, wants and goals, and identifying what tasks or occupations were limited in achieving those goals (Fisher & Bray Jones, 2017). With her medical status more stable, Karina was able to participate in and demonstrate her abilities in these desired areas of occupation. Karina's communication abilities were improving with speech therapy, and she expressed a desire to engage in activities that fostered her spiritual well-being. Since being hospitalized, she was not able to attend her youth group, so the OT decided to use neurodevelopmental treatment techniques and a weight-bearing splint to facilitate Karina making a liturgical flag, something she previously used in dance routines, and which she used to dance for her family and in photographs she sent to her friends. Although the current research regarding the use of NDT strategies in pediatric motor control recovery is mixed, these strategies have some support in the literature and were appropriate for the acute care setting where there were space and time limitations. While participating in this meaningful preferred occupation, Karina was provided tactile discrimination activities (e.g., feeling and identifying materials with her let hand) as a means to promote somatosensory retraining (Turville et al., 2019). By combining elements of NDT with principles based on sensory integration, the therapist facilitated improvements in Karina's LUE motor control, overall fine motor skills, functional problem-solving skills, and communication abilities. The OT also collaborated with speech therapy, as Karina was very driven to sing religious songs, which was an excellent motivator during her language rehabilitation sessions.

After several weeks of intensive therapy and medical interventions, Karina was demonstrating improved global functioning. She was actively participating in therapy and showing recovery from her brain injury from a motor, cognitive and behavioral standpoint, presenting at Rancho Level VI (confused, appropriate, moderate assistance). She had stabilized medically, and the interdisciplinary team was recommending that Karina transfer to an inpatient rehabilitation facility to maximize her progress with the goal of returning to baseline functionality.

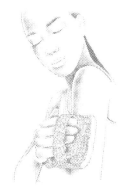

Figure 11.2 As Karina Progressed With her Functional Skills, the Occupational
          Therapist Encouraged Her to Use Different Textured Materials for
          Washing Her LUE to Promote Somatosensory Retraining

*Karina transferred to the pediatric inpatient rehabilitation (IPR) facility 5
weeks after her initial admission. Upon admission to the IPR setting Karina was
evaluated by OT, PT and Speech-Language Pathology to appraise her current
level of functioning, establish goals, and determine therapeutic plans of care.
The purpose of inpatient rehabilitation is to shift the focus from acute medical
stabilization to assessment of a child's functional level, potential for improvement,
family goals and values, and needs for a safe discharge back to community living.
After three weeks, Karina discharged and returned to her home and community
life. At the time of discharge from inpatient rehabilitation, Karina was on the
road to independence. Although she still required the use of adaptive equipment
and strategies, she demonstrated the ability to live a much more independent life.
Outpatient occupational therapy was arranged closer to home to continue to work
towards her goals.*

Conclusion

The pediatric acute setting presents a unique context for the delivery of occupational therapy services, and while it may not be a traditional environment to provide treatment based upon sensory
processing principles, it is imperative that occupational therapy
practitioners consider the influence of sensory processing on an
individual's recovery and engagement in meaningful occupations.
Controlling and adapting the sensory environment, while providing
sensory-based activities informed by assessment and based upon best
available evidence, can positively enhance therapeutic sessions and
amplify outcomes in this setting. The evidence in the use of sensory-
based interventions in this setting continues to show mixed efficacy,

perhaps due to the medical acuity, the constraints of the setting, and/ or the quality and breadth of research in this area to date. As occupational therapists working in this setting, regardless of treatment approach, it is imperative to monitor and document responses to interventions to determine the effectiveness of services. In Karina's case, like all others in the hospital setting, multiple team members contributed to her care and recovery.

References

Adolph, K. (2008). Learning to move. *Current Directions in Psychological Science*, *17*(3), 213–218.

American Occupational Therapy Association. (2017). The practice of occupational therapy in feeding, eating, and swallowing. *American Journal of Occupational Therapy*, *71*(7112410015).

Bernard, S., Loeslie, V., & Rabatin, J. (2016). Use of a modified Frazier water protocol in critical illness survivors with pulmonary compromise and dysphagia: A pilot study. *American Journal of Occupational Therapy*, *70*(1), 7001350040p1–7001350040p5.

Cameron, S., Ball, I., Cepinskas, G., Choong, K., Doherty, T. J., Ellis, C. G., Martin, C. M., Mele, T. S., Sharpe, M., Shoemaker, J. K., & Fraser, D. D. (2015). Early mobilization in the critical care unit: A review of adult and pediatric literature. *Journal of Critical Care*, *30*(4), 664–672.

Chang, P. F. J., Baxter, M. F., & Rissky, J. (2016). Effectiveness of interventions within the scope of occupational therapy practice to improve motor function of people with traumatic brain injury: A systematic review. *American Journal of Occupational Therapy*, *70*(3), 7003180020p1–7003180020p5.

Cole, A., & Cox, T. (2019). Treatment of glenohumeral subluxation: A review of the literature and considerations for pediatric population. *American Journal of Physical Medicine & Rehabilitation*, *98*(8), 706–714.

Dang, B., Chen, W., He, W., & Chen, G. (2017). Rehabilitation treatment and progress of traumatic brain injury dysfunction. *Neural Plasticity*, *2017*.

Dieruf, K., Poole, J. L., Gregory, C., Rodriguez, E. J., & Spizman, C. (2005). Comparative effectiveness of the GivMohr sling in subjects with flaccid upper limbs on subluxation through radiologic analysis. *Archives of Physical Medicine and Rehabilitation*, *86*(12), 2324–2329.

Edwards, B. (2020). Considerations for using sensory-based approaches in the pediatric acute hospital setting. *SIS Quarterly Practice Connections*, *5*(3), 9–10.

Fisher, A., & Bray Jones, K. (2017). Occupational therapy intervention process model. In *Perspectives on human occupation: Theories underlying practice* (pp. 237–286). FA Davis.

Fleming, M. H. (1991). The therapist with the three-track mind. *American Journal of Occupational Therapy*, *45*(11), 1007–1014.

Hua, F., Xie, H., Worthington, H. V., Furness, S., Zhang, Q., & Li, C. (2016). Oral hygiene care for critically ill patients to prevent ventilator-associated pneumonia. *Cochrane Database of Systematic Reviews*, *10*.

Huang, Y. C., Leong, C. P., Wang, L., Wang, L. Y., Yang, Y. C., Chuang, C. Y., & Hsin, Y. J. (2016). Effect of kinesiology taping on hemiplegic shoulder pain and functional outcomes in subacute stroke patients: A randomized controlled study. *European Journal of Physical and Rehabilitation Medicine*, 52(6), 774–781.

Jyotikant, S. R. (2016). A comparative study of effectiveness between electrical stimulation and splinting techniques used along with neurodevelopmental treatment for improving hand function in hemiplegic patients. *International Journal of Physiotherapy and Research*, 4(1), 1360–1364. doi:10.16965/ijpr.2015.20

Lancioni, G. E., Bosco, A., Belardinelli, M. O., Singh, N. N., O'Reilly, M. F., & Sigafoos, J. (2010). An overview of intervention options for promoting adaptive behavior of persons with acquired brain injury and minimally conscious state. *Research in Developmental Disabilities*, 31(6), 1121–1134.

Lombardi, F., Taricco, M., De Tanti, A., Telaro, E., & Liberati, A. (2002). Sensory stimulation of brain-injured individuals in coma or vegetative state: Results of a Cochrane systematic review. *Clinical Rehabilitation*, 16(5), 464–472.

Loret, C. (2015). Using sensory properties of food to trigger swallowing: A review. *Critical Reviews in Food Science & Nutrition*, 55(1), 140–145.

Lundine, J., Bates, D. G., & Yin, H. (2015). Analysis of carbonated thin liquids in pediatric neurogenic dysphagia. *Pediatric Radiology*, 45(9), 1323–1332.

McCullough, G. H., & Kim, Y. (2013). Effects of the Mendelsohn maneuver on extent of hyoid movement and UES opening post-stroke. *Dysphagia*, 28(4), 511–519.

Megha, M., Harpreet, S., & Nayeem, Z. (2013). Effect of frequency of multimodal coma stimulation on the consciousness levels of traumatic brain injury comatose patients. *Brain Injury*, 27(5), 570–577.

Mendell, D. A., & Arvedson, J. C. (2016). Dysphagia in pediatric traumatic brain injury. *Current Physical Medicine and Rehabilitation Reports*, 4(4), 233–236.

Merkel, S., Voepel-Lewis, T., & Malviya, S. (2002). Pain assessment in infants and young children: The FLACC scale: A behavioral tool to measure pain in young children. *AJN The American Journal of Nursing*, 102(10), 55–58.

Meyer, M. J., Megyesi, J., Meythaler, J., Murie-Fernandez, M., Aubut, J. A., Foley, N., Salter, K., Bayley, M., Marshall, S., & Teasell, R. (2010). Acute management of acquired brain injury Part III: An evidence-based review of interventions used to promote arousal from coma. *Brain Injury*, 24(5), 722–729.

Padilla, R., & Domina, A. (2016). Effectiveness of sensory stimulation to improve arousal and alertness of people in a coma or persistent vegetative state after traumatic brain injury: A systematic review. *American Journal of Occupational Therapy*, 70(3), 7003180030p1–7003180030p8.

Schell, B. A., & Cervero, R. M. (1993). Clinical reasoning in occupational therapy: An integrative review. *American Journal of Occupational Therapy*, 47(7), 605–610.

Turville, M. L., Cahill, L. S., Matyas, T. A., Blennerhassett, J. M., & Carey, L. M. (2019). The effectiveness of somatosensory retraining for improving sensory function in the arm following stroke: A systematic review. *Clinical Rehabilitation*, 33(5), 834–846.

Wieczorek, B., Ascenzi, J., Kim, Y., Lenker, H., Potter, C., Shata, N. J., Mitchell, L., Haut, C., Berkowitz, I., Pidcock, F., Hoch, J., Malamed, C., Kravitz, T., &

Kudchadkar, S. R. (2016). PICU Up! Impact of a quality improvement intervention to promote early mobilization in critically ill children. *Pediatric Critical Care Medicine: A Journal of the Society of Critical Care Medicine and the World Federation of Pediatric Intensive and Critical Care Societies, 17*(12), e559.

Witt, W. P., Weiss, A. J., & Elixhauser, A. (2015). *Overview of hospital stays for children in the United States, 2012* (Statistical Brief# 187). Healthcare Cost and Utilization Project (HCUP) Statistical Briefs. Agency for Healthcare Research and Quality (US), Rockville (MD); 2006. PMID: 25695124.

12 Mealtime Participation

Feeding and Eating Issues in Children With Neurodevelopmental Disorders

Stefanie C. Bodison and Joan Surfus

Mealtime is a significant occupation for humans of all ages. It not only provides needed nourishment for the human body to grow and develop, but also offers an opportunity for people to connect with one another (Ernsperger & Stegen-Hanson, 2004; Franklin & Roger, 2002; Pedersen et al., 2004). Beginning as early as the first moments of life, when the infant effectively receives the initial "meal" shortly after birth, either via breast, bottle, or alternative means, the relationship between sustenance and emotional comfort is created and will continue to sweeten for the rest of life. Mealtime is the one occupation that most infants begin to master on the first day of life and that which they continue to participate in until their last.

Successful mealtime experiences can be defined by multiple factors including the level of social connectivity experienced; the amount of independence exerted during a meal over such things as food choices and ability to self-feed; the nutrition received; and the amount of food remaining after the meal. Occupational therapists working with children who have challenges in their mealtime experiences recognize there are various components of mealtime to consider. These include but are not limited to the child's gross motor ability to sit upright at an eating surface and demonstrate enough fine motor control to handle the food and bring it to their mouth; the child's oral motor ability to break down the food and move it into swallowing position; the child's ability to swallow the food safely and without delay; and finally, the gastrointestinal system's ability to process the food so that what has been consumed can be converted to energy. In addition to the child's personal factors, feeding is imbued with social and relational meaning, and so sociocultural, emotional and environmental factors can also influence the occupation of mealtime (AOTA, 2017).

When there are problems with feeding and eating for any child, it can disrupt the natural occupations of life and significantly impact both physical and social-emotional growth. When the feeding and eating challenges experienced by the child are inconsistent, complex, fluctuating

DOI: 10.4324/9781003050810-15

and/or seem behaviorally driven, occupational therapists have the difficult task of discerning what might be causing the mealtime challenges and deciding how to assist. There are multiple theories regarding the underlying feeding and eating struggles of children with neurodevelopmental disorders, as well as thoughts about the types of interventions to employ. While there are many resources offering strategies and approaches to intervene, there are few that provide a clinical reasoning process required to determine the most appropriate ways to intervene, with an emphasis on the use of combined intervention approaches.

The purpose of this chapter is to provide a stepwise approach to the evaluation and intervention planning of the feeding and eating abilities of children with neurodevelopmental disorders. To do so, the content herein has been divided into two overlapping sections: 1) comprehensive evaluation of feeding and eating abilities; and 2) intervention planning using a combination of approaches through the use of a case vignette to reinforce the clinical reasoning process.

Before we begin, however, we have a few words about diagnoses and important considerations about medical precautions. We have attempted to focus this chapter on children with a variety of neurodevelopmental disorders, and not one in particular. While there may be subtle nuances of intervention foci or approaches that may arise when treating a child with a specific diagnosis such as autism spectrum disorder or Down's syndrome, we believe that the evaluation process presented here will aid in uncovering the foundation of the feeding and eating issues regardless of diagnosis. Additionally, proficiently addressing the oral motor and feeding abilities of the child with special needs requires ongoing post-professional education and mentoring (AOTA, 2017). It is recommended that the reader is aware of any state and/or local licensure requirements governing their practice area, so that the necessary post-professional training is obtained prior to intervening with clients.

Finally, foundational to the assessment of feeding and eating skills and its impact on mealtime participation is the knowledge of typical feeding and eating development. While a detailed analysis of the development of oral motor skills, including the swallowing reflex, lies outside the scope of this chapter, it is imperative that clinicians have a working understanding of these developmental processes, so that they can compare what the child is doing to what might be developmentally expected or appropriate.

Comprehensive Evaluation of Feeding and Eating Abilities

Grounded in the foundational knowledge of typical sensory and motor development, we progress to a description of a comprehensive evaluation of the child's feeding and eating skills including identification of sensory impairments and how they impact mealtime participation. This comprehensive evaluation involves several components: 1) completion by the parent/caregiver of a three-day diet record prior to the in-person evaluation; 2) a detailed interview with the parent/caregiver to gain insight into past and current functional abilities; 3) an observation of the mealtime experience with the child and parent/caregiver; and 4) a hands-on evaluation of feeding and eating abilities. Each of these four elements will be discussed in greater detail, with tools offered to assist the clinician in gathering the needed data. It is important to note that the comprehensive occupational therapy evaluation suggested here, in best practice, occurs as part of a larger multidisciplinary team evaluation. Whenever possible, it is helpful if the occupational therapist has the opportunity to collaborate with the child's pediatrician, other team members (i.e., speech-language pathologist, physical therapist), and advocate for the inclusion of a registered dietitian, psychologist, and gastroenterologist in the child's care as well. Several children's hospitals and outpatient centers across the United States of America offer this interdisciplinary team approach, and whenever possible, clinicians should strive to develop their own team, or multidisciplinary community relationships, to ensure the best care for the child.

Completion of the Three-Day Diet Record

One of the most useful ways clinicians can gain insight into the child's eating and feeding challenges is through a three-day diet record that the parent/caregiver completes prior to the in-person evaluation. This three-day diet record provides the clinician with insight into the types, quantities and textures of foods eaten, and the environmental factors that may be hindering or contributing to success. This diet record also highlights if there are food preferences in the types of foods eaten, and the texture, shape, color, or brand of food item consumed. An example of a three-day diet record is provided in Figure 12.1. The three-day diet record is not difficult to create, nor should it be difficult for the family to complete. It is critical to communicate to families the importance of filling in all foods offered as well as the amounts consumed, and to consistently do so for three consecutive days. The three-day diet record is a simple yet informative way to gather data that will assist the clinician in ruling out issues related to food selectivity, sensory sensitivity, and general nutritionally positive or negative behaviors. A review of foods eaten or not eaten assists with forming and supporting a hypothesis for why certain foods are eaten and others refused.

Time	Type of food and method prepared (fried, baked, etc.)	Amount Offered?	Amount Eaten?	Setting H= Home C= Community S= School Time to complete meal
7:30 am	Wheat toast Peanut Butter Apple Yogurt	1 slice 1 Tbs ½ apple 1 small container	½ slice ½ Tbs 2 bites ½ container	H 20 minutes to eat the small amount consumed

Figure 12.1 Example of a Portion of a Three-Day Diet Record

Interview of the Parent/Caregiver

The next critical element of the comprehensive occupational therapy evaluation of eating and feeding skills revolves around the parent/caregiver interview. A sample list of questions is provided in Table 12.1 to provide some guidance in this interview process. Ultimately, the goal is to better understand the child's feeding and eating progression so that potential problems can be uncovered. The interview guide in Table 12.1 is not meant to be an exhaustive list of topics, nor is it anticipated that every question will apply verbatim. The guide is designed to assist clinicians in obtaining the data necessary, while stimulating the clinical reasoning process so that additional questions can be generated as needed.

Table 12.1 Feeding and Eating Questions to Guide the Parent/Caregiver Interview

Parent Questions	How it guides clinical reasoning
1. "What are your concerns about (child's name)'s feeding/ chewing/ swallowing/ mouth?" and if there are older siblings; "Is this child's feeding/ chewing/swallowing different than your other children? How?"	Helps direct to the areas one may want to concentrate on during assessment.

(Continued)

Table 12.1 (Continued)

Parent Questions	How it guides clinical reasoning
2. "Were there any problems during pregnancy, during or after (child's name)'s birth?	Difficulties during these times may identify whether a child is "at risk" for feeding/oral motor problems.
3. Did he/she have any illnesses or respiratory infections?	Frequent respiratory infections may suggest feeding/swallowing difficulties.
4. Did your child spit up often/ have reflux?	
5. Was he/she very fussy/colicky?	
6. What about now?"	
7. "How was _____ fed as an infant?"	Some mothers attempt to breast feed, but switch to a bottle because the infant is having difficulty.
8. "Did he/she have any difficulties breast feeding/ bottle feeding?"	This will also give information regarding early feeding difficulties
9. "How long did/ does it take _____ to eat?"	An infant/child needing longer than 20–30 minutes to eat a meal may suggest feeding problems.
10. "How often did he/she eat as a baby?"	Frequent nursing/bottle feeds suggests that the child was not getting enough nutrition possibly due to an inadequate suck
11. "Did/ does your child have any problems gaining weight or growing?"	Helps assure that the child is meeting his/her nutritional needs.
12. "When did _____ start eating table foods?	Provides insights into table food behaviors
13. Did he/she have any trouble when they were introduced?"	
14. "How does your child drink? Cup? Bottle? Straw? Sipper cup?"	Helps identify current oral motor skills.
15. "Does _____ mind having his/her teeth brushed, face washed?"	Helps identify sensory concerns
16. "Does _____ seem to know where his/her mouth, lips, tongue, teeth are?	
17. Does your child mind getting dirty?"	
18. "Is your child a messy eater?"	
19. "Do they notice food/liquid on their face/lips?"	
20. "Do they mind touching food or having food on their face?"	

Observation of the Mealtime Experience

As part of the evaluation process, it is important to observe the child and parent during a mealtime exchange to better understand the types and quantities of food presented to the child, the parental/caregiver expectations, and the naturally occurring feeding and eating behaviors exhibited by the child. In our clinical practices, we attempt to observe the child during mealtimes under two conditions: once during a more naturally occurring mealtime in the child's home and the other, during the in-person evaluation at our clinical site.

The most ideal way to observe the child and caregiver at home is in-person. However, if it is not possible for the clinician to visit the child's home, the next best option is to instruct the child's parent/caregiver to video record the mealtime, with the camera angled in a way to capture the child and parent interaction. The goal here is less about assessing the child's oral motor skills, and more about assessing the environmental factors and child/parent interactions that are both optimally and sub-optimally supporting the mealtime experience. During the in-person evaluation within the clinical setting, the clinician should observe the child and caregiver interaction during a meal that the family brings with them. The observation of this interaction, coupled with caregiver inter-view and three-day diet record, may reveal caregiver and/or child stress during the mealtime experience. Caregivers of children with feeding difficulties present with stress around feeding behaviors at higher rates than those of typically developing children, and this stress can further hinder the mealtime experience (Carpenter & Garfinkel, 2021). During this interaction, it is important that the clinician merely observe, rather than intervene for at least 10–15 minutes. Again, this is an opportunity to understand the optimal and sub-optimal factors supporting the meal-time experience. Once the 10–15 minutes have expired, the clinician can then interview the parent about some of the observed interactions to gain a better understanding about the types of eating behaviors observed.

Hands-on Evaluation of Feeding and Eating Abilities

To aid in the evaluation of feeding and eating skills during the in-person assessment period, we have developed a quick, criterion referenced observational tool designed to provide clinicians with a straightforward way to analyze the impact of anatomical, neuromotor and sensorimotor functions on eating and feeding. We call this tool the *Eating Sensory, Neu-romotor, Anatomical Scale for Kids (E-SNACK)* (Table 12.2). We have cho-sen to focus on the anatomical, neuromotor and sensorimotor aspects of feeding and eating skills because they serve as the foundation for all mealtime behaviors. The E-SNACK does not compare the child's scores to a typically developing population, only helps to organize evaluation

Table 12.2 The Eating Sensory, Neuromotor, and Anatomical Scale for Kids (E-SNACK)

	Anatomical Structures	Neuro-motor	Sensori-motor	Notes
Mouth at Rest				
Swallowing				
Biting				
Chewing				
Food Intake				
Liquid Intake				
Total				
Score				

Source: ©2010 Stefanie C. Bodison OTD, OTR/L, SWC & Joan Surfus, OTR/L, SWC

data and appraise the child's feeding performance. The scoring system is meant to be an easy guide to help clinicians determine which developmental skill is most impacting the feeding process at a given point in time.

When performing the hands-on evaluation of the child's eating and feeding abilities using the E-SNACK, you will want to have the following items available: pureed food (e.g., apple sauce, pudding), chewy food (e.g., dried fruit, licorice), soft cookie (e.g., graham cracker), hard cookie (e. g. pretzel, biter cookies), cups, straws, sipper tops or bottle (as needed), spoons, bowls, toothbrush/tongue depressor, and a pen-light. With these materials present, you will do the following activities, and appraise the child using the E-SNACK as discussed later.

1. Look at child walking, sitting, transitioning between movements:

   - How are the movements? Smooth? Jerky?
   - How is the child's head and trunk control?

2. Observe the child's mouth at rest:

   - Are features symmetrical?
   - How does tone look? Tense? Loose/floppy? Average?
   - How is the child holding his/her mouth?

3. Ask child to do each of the following (or imitate you):

   - open and close mouth
   - pucker lips (blow or kiss)
   - retract lips (smile or say "eee")
   - click teeth

- stick out tongue
- move tongue side to side
- put tongue up and down behind teeth

4. Observe child breast feeding, bottle feeding, or both (if relevant):

- Does the child form a lip seal around the nipple?
- Is the child able to express liquid successfully for 3 or more sucks without stopping?
- Is there any leakage of liquid around the nipple during suck or swallow?
- Is there any tongue protrusion from his/her mouth when swallowing?

5. Have parent/caregiver feed child or allow child to feed him/herself using a spoon and pureed food.

- Does the child open his/her mouth in a graded fashion to allow for feeding?
- Are lips closed around spoon?
- How is food retrieved off spoon? (e.g., lip action, tongue licking, etc.)
- Once food is in the child's mouth, is he/she able to move it back and swallow?
- Is there any tongue protrusion, loss of food around the lips, or residual food in the mouth after swallowing?
- Does child cough or exhibit a wet, gurgly vocal quality after swallow?

6. Have child drink from an open cup on their own or with assistance if needed.

- Does child grade opening their mouth for the cup?
- Do lips close around cup?
- Does child bite edge of cup or place tongue under rim to stabilize it?
- Is there any leakage of liquid?

7. Have child eat a soft cookie, a hard cookie, and chewy food. For each item look for the following:

- Does the child try to bite the food item? If so, where is the item placed for biting? (e.g., front teeth, molars)
- How is the child chewing? In the front? With an up and down "munching" pattern? Is the jaw moving at angles or in a "rotary" and grinding pattern?
- Does the child transfer the food to either side of his/her mouth using tongue movements only?

- Are there any excessive head or body movements when biting or chewing? (e.g., turning head to one side to move food to that side.)
- Is there any tongue protrusion, loss of food around the lips, or residual food in the mouth after swallow?

8. Give the child a cup with a regular straw.

- Is the child able to make a lip seal around the straw?
- How deeply does the child place the straw in his/her mouth?
- Does the child bite on the straw or rest it on his/her tongue?
- Is the child able to draw liquid through straw and into his/her mouth?
- Does there appear to be any excess movements in the lips, tongue, jaw or cheeks when sucking? (e.g., jaw sliding, tongue thrust.)
- Is there any loss of fluid around the straw or out of mouth during swallow?
- Does the suck and swallow appear effortless and is the child able to synchronize sucking with swallowing easily?

9. Use the toothbrush and tongue depressor to check oral sensation, help with placement of food, or give a "target" to have the child aim at with tongue. The penlight can be used to examine the inside of the mouth and check for any structural abnormalities, to observe for elevation of the soft palate when vocalizing, and to check for residual food in the mouth after swallowing.

Intervention Planning and Case Vignette

As a clinician utilizing a family-centered approach, it is important to recognize that organic feeding issues do not arise simply because the child wants to be defiant. Generally speaking, all children want to eat. It is typical, from the moment of birth, to have an internal drive to eat. It is typical to want to enjoy a mealtime experience. While the reasons for delays or disruptions in feeding behaviors are varied, it is rare to see an actual situation where a child develops avoidant feeding behaviors simply to control the family unit or manipulate specific situations. It is the authors' opinion that feeding issues arise for any number of issues assessed via the E-SNACK and could ultimately contribute to avoidant and/or maladaptive behaviors.

When planning for intervention, it is important to understand that each theory or frame of reference utilized must relate to an identified problem area. Appendix B provides an example of ways in which therapists can consider how to combine principles of sensory integration with other treatment approaches, based upon those areas of challenge affecting function; in this case, affecting feeding and mealtime occupations. Therefore, our intent with the case study is to show how the evaluation data comes together to illuminate the potential areas of concern to be addressed during an occupational therapy intervention period using blended approaches.

Case Example

In this case example, the child presents with Down's syndrome which led the clinician to hypothesize that both neuromotor and sensory integration theories would be pertinent in the evaluation and likely, intervention processes. If the clinician only chooses one theory, the child's progress would be limited, because neither theory is adequate enough in isolation to fully address the child's concerns.

Background Information and Reason for Referral

Noah, a 1-year-10-month-old, lives with his parents and older sibling (4 years old). He was born at 37 weeks without complications. During pregnancy, his mother developed gestational diabetes and was treated with insulin. Noah has a diagnosis of Down's syndrome and has mild to moderate delays in his motor and speech development. Noah's mother reports that he has a breathing machine for treatments with Pulmicort and Albuterol, for "congestion."

Noah breast fed for the first two months of life but parent reports that he "sucked slow" because he was tired and would stop sucking all together before "finishing" his meal. This fatigue was also reported with bottle drinking. He was introduced to pureed foods around 6 months of age but ate very little. When transitioning to more solid/lumpy food, he was unable to handle this texture and his mother reports he would spit the food out. It was around this presentation of solid/lumpy foods that Noah began to refuse many foods presented. Currently, Noah eats very smooth purees and continues to struggle with solids and mixed textures. Noah does not mind having his face washed or teeth brushed and parent reports that he often does not notice food left on his face, lips, or hands. He eats in his highchair for meals; however, Noah drinks a high calorie nutritional drink by bottle while lying flat on his back. His mother also reports problems with constipation.

Summary of 3-Day Diet Record

Noah's three-day feeding diary revealed adequate calories (due to provision of nutritional drink) but food repertoire is extremely limited. His mother reports that he eats two, 6-ounce yogurts, two 4-ounce servings of pureed chicken & vegetable soup (homemade), one 4-ounce serving of pureed fruit. In addition, he drinks three, 8-ounce servings of the nutritional drink. The most water he has taken is up to 4 ounces in one day.

Results from Observation of Caregiver/Child Feeding Interaction

The caregiver provided a videotaped interaction for review. During the observation, Noah was observed sitting in his highchair, and throughout the feeding interaction, his mother continually adjusted multiple pillows that were being used to prop him up and keep his trunk centered. When the pillows became misaligned, Noah would fall to the side or slide out of his highchair. Noah did not attempt to self-feed by bringing his hands to his mouth with or without the spoon, but he did participate in the feeding activity by opening his mouth as the spoon was approaching. The mealtime appeared to be calm, and Noah was positively engaged with his mother throughout the interaction.

Assessment of Feeding and Eating Skills

Table 12.3 describes the results of Noah's assessment using the E-SNACK.

Postural Control and Self-Feeding Skills

Noah is not yet sitting independently with good stability. He props himself, prefers to lean on someone, or lies on his back. When in a supported seated position, Noah sits with posterior pelvic tilt, trunk flexion and "fixes" his neck/head in hyper-extension for greater stability. When presented with a bottle, he will lay down on his back (flat), hold the bottle, and drink it. This position allows him to be independent with taking/holding the bottle but puts him in a poor position for feeding or developing advanced feeding skills. He is beginning to finger feed, but unable to manage the food (e.g., cereal) and is not yet utilizing a spoon.

Anatomical Structures

Teeth are present and appear healthy. No reported problems. No structural anomalies noted. No limitation in range of motion of any body or oral structures.

Neuromotor

Noah is able to manage smooth purees, clearing from a spoon presented by an adult. When presented with a thicker puree (mashed vegetable and chicken soup), Noah took the bite but was unable to manage it and

Table 12.3 Noah: The Eating Sensory, Neuromotor, and Anatomical Scale for Kids (E-SNACK)

3 – Within Functional Limits 2 – Minimal/No negative impact on functional performance 1 – Significant impact on functional performance NA – Not assessed

	Anatomical Structures	*Neuro-motor*	*Sensori-motor*	*Notes*
Mouth at Rest	3	2	3	Open mouth posture, decreased active movement of lips. Low tone in cheeks. Decreased stability at head/neck, as noted by "fixing" with his neck slightly in a hyper extended position for greater stability when eating.
Swallowing	3	1	2	No known anatomical deficits. Decreased coordination with oral transit, especially with thin liquids (water), which must be given via eyedropper. He is able to manage nutritional drink and smooth purees without signs of swallowing difficulty.
Biting	3	1	1	Dentition is present with no reported issues. Not aversive to presentation of solids; he is not able to bite from a whole, soft or meltable solid (e.g., baby rice crackers, puffs) when presented to front teeth and holds his jaw open without initiating biting. Lack of ability to stabilize jaw as well as inability to "figure out" how to take a sustained bite.
Chewing	3	2	1	When food is placed laterally between his teeth, Noah uses a munching pattern with poor grading of jaw movements and loss of food from mouth; poor lateralization and ability to form a cohesive bolus noted. Not aversive to the texture of the food placed.
Food Intake	3	1	1	Poor lip closure on the spoon. Poor tongue control with tongue pushing spoon and food out of mouth. Inability to manage solids or mixed textures. Able to use fingers to pick up small objects (e.g., cheerios) but does not bring to mouth, and not able to manage orally. Not yet scooping or bringing loaded spoon to mouth.
Liquid Intake	3	1	1	Only taking liquids from eyedropper or bottle. Unable to drink from an open cup, sippy cup, or straw.
Total Score	18	8	9	

Source: ©2010 Stefanie C. Bodison OTD, OTR/L, SWC & Joan Surfus, OTR/L, SWC

with an anterior-posterior motion of his tongue, most of the food spilled from his mouth. When a meltable solid is placed laterally between his teeth he uses a munching pattern.

Sensorimotor

When presented with a piece of graham cracker to front teeth he did not initiate a bite. When presented between lateral teeth, Noah utilized a munching pattern with difficulties grading his jaw movements i.e., opening his jaw to wide or not enough. He munched successively, but had difficulty moving the food to form a bolus. He demonstrated better chewing and management on the left than the right. If the bite went to the middle of his tongue, he was unable to lateralize the food to his side teeth. Noah appears to be hyporesponsive to tactile and proprioception as well as has difficulties with poor motor planning.

Respiratory Function

Utilizes breathing machine for treatments with Pulmicort and Albuterol as needed for "congestion"

Summary of Findings

Noah's strengths include his interest in social interactions with others, and his ability to interact with simple cause and effect toys. Additionally, Noah's family is very supportive and involved in supporting his development. His abilities in feeding and eating are impacted by his deficits in neuromotor (strength and stability) and sensorimotor (praxis and processing tactile and proprioceptive input) skills.

More specifically, Noah is unable to maintain upright posture during mealtime and has a history of fatigue with respect to oral functions, both of which impact his ability to successfully perform and participate in the occupation of feeding. Although he has difficulties with managing foods of varying textures, Noah does not appear to be aversive to the textures of foods or toys but has an inability to feel the food in and around his mouth and move and manage the solid food when it is in his mouth. This, coupled with his observed play skills, indicates there is difficulty in the area of praxis. Noah appears to have difficulty planning and executing the motor movements needed to successfully handle increasingly more complex foods.

Difficulties in these areas decrease independence in the areas of self-feeding (finger feeding, tool use, etc.), eating age-appropriate foods (chewing/drinking/swallowing), and age-appropriate play. Noah has a limited repertoire in his diet, which impacts his willingness to eat a variety of foods and impacts his nutritional balance.

Occupational Therapy Goals

In an effort to monitor Noah's response to therapy, the following goals were developed to track progress through occupational therapy services:

1. Increase the ability to form a cohesive bolus with thicker purees (e.g., oatmeal, thicker pureed soup).
2. Improve postural control as needed for maintaining upright sitting (in his highchair), grasping a utensil, holding an open cup and the ability to bring either to his mouth.
3. Increase the ability to transition to open cup and manage liquids.
4. Increase oral somatosensory processing and praxis to safely manage textures.

Intervention Strategies

Based on Noah's age and social engagement strengths, occupational therapy intervention will focus on using play-based activities while combining principles of sensory integration (SI), biomechanical and neuromotor

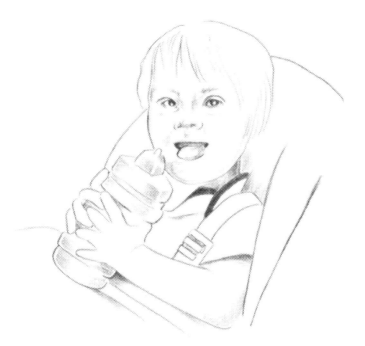

Figure 12.2 Addressing Positioning During Feeding: The High Back of the High Chair Helps Support His Trunk and Head; the Closeness of the Tray also Lends Support to His Forearms

approaches to address underlying postural control, strength, somatosensory processing, and praxis issues impacting oral motor feeding/eating skills. Additionally, services also provide for task-specific opportunities of feeding and mealtime, while also employing parent education and training through a coaching approach (Kraversky, 2019).

For example, the therapist uses a social interaction game for Noah on a platform swing, providing vestibular and proprioceptive information combined with trunk strengthening opportunities (Gupta et al., 2011). Other play-based activities combining elements of SI, neuromotor and biomechanical approaches focus on intra and extra-oral input (e.g., stretching, vibration, oral play) to increase jaw/tongue strength and stability, tactile discrimination and proprioception while facilitating graded control. For example, using a textured wash cloth to provide tactile input with quick stretching of extraoral musculature, using a vibrating textured toothbrush for teeth brushing, or a textured chewy toy dipped into pureed food to have Noah initiate biting/chewing on when placed between different teeth (front, lateral).

The therapist will also provide Noah opportunities to practice oral motor and feeding skills during in-person sessions. This starts by positioning Noah in a high chair with attention to supporting ideal pelvic, trunk and neck alignment needed to facilitate optimal oral motor control. It may include gradual introduction of solids with initial placement laterally, as a means to promote motor planning and bolus formation. With increased repetitions and development of skills, the therapist may challenge Noah by varying the placement of solid foods or use of different textures and consistencies.

Telehealth will also be used to provide in-home coaching for the caregivers during mealtime. These sessions will focus on carry-over of activities within the clinic setting, empowering caregivers in their abilities to support Noah's mealtime skill development. By combining these intervention approaches and service delivery models, the therapist can provide a holistic plan to meeting Noah's mealtime goals.

References

American Occupational Therapy Association. (2017). The practice of occupational therapy in feeding, eating, and swallowing. *American Journal of Occupational Therapy, 71*(7112410015), 10–5014.

Carpenter, K. M., & Garfinkel, M. (2021). Home and parent training strategies for pediatric feeding disorders: The caregivers' perspective. *The Open Journal of Occupational Therapy, 9*(1), 1–21.

Ernsperger, L., & Stegen-Hanson, T. (2004). *Just take a bite: Easy, effective answers to food aversions and eating challenges.* Ingram Publishing Services.

Franklin, L., & Roger, S. (2002). Parents' perspectives on feeding medically compromised children: Implications for occupational therapy. *Australian Occupational Therapy Journal, 50*, 137–147.

Gupta, S., Rao, B. K., & Kumaran, S. D. (2011). Effect of strength and balance training in children with down's syndrome: A randomized controlled trial. *Clinical Rehabilitation, 25*(5), 425–432.

Kraversky, D. G. (2019). Occupational performance coaching as an ultimate facilitator. *OT Practice, 24*(11), CE1–7. www.aota.org/~/media/Corporate/Files/Publications/CE-Articles/CE_Article_November_2019.pdf

Pedersen, S. D., Parsons, H. G., & Dewey, D. (2004). Stress levels experienced by the parents of eternally fed children. *Child: Care, Health, and Development, 30*(5), 507–513.

13 The Context of Play

Erna Imperatore Blanche and Lisa A. Test

Sylvia, an occupational therapist, prepares to perform an evaluation on Randy, a 7-year-old boy referred to treatment because of motor performance and social participation difficulties. She greets the child in the waiting room and while establishing rapport asks him about his play preferences at home and school. He likes Legos and board games, so Sylvia offers to start the evaluation either in the fine motor room or in the gym. He chooses to start in the gym but when he arrives at the gym door, he notices that other children and their therapists are in the large room and flatly refuses to go in. He appears interested in watching the children, but even after gentle coaxing, he does not enter the room. Sylvia decides then to test fine motor skills first and bring him back to the gym later to assess gross motor skills, the reason he has been referred to occupational therapy. After the children in the room leave, Sylvia tries again to bring him into the large room, this time the child climbs on a large piece of equipment and surveys the environment from there. Sylvia throws a bean bag at him to evaluate his ability to catch and throw it, but Randy refuses to even attempt to catch it. Sylvia throws another beanbag to the child that lands on his leg. Randy, not wanting to engage, throws it back at her. At that point, Sylvia realizes she can assess the child's motor planning skills by having him throw bean bags back at her. With a smile, she throws another bean bag, this one lands on his lap, now the child is faster in responding. Sylvia then throws more beanbags making sure they land on different parts of the body; Randy is now engaged in throwing them back at her. His active cooperation increases with each time he throws the beanbags back at her and at times he even attempts to catch them. After a few minutes, he puzzledly looks at her and asks in a bemused way "how old are you?" Sylvia laughs and answers, I will tell you before you go. The exchange changes Randy's cooperation, from there on he tries different activities and allows Sylvia to complete the evaluation. When it is time to put his shoes back on, he remembers "how old are you?" Sylvia responds: "guess," the child then answers, "you are a teenager." Sylvia then answers, she is 45.

Play is considered a context, an occupation, and an experience (Parham, 2015). As a context, it includes the circumstances that allow an occupation or activity to occur. Creating a context of play in a session is complex. It depends on the clinician's attitude and skill, the novelty of a physical environment that invites exploration and play, and the child's

DOI: 10.4324/9781003050810-16

motivation to engage in occupations with specific experiences. In this chapter, we will view play as an occupation with specific experiences that are promoted in a context created by the intervener. In the previous excerpt, Sylvia, when throwing beanbags at the child, was able to create an incongruous context in which being silly, non-serious, and spontaneous was allowed. Incongruous because adults don't engage in pillow fights or beanbag fights. The incongruity peaked the child's curiosity and active participation allowing Sylvia to do her job. In this excerpt, the novelty of the physical environment was present, but it required a skilled therapist to spontaneously utilize the opportunity created by a beanbag accidentally falling on the child's leg to pique the child's motivation and curiosity. His appraisal of the therapist's age points to the incongruity between size and her behavior. Her size was not the one of a child; her behavior was not the one of an adult. Hence she had to be a teenager.

As an occupation, play is complex. In occupational therapy, the most influential description of the complexity of play is by Reilly (1974) who used a general systems approach to illustrate it. The complexity of play, when viewed as an occupation, has form, function, and meaning (Clark et al., 1991). The form of play is what practitioners and researchers observe and decide to label as an enjoyable occupation or play. This view is the one also used in some evaluation tools that assess play. For example, Bundy's *Test of Playfulness* (Bundy et al., 2001; Skard et al., 2008) and Knox's *Revised Knox Play Scale* (Knox, 2008) focus on observations of behaviors labeled as play. This view abounds in the literature on play. A second way of studying play as an occupation is by its function or the purpose it serves. An example is using play as a tool to promote developmental skills. The function of play has also been linked to wellbeing and quality of life (Eicher-Catt, 2016; Royeen, 1997). This view of play focuses on using the motivational aspects of pleasurable occupations to target other skills. It is an often-used function of play in clinical practice. Creating a context for deriving pleasure from an activity also serves the function of play in the intervention process. The third way of studying play as an occupation is by its meaning. The meaning of play for everyone emanates from the experience derived from it (Blanche, 2002). When creating a play experience to target skill development, it is imperative to understand the elements that create the meaningfulness of that experience in the context of the intervention process. In this chapter, we will discuss play and its role in approaches that are often blended with sensory integration interventions. Creating a context where play can occur requires an understanding of the experience of play. We will start with a review of what constitutes that experience, continue with Ayres' view of play, and conclude by providing examples of its centrality in the intervention process. We emphasize the notion that to use play in the intervention process, it is important to understand its experiential characteristics so these can be incorporated into intervention not only

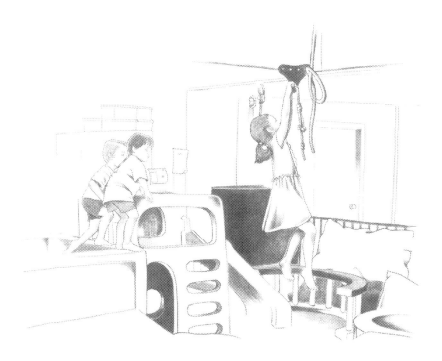

Figure 13.1 SI Sessions Offer Many Characteristics of Play: Freedom, Fun, Spontaneity, Excitement, and Active Engagement With Others and the Environment

as a context but also as an end in itself as learning to play is ultimately important throughout life.

Elements of Play as a Context in Treatment

To fully understand the experiential characteristics of play, we will go back to the seminal work of theoreticians describing play across the lifetime and its application to disability. According to those theorists, play includes a number of characteristics including fostering a sense of freedom (Marcuse, 1966, 2015); intrinsic motivation, and being engaged for the purpose of enjoyment (Caillois, 1961; Huizinga, 1955); spontaneity (Lieberman, 1977); bracketed outside ordinary life and thus requires a momentary suspension of reality (Bateson, 1955, 1972; Marcuse, 1966, 2015; Singer & Singer, 1990; Turner, 1982, 1987); may be linked to creativity (Huizinga, 1955); physically or mentally active (Sutton-Smith & Kelly-Byrne, 1984); and play involves tension and higher levels of arousal (Huizinga, 1938, 1955, 1995). The unique combination of these experiences differentiates what we call play from other activities (Blanche, 2002). In the encounter of Sylvia and Randy, most of these play experiences were systematically targeted. The activity was spontaneous, the child felt free to throw beanbags to an adult, it was outside ordinary life, it was active, and it became an enjoyable activity.

In addition to Reilly (1974), occupational scientists and occupational therapists making significant contributions to the study of the experiences of play include Knox (1996), who studied playfulness in children and described the playful child as being curious, imaginative, socially and verbally flexible, joyful, physically active, creative, and in control over the play situation; Bundy (1997; Bundy et al., 2001) who described playfulness as including specific characteristics of intrinsic motivation, internal sense of control, and freedom to suspend reality; Primeau (1998), who studied the play of children in the context of family life and found that the experiences of play were often intertwined during daily routine for both parents and children as long as a context was created; Parham (2015) who contributed to the theoretical description of play as well as to its use in clinical practice; and Blanche (2002) who identified different forms of play motivated by distinct experiences and Blanche and Knox (2008) who applied these to clinical practice with children with disabilities.

Ayres' View of Play as Part of the Therapeutic Process

Ayres clearly understood the importance of creating a context of play in the intervention process, even when she did not fully explain how to elicit it. In relationship to play, Ayres identified three important elements: (1) creating environments that invite the child to actively engage in play, (2) providing a safe context that was separate from everyday life and in which failure had no repercussions, and (3) promoting intrinsic motivation and enjoyment while performing an activity (Ayres, 1972, 1979; Ayres & Robbins, 2005). These principles resonate with the ones described in the classic literature on play. They are easier to address in a clinic setting, and somewhat harder to incorporate in hospital settings, school-based practice, or telehealth.

Creating an Environment

The creation of a physical environment that invites active play is the simplest one of these elements. Proof of this is that pediatric settings have been altered since the inception of sensory integration. Fredricks (2011) describes four task characteristics that facilitate engagement, for this author tasks need to be varied, interesting, meaningful, challenging and that promote autonomy. These are characteristics that also trigger the intrinsic motivation to play.

The environment can also serve a child's motivation for different types of play experiences. For example, high intensity activities may include physical activity and intense sensory experiences, while low intensity activities may promote relaxation and include seated activities and simple games. Creative activities can include building with blocks or painting a picture, while mastery can be attained when refining a recently acquired motor skill.

However, the physical environment is not the only element that invites active engagement. Play is active (Hanline & Fox, 1993; Sutton-Smith & Kelly-Byrne, 1984) either physically or cognitively (Blanche, 2002). Therefore, promoting active play is part of the art of therapy that requires a skilled practitioner who is able to read the child's motivation to play, generate curiosity, and modify the environment for the child to "want" to actively participate.

The use of the physical environment to invite play is more difficult in other environments such as schools. For example, the use of the physical environment to invite the child to play is limited in Telehealth, thus the clinician has to become more creative in using existing materials to motivate the child to engage in the session. The use of innovative materials can tap the child's curiosity, sense of adventure, creativity, or increase mastery over a novel task. Creating an environment of play in telehealth requires the therapist to (1) prepare the session with novel activities and toys that keep the child's interest in staying engaged; (2) be flexible to change the activity if siblings or other children are present during the session; and (3) be attuned to the elements in the home environment that can be used during the session.

Creating an environment of play in the educational environment requires the therapist to be knowledgeable of development and curricula expectations. A clinician can assist in designing the classroom and play yard to allow for choice-making and fostering intrinsic motivation. For example, in the block area of a preschool classroom, there might be images of different block designs that might foster the child's imagination and generate ideas. Table 13.1 offers tips on arranging the environment in multiple situations.

Safe Context

The creation of a safe context in which the child can try and fail requires bracketing the experience outside ordinary life. This is a central theme in play theory (Bateson, 1955, 1972). Creating a safe context for play is couched in the therapeutic alliance between child and therapist and should be considered as interrelated. Several approaches capitalize on the creation of the therapeutic alliance in play. Developmental, Individual Difference, Relationship-Based Model (DIR) is the closest to sensory

Table 13.1 Tips for Arranging the Physical Environment to Foster Play

---

- Provide choices that include multiple sources of sensory input
- Create an inviting and challenging environment by using novel tasks or materials
- Offer at least three choices of activities/equipment to promote intrinsic motivation
- Use color – do not overdo it – if mats are one color, you can have equipment in contrasting colors
- Use smaller spaces if the child has difficulty choosing, control the environment
- Offer choices of non-structured material that can make the activity successful and fun (e.g., foam, Play-Doh)
- Make the environment physically and socially safe – use mats and crash pads that make falling a fun activity and do not over correct.
- Change the environment often – novelty invites exploration and play

---

integration as it capitalizes on the safe context and the therapeutic alliance in a more explicit manner than most other approaches (Hess, 2013; Schoen et al., 2018).

Ayres may not have been explicit about an alliance in her descriptions of the therapeutic process, but she embedded it implicitly in her descriptions of sensory integration treatment. For example, Ayres (1972) describes self-fulfillment as the child's objective in the treatment session and highlights the cooperation with the child as crucial in attaining the therapeutic objectives. The therapeutic alliance is central in cooperative play, as the therapist needs to fully understand the child's limitations and motivations; create a sense of freedom of choice within a structure already provided by the physical environment; and respond to and build on a child's choice (Ayres, 1972; Bundy & Hacker, 2020). Understanding the child's motivations requires the clinician to read the child's verbal and nonverbal cues (i.e., facial and body expressions and movements) and respond to these accordingly. Table 13.2 provides tips for interacting with the child.

Table 13.2 Tips for Interacting With the Child to Foster Play

---

- Laugh at yourself – be silly
- Accept the child's suggestions – the best ideas come from the children
- Do not overcorrect, just enough to provide feedback – make it fun
- Be spontaneous – you can move on if something doesn't work
- Allow freedom
- Do not be afraid of challenging the child's skills
- Be accepting of failure and mistakes, including your own.

Intrinsic Motivation

The use of intrinsic motivation in the treatment session requires an experienced practitioner who can incorporate this as a central experience of play during the length of a session. The intrinsic motivation to play is in the enjoyment derived from the process of engaging in the activity and includes many forms of play (Blanche, 2002; Caillois, 1961; Huizinga, 1938, 1955, 1995). Tapping into intrinsic motivation requires understanding the child' interests, desires, strengths, and weaknesses. If the child was not motivated to come to therapy, then it was time to consider a different approach. It is this element of intrinsic motivation and child directedness that interveners have the most difficulty following. On one extreme are clinicians who just let the child choose anything they want during the session, and on the other extreme are those that plan and direct the child to pre-determined activities.

A session that is "child-directed" means that the child "directs" from what the intervener has provided as choices for the child. The context

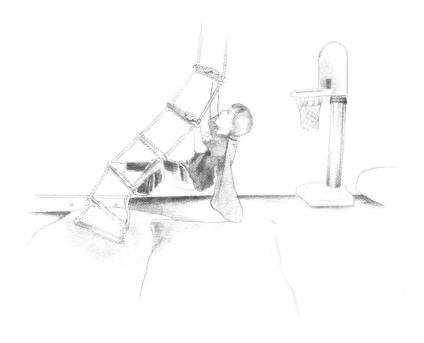

Figure 13.2 This Picture Illustrates Fantasy Play as the Child Is Pretending to Be a Superhero Climbing Onto a Building

Table 13.3 Tips for Fostering Intrinsic Motivation

TIPS for Reading the Child's Motivations	TIPS for Responding to the Child's Actions
• Listening to the child's verbalizations (i.e., words, pitch, tone) • Attending to the child's facial expressions (i.e., anger, pain, joy, surprise) • Observing the child's body movements (i.e., tensing, fast/slow movements)	• Asking questions about preferences • Clarifying the child's preference • Stabilizing equipment • Modeling an action for the child to imitate • Facilitating the child's movement • Guiding • Offering alternatives • Waiting for a response • Letting go • Altering the challenge by making a task easier or more difficult

for using intrinsic motivation in the session requires the creation of an environment in which the child is free (Ayres, 1972). The context of play is not necessarily total freedom to be "child-directed," but freedom for the child to choose and stay in activities that allow the therapist to organize and elicit adaptive responses. A therapist can convert any activity into play by arranging the environment and modifying his/her interaction skills (see Table 13.3).

Intrinsic motivation is also central in DIR. Other intervention approaches are starting to incorporate the child's choices in the therapeutic session and hence at least that element of play is enforced. In DIR/Floortime intervention, two of the central principles are following the child's lead and mastery of functional emotional developmental capacities (Hess, 2013). This aligns with the principles of sensory integration. The practitioner is charged with combining these approaches to facilitate active engagement and play. For example, a child with autism might have an interest in lining up blocks in a repetitive manner. The skilled practitioner might enter into the child's world and expand on this child's interest. Perhaps the line of blocks becomes a train or a tractor. Maybe the blocks are hidden in a sandbox and the child needs to use his tactile skills to find the blocks in order to make a train. Intrinsic motivation can be incorporated in other intervention approaches and other therapeutic contexts.

Centrality of Play: Promoting Play and Leisure Across the Lifespan

The centrality of play and leisure in life and the intervention process and their link to meaningful engagement and quality of life is part of the International Classification of Function (ICF) model and is advocated by many (Majnemer, 2009; Perenboom & Chorus, 2003). For many play theorists, leisure is an extension of play (Blanche, 2002; Bundy, 1997; Reilly, 1974). As clinicians, we can promote play and leisure at the individual, family, and community level. At the individual level, clinicians guided by the Reasoning in Action Model (RAM) model can discern the factors affecting the child's ability to function, to play, and to interact with the environment.

At the family and the community level, the clinician must collaborate with both the child and the family to create an environment that fosters play and leisure, being conscious of the cultural context. In the same way as the clinician reads the child's motivation for preferred play activities, the clinician needs to identify the family's preferred play and leisure activities. For example, some families like to go camping, others like to go to museums, while others may prefer sport activities. Fostering the child's intrinsic motivation is important when helping families incorporate all members into leisure activities. Play can also be embedded in the context of the family routines (Primeau, 1998). In her qualitative research, Primeau (1998) explored parents' inclusion of their children's play activities. Some families played with their children while doing housework or included their children in the activity. Because the use of telehealth in the intervention provides an opportunity to enter into the family's home and daily routine, clinicians can then find ways to create opportunities in which play is possible, such as including play in household routines.

Play in the community often includes outdoor play, which is a context often ignored in the creation of treatment settings (Wilkinson et al., 2019). For children, toys and outdoor play are significant elements of what they consider play (Nicholson et al., 2014), therefore outdoor activities need to be included when fostering play in the community. The choice of preferred toys can include open ended materials such as blocks and Play-Doh and loose parts such as boxes, shovels, art materials that can be manipulated and moved (Wilson, 2004). Access to nature and outdoor activities and the natural environment afford many opportunities to provide sensory experiences for a child to learn about their body in relation to space and can have a positive effect on stress, functional behavior, and health (Kumari Sahoo & Senapati, 2014; Mygind et al., 2019). Outdoor play and therapy can also take different forms as interventions in farms (Protopapadaki, 2019) or interventions that include play and the promotion of creative expression in outside and inside spaces (Vliagofti et al., 2019). Therefore, clinicians need to assist families in identifying the best community outings that can be included in the child's repertoire of daily activities. Chapter 8 emphasizes the benefits of nature on health and wellbeing.

Table 13.4 Play as Context in Intervention

Disability/Foci	Research
ADHD	Play-based interventions promote social play, social skills, parent-child relationships (Barnes et al., 2017)
Autism	Imitation and modeling, combined with adult-structured/child directed approaches improve play (Kuhaneck et al., 2020)
Cerebral Palsy	Virtual reality, play based intervention fosters self-efficacy (Reid, 2002)
Early Intervention	Occupational therapist – led community playgroup effective in increasing playfulness of children enrolled in early intervention (Fabrizi, 2016)
Hospital	Play interventions reduce anxiety and negative emotions in hospitalized children (Li et al., 2016)
Physical Disability/Developmental Coordination Disorder	Scaffold activity and/or environment to increase participation (Poulsen et al., 2004)
School-Based	Opportunities for natural outdoor play (e.g., nature-based elements and multisensory garden) promote self-regulation and attention (Kemple, 2016)

The research on the use of play as a therapeutic tool with children with disabilities supports its inclusion in the intervention process. These studies highlight the importance of creating a context of play for promoting the development of functional skills. Table 13.4 provides some examples of research studies in which play has been used as a context in the intervention.

However, the context of play is not only important in the acquisition of functional skills, but also as a milieu in which children learn to develop the ability to enjoy occupation with experiences that give meaning to life. Our responsibility is not only to use play but also to help children develop play skills. Therefore, using play as a context, targets developmental skills as well as the ability to play. Only when we are able to help children develop their ability to engage in play can we say we have been successful interveners.

References

Ayres, A. J. (1972). *Sensory integration and learning disorders.* Western Psychological Services. https://doi.org/10.1177/002221947200500605

Ayres, A. J. (1979). Sensory integration therapy. In *Sensory integration and the child* (p. 1352156). Western Psychological Services.

Ayres, A. J., & Robbins, J. (2005). *Sensory integration and the child: Understanding hidden sensory challenges*. Western Psychological Services.

Barnes, G., Wilkes-Gillan, S., Bundy, A., & Cordier, R. (2017). The social play, social skills and parent – child relationships of children with ADHD 12 months following a RCT of a play-based intervention. *Australian Occupational Therapy Journal, 64*(6), 457–465. https://doi.org/10.1111/1440-1630.12417

Bateson, G. (1955). A theory of play and fantasy; A report on theoretical aspects of the project of study of the role of the paradoxes of abstraction in communication. *Psychiatric Research Reports, 2*, 39–51.

Bateson, G. (1972). A theory of play and fantasy. (1955) In: Steps to an ecology of mind. *New York Times*.

Blanche, E. I. (2002). Play and process: Adult play embedded in the daily routine. In J. Roopnarine (Ed.), *Conceptual, social-cognitive, and contextual issues in the field of play* (pp. 249–278). Ablex Publishing.

Blanche, E. I., & Knox, S. H. (2008). Learning to play: Promoting skills and quality of life in individuals with cerebral palsy. *Clinics in Developmental Medicine, 178*(1), 357–370.

Bundy, A. C. (1997). Play and playfulness: What to look for. In L. D. Parham & L. S. Fazio (Eds.), *Play in occupational therapy for children*. Mosby.

Bundy, A. C., & Hacker, C. (2020). The art of therapy. In A. C. Bundy & S. J. Lane (Eds.), *Sensory integration theory and practice* (3rd ed.). F.A. Davis.

Bundy, A. C., Nelson, L., Metzger, M., & Bingaman, K. (2001). Validity and reliability of a test of playfulness. *The Occupational Therapy Journal of Research, 21*(4), 276–292. https://doi.org/10.1177/153944920102100405

Caillois, R. (1961). *Man, play and games* (M. Barash, Trans.). Free Press of Glencoe.

Clark, F. A., Parham, D., Carlson, M. E., Frank, G., Jackson, J., Pierce, D., Wolfe, R. J., & Zemke, R. (1991). Occupational science: Academic innovation in the service of occupational therapy's future. *American Journal of Occupational Therapy, 45*(4), 300–310. https://doi.org/10.5014/ajot.45.4.300

Eicher-Catt, D. (2016). Learning to take play seriously: Peirce, Bateson, and Huizinga on the sacrality of play. *Semiotica, 2016*(212), 259–276. https://doi.org/10.1515/sem-2016-0135

Fabrizi, S. (2016). Measuring the effectiveness of occupational therapist – Led playgroups in early intervention. *American Journal of Occupational Therapy, 70*(4_Supplement_1), 7011520295p1–7011520295p1. https://doi.org/10.5014/ajot.2016.70S1-PO3065

Fredricks, J. A. (2011). Engagement in school and out-of-school contexts: A multidimensional view of engagement. *Theory into Practice, 50*(4), 327–335. https://doi.org/10.1080/00405841.2011.607401

Hanline, M. F., & Fox, L. (1993). Learning within the context of play: Providing typical early childhood experiences for children with severe disabilities. *Journal of the Association for Persons with Severe Handicaps, 18*(2), 121–129. https://doi.org/10.1177/154079699301800205

Hess, E. B. (2013). DIR®/Floortime™: Evidence based practice towards the treatment of autism and sensory processing disorder in children and adolescents. *International Journal of Child Health and Human Development*, 6(3), 267–274.

Huizinga, J. (1955, first published 1938). *Home Ludens: A study of the play-element in culture*. Beacon Press

Huizinga, J. (1995). The nature of play. In *Philosophic inquiry in sport*. Human Kinetics.

Kemple, K. M., Oh, J., Kenney, E., & Smith-Bonahue, T. (2016). The power of outdoor play and play in natural environments. *Childhood Education*, 92(6), 446–454. https://doi.org/10.1080/00094056.2016.1251793

Knox, S. (1996). Play and playfulness in preschool children. *Occupational Science: The Evolving Discipline*, 80–88.

Knox, S. (2008). Development and current use of the revised Knox preschool play scale. In *Play in occupational therapy for children* (pp. 55–70). Mosby. https://doi.org/10.1016/b978-032302954-4.10003-0

Kuhaneck, H., Spitzer, S. L., & Bodison, S. C. (2020). A systematic review of interventions to improve the occupation of play in children with autism. *OTJR: Occupation, Participation and Health*, 40(2), 83–98. https://doi.org/10.1177/1539449219880531

Kumari Sahoo, S., & Senapati, A. (2014). Effect of sensory diet through outdoor play on functional behaviour in children with ADHD. *Indian Journal of Occupational Therapy (Indian Journal of Occupational Therapy)*, 46(2).

Li, W. H., Chung, J. O. K., Ho, K. Y., & Kwok, B. M. C. (2016). Play interventions to reduce anxiety and negative emotions in hospitalized children. *BMC Pediatrics*, 16(1), 36. https://doi.org/10.1186/s12887-016-0570-5

Lieberman, J. N. (1977). *Playfulness*. Academic Press.

Majnemer, A. (2009). Promoting participation in leisure activities: Expanding role for pediatric therapists. https://doi.org/10.1080/01942630802625163

Marcuse, H. (2015). *Eros and civilization: A philosophical inquiry into Freud*. Beacon Press. (Original work published 1966)

Mygind, L., Kjeldsted, E., Hartmeyer, R., Mygind, E., Stevenson, M. P., Quintana, D. S., & Bentsen, P. (2019). Effects of public green space on acute psychophysiological stress response: A systematic review and meta-analysis of the experimental and quasi-experimental evidence. *Environment and Behavior*. https://doi.org/10.1177/0013916519873376

Nicholson, J., Shimpi, P. M., Kurnik, J., Carducci, C., & Jevgjovikj, M. (2014). Listening to children's perspectives on play across the lifespan: Children's right to inform adults' discussions of contemporary play. *International Journal of Play*, 3(2), 136–156. https://doi.org/10.1080/21594937.2014.937963

Parham, L. D. (2015). Role of play in assessment. In D. Pronin Fromberg & D. Bergen (Eds.), *Play from birth to twelve. Contexts, perspectives and meanings* (pp. 233–243). Routledge.

Perenboom, R. J., & Chorus, A. M. (2003). Measuring participation according to the international classification of functioning, disability and health (ICF). *Disability and Rehabilitation*, 25(11–12), 577–587. https://doi.org/10.1080/0963828031000137081

Poulsen, A. A., & Ziviani, J. M. (2004). Can I play too? Physical activity engagement of children with developmental coordination disorders. *Canadian Journal of Occupational Therapy*, 71(2), 100–107. https://doi.org/10.1177/000841740407100205

Primeau, L. A. (1998). Orchestration of work and play within families. *American Journal of Occupational Therapy, 52*(3), 188–195. https://doi.org/10.5014/ajot.52.3.188

Protopapadaki, M. (2019). *Sensory integration intervention on a green care farm.* Presentation at the European Sensory Integration Congress, Thessaloniki, Greece, June 22, 2019.

Reid, D. T. (2002). Benefits of a virtual play rehabilitation environment for children with cerebral palsy on perceptions of self-efficacy: A pilot study. *Pediatric Rehabilitation, 5*(3), 141–148. https://doi.org/10.1080/1363849021000039344

Reilly, M. (1974). *Play as exploratory learning: Studies of curiosity behavior.* Sage

Royeen, C. (1997). Play as occupation and as an indicator of health. *The Essence of Play: A Child's Occupation,* 1–14.

Schoen, S. A., Miller, L. J., & Flanagan, J. (2018). A retrospective pre-post treatment study of occupational therapy intervention for children with sensory processing challenges. *The Open Journal of Occupational Therapy, 6*(1), 4. https://doi.org/10.15453/2168-6408.1367

Singer, D. G., & Singer, J. L. (1990). *The house of make-believe.* Harvard University Press.

Skard, G., & Bundy, A. C. (2008). Test of playfulness. In *Play in occupational therapy for children* (pp. 71–93). Mosby. https://doi.org/10.1016/b978-032302954-4.10004-2

Sutton-Smith, B., & Kelly-Byrne, D. (1984). The masks of play. In B. Sutton-Smith & D. Kelly-Byrne (Eds.), *Masks of play* (pp. 184–197). Leisure Press.

Turner, V. (1982). *From ritual to theatre: The seriousness of human play.* Performing Arts Journal Publications.

Turner, V. (1987). *The anthropology of performance.* PAJ Publications.

Vliagofti, O., Iliadis, K., Theodorakis, M., Tsiara, K., Karamani, I., Blioumis, K., Papaplioura, E., Papakonstantinou, E., Papathanasiou, G., Tsiogka, E., Koutsioyki, A., Papadopoulou, A., Florou, M., Zachou, E., Florou, P., Florou, D., Papagoras, C., Tragias, G., & Dimou, S. (2019). *A presentation of the camp based community program of "kivotos" center.* Presentation at the European Sensory Integration Congress, Thessaloniki, Greece, June 22, 2019.

Wilkinson, K., Rossi, J., Scott-Cole, L., Silvia, R., Allman, C., Kennedy, A., King, S., Langan, J., Lasnicki, S., Miller, A., Schutt, K., & Wilcox, H. (2019). Outdoor play in pediatric OT practice. *American Journal of Occupational Therapy, 73*(4_Supplement_1), 7311515352P1–7311515352P1. https://doi.org/10.5014/ajot.2019.73s1-po5020

Wilson, R. (2004). Why children play under the bushes. *Early Childhood News, 16*(2), 14.

14 The STAR Frame of Reference

Sensory Integration/ Processing, Regulation, and Relationship

Virginia Spielman, Sarah A. Schoen, and Michele Parkins

Program: The STAR Frame of Reference (FoR)/STAR PROCESS

Type of program: Interdisciplinary clinic-based program with parent coaching.

Clients/patients/population served: Individuals impacted by differences in sensory integration and processing.

Ages: Life span application (this chapter focuses on the pediatric population).

Diagnoses or functional issues: Challenges with participation and function caused by differences in sensory integration and processing.

Context: Clinic based interdisciplinary work, predominantly takes place in the sensory gym with an emphasis on parent empowerment and protected time for parent education. The parent-child relationship is considered the "greatest context of all".

Number of sessions (per week, month, etc.): 3–5 sessions per week of 50–90 minutes in length, for a 20–30-week period (must be tailored to the family's individual needs and availability).

Program Goals/Objectives: The central objective of the STAR FoR is to support development of self-organized, self-directed clients through addressing differences in sensory integration and processing and their impact on relational health and capacity to regulate. The parent-child relationship is prioritized, and client self-actualization is facilitated through relationship-based therapeutic play. Goals focus on meaningful function and participation in daily life, formation of positive relationships, self-determination, and development of positive self-identity.

Type of Interventions:

STAR FoR includes: Sensory Integration (SI) theory and Developmental Individual Difference and Relationship-based (DIR) model

DOI: 10.4324/9781003050810-17

The mechanisms of sensory integration and processing underlie the human capacity for meaning making (Mueller & Tronick, 2020). How we experience sensations, feel feelings, take note of our own bodies, exchange signals with others and *make sense* of our world is all dependent on the neurobiological processes of sensory integration. For the purposes of this chapter and to "put it simply": in order to develop relational capacity, meaningful occupational engagement, and attain self and community actualization – we must first develop body schema, mastery of sensory motor cause and effect, sense of bodily location in space and time, and a multi-sensory map of the world around us. Sensory integration and processing in the context of human relationships and experience constructs our inner emotional (psychical) schema (see Ayres, 1972, p. 266).

The dynamic relationship between sensory motor and social emotional development can be theoretically represented with the combination of Ayres Sensory Integration (ASI™) and the DIR (Developmental Individual Difference and Relationship-based) model. The theories align with one another in many ways, paying particular attention to the manner in which individual differences (for ASI™ differences in sensory integration) support or derail development. Philosophically, both emphasize client autonomy and self-actualization, and prioritize respecting and honoring the dignity of the child or person being helped (Ayres, 1972; Greenspan & Wieder, 2006b). Clinically these theories emphasize tapping into internal motivation and following the child's lead with the goal of supporting self-organization and agency of the integrated child (Ayres & Robbins, 2005; Greenspan & Wieder, 2006a). It is also interesting to note that both theories, unusually for the time at which they were written, emphasized the importance of understanding what underlies "behaviors" (Greenspan & Wieder, 2006a; Lane et al., 2019).

Individual differences in sensory integration and processing impact human development in almost every domain. This is exemplified when a caregiver and baby engage in early interactions exchanging continuous socio-sensory signals. This interpersonal experience is distinctly sensory *and* distinctly affective, both at the same time, laying the foundation for strong attachment relationships. In this socio-sensory space, co-regulation is constantly taking place. Co-regulation is the transactional process of supporting and shifting state of arousal through interactions between social partners. Sensation supports the formation of relationships that enable access to co-regulation experiences and lays the foundation for self-regulation. In the context of these exchanges, the baby learns that his actions and gestures/vocalizations have an impact on his world. Thus, the beginning of sense of agency emerges. Providing therapy that supports the social emotional response of the caregiver and child along with the neurobiological response of the sensory system, provides a comprehensive, dynamic approach to the dual sensory motor and social emotional differences in development.

In application of both DIR/Floortime and ASI™ there is a fundamental focus on playful interaction and connection to bring success (Greenspan & Wieder, 1998; Parham et al., 2007). Both have a focus on foundations to support higher level capacities: ASI™, considering the integration of all sensory systems to support production of an adaptive response, often observed in the form of a higher-level motor response (Spitzer & Smith Roley, 2001); DIR considering the integration of functional emotional capacities to support observable higher level social emotional development (Wieder, 2017). A focus on these foundations provides a shared base from which the clinician can launch deeper into this powerful and dynamic therapeutic combination. Through blending of the two frameworks, the clinician deliberately facilitates both sensory motor development and relational health, ameliorating attachment processes – which are commonly interrupted by individual differences (Cermak, 2001; DeSantis et al., 2004; Whitcomb et al., 2015).

DIR is a model of human development, which emphasizes the development of Functional Emotional Developmental Capacities and provides a framework of strategies to support growth in this domain (Greenspan et al., 2001; Wieder, 2017). The DIR model harnesses the power of sensori-affective signaling between communication partners. In Floortime™ therapy, this input comes from an attuned and mindful therapist, ideally with the parents in the room participating as play partners and learning how to apply these techniques all the time every day. Sensory integration and processing impact functional emotional development at every level – for better or worse. The converse is also true; supporting functional emotional growth facilitates change in sensory processing capacities.

Program Description: The Star FoR

The STAR FoR is suited for application by interdisciplinary teams, the FoR assumes the individual is a complex, dynamic system influenced by, and able to influence, the contexts in which they exist. Contexts include family relationships, and the nested environmental ecologies within which the family system is located. The STAR PROCESS is the therapeutic application of the STAR FoR and incorporates strategies from Ayres Sensory Integration therapy (ASI®) and DIR/Floortime (Miller et al., 2019a). The STAR PROCESS will be discussed later.

A hallmark of the STAR FoR is the application of ASI® therapy related to two other domains of development: Regulation and Relationship. The importance of the mutually reliant and bi-directional processes between all three domains, as the foundation for positive identity development

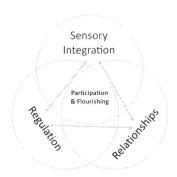

Figure 14.1 The Three Foundational Domains of the STAR Frame of Reference

and psychological well-being, is the emphasis. To that end, the STAR FoR emphasizes autonomy and self-actualization and is therefore a strengths-based approach that privileges the parent-child relationship.

Referral and Presenting Problems

The assessment process begins with completion of an extensive history form and participation in an in-person, video chat or telephone intake meeting. Preliminary information is obtained about the child and family, and includes a family history, medical history/current information, and description of performance at home, school and in the community. The objective is to obtain a holistic picture of the child's presenting problems, parental perceptions of these problems and of the parent's priorities for treatment.

Interdisciplinary Collaboration

The STAR FoR employs an interdisciplinary, family-centered approach that includes a range of clinicians such as occupational therapists, speech, and language pathologists, feeding specialists, mental health professionals (psychologists, counselors, marriage family therapists, etc.) and teachers. This approach to therapeutic support promotes integrated models of care with collaboration across all disciplines. Treatment sessions and parent education meetings frequently involve more than one discipline. Knowledge is shared, synthesized, and applied as one integrated program.

Assessment

Families seeking assessment very commonly present with functional challenges in regulation and relationships. Thereby, assessment necessitates deep consideration of the connection between sensory processing, regulation, and relationships within the context of the individual family unit. Assessment is an essential feature of understanding the underlying nature of the child's presenting problem. A social emotional component to the assessment process is included as standard practice. The assessment process includes standardized testing of sensory integration and processing as well as structured and unstructured clinical observations in the occupational therapy gym of sensory-motor abilities, problem solving skills, capacity for engagement and relationship, and play. Norm-referenced parent and teacher report measures are used to supplement the examiner-administered scale with tools that examine sensory processing patterns, associated adaptive behavior and behavior problems, social emotional growth, and parent efficacy. Results are used to inform and facilitate treatment planning and evaluation reports include a description of the child's/family's strengths that support success in therapy.

Impact Statements

Impact statements are a defining characteristic of evaluation reports utilizing the STAR FoR. These statements are designed to help families/professionals understand the proposed link between sensory integration and processing differences and presenting problems, thereby clearly connecting sensation, regulation, and relationship. The goal is for parents and professionals to understand the association of these underlying mechanisms with function and participation. See Box 14.1.

Goal Attainment Scaling

Functional goals are established during a parent only meeting following the evaluation and are based on parent/child priorities. Using the format

---

Box 14.1

Example Impact Statement

Impact of dyspraxia on ability to participate in pretend play and play routines with peers. Tiffany's challenges with movement planning and execution affect her ability to create a plan of action in her play with peers. She has difficulty learning new games, following directions and anticipating the results of her or other people's actions. As a result, she has difficulty following play schemes created by others causing her considerable stress and fatigue. Accordingly, Tiffany avoids playground activities, and organized sports with peers as well as imaginary play that isn't rooted in what is familiar and rehearsed.

of Goal Attainment Scaling, progress is monitored and quantified at the end of the program (Kiresuk et al., 2014) through a final parent meeting.

Parent Meetings

Imperative to the STAR FoR is the inclusion of parent only education/collaboration meetings. By creating this separate time, it is never necessary to talk about the child in front of them and the playful flow of sessions does not need to be interrupted. A minimum of three meetings are scheduled throughout intervention that focus on training parents/caregivers to be active participants in the treatment process and in developing a sensory lifestyle. The term sensory lifestyle refers to the cultivation of proactive strategies to support sensory health all the time every day. This involves increased awareness of the sensory needs of every family member, ongoing options for nourishing the sensory systems throughout the day, environmental accommodations suited to every context and more (Bialer & Miller, 2011).

Intervention

The **STAR PROCESS** is designed to address relationship, regulation and sensory processing/integration challenges that are interfering with functioning in daily life across the lifespan. In pediatric populations it is most often an intensive, short term intervention. A common template for program intensity and frequency is 30 sessions that are attended three to five times a week. Additionally, it is preferred that programs include psychoeducational sessions with a clinical psychologist or other mental health professional who informally explores the parent-child relationship and family systems.

The foundation of therapy is the integration of sensory, regulation and relationship strategies in an intentional, ongoing basis, within the context of play. Regulation refers to the individual's capacity to shift and maintain states concordant with the demands of the environment. In a balanced nervous system "regulation" toggles between unconscious and conscious as we shift between states according to internal and external context-dependent demands. Factors that impact regulation include emotion, social, cognitive, language, physical health, sensory processing, and sensorimotor. This definition of regulation is distinctly different from self-control, self-governance and more executive function related definitions of the term (Burman et al., 2015). The most commonly visible manifestation is in the form of a "behavioral" reaction or an emotional reaction. The third domain, relationship, requires an understanding of attachment processes and a trauma informed lens.

Play naturally supports human development across all domains, including motor, cognitive, social, emotional, etc. (Yogman et al., 2018). Play is child-led, and the therapist's job is to exploit every therapeutic opportunity within the play scheme without compromising fun or entering into power struggles. Therapeutic play resides in the Zone of Proximal Development (Vygotsky, 1978), the just right challenge (Ayres, 1972) or *the just right success* (Bialer & Miller, 2011). Therapeutically, scaffolded interactions and activities support growth and development of the self-organized child.

When using the STAR FoR each child and family's unique narrative is considered in parallel with the child's strengths and challenges within the family. Sessions are characterized by creating a supportive positive relationship with the child, connecting through attunement, transactional supports, ensuring opportunities for success and active collaboration, and experiences of joy and playfulness for all involved. Highly developed reflective practice including clinical reasoning in the moment, and reflection in action and on action, are paramount.

Process Reflects Application of the FoR and Embodies the Following Seven Principles

Play. Therapy occurs within the context of play. The therapist assumes the role of play partner and creates motivation by tapping into the child's preferred play activities. This is later transferred to the parent-child dyad through coaching the parent.

Relationship. Intervention focuses on the parent-child relationship. Intentional support is provided for three primary relationships: therapist-child, therapist-parent and parent-child. Parents are a central part of the therapy session with the goal of creating opportunities for success between the parent and the child.

Organization. At all times, each session focuses on helping the child attain the optimal level of arousal to support participation and learning. An organized, regulated state is achieved first through co-regulation and then moves to strategies for increasing self-regulation capacity. An important component of this work includes tuning in to the 'wisdom of the body' and attending to interoceptive sensory signals relating to arousal and state of internal well-being. An individual must first experience regulation (a state of calm, alert, availability) in order to learn self-regulation (Shanker, 2010). Individualized relationship-based supports are an important part of this process, such as safety, consistency, predictability, and environmental accommodations (reducing visual distractions, mitigating auditory overwhelm, minimizing smells/perfumes etc.) and ensuring hydration and dietary needs are met. These strategies can be augmented by the application of cognitive strategies like visual schedules and social stories; visual scales and reference tools can further support regulation as well as helping the child identify their own arousal level.

Collaboration. Collaboration occurs with the child, the parent as well as with other professionals on the multidisciplinary team both inside the treatment space and in all other contexts.

Emotional regulation. Emotional regulation and awareness are supported as the therapist (and consequently the parent) attunes to the child's emotional state and the emotions that underlie their behavior. As sensory processing improves, and awareness of internal body states, the child's understanding and recognition of their own emotions is supported.

Sensation. Addressing the child's sensory processing and integration challenges is ongoing throughout intervention. Therapy requires active participation and involves static and dynamic equipment in a therapy gym that provide sensory rich experiences especially in tactile, vestibular, and proprioceptive domains. Every session in the sensory gym includes all the components of ASI™ and meet fidelity requirements (Parham et al., 2007). These deliberate considerations of relationship, environment and individual, through the lens of ASI™ facilitate a truly transactional approach to client-centered support.

Success. The child and parent are always scaffolded to experience success. Success ensures mastery of the environment and forms the basis for the development of self-esteem and self-confidence.

Groups

Group therapy at STAR Institute commonly follows the completion of a 1:1 program but can also stand alone or precede more intensive programs. Groups utilizing the STAR FoR focus on the three domains of sensory processing, regulation, and relationships. Through this strengths-based, collaborative process, STAR Groups utilize shared occupations to build attention, social competence, emotional regulation, and self-organization.

Application of the STAR FoR to a groups program is characterized by foundational characteristics listed in Table 14.1.

Table 14.1 Foundational Characteristics of the STAR Frame of Reference

Requirement	Description/Strategies
Strength Based	Presume competence
	Reframe 'behavior' and facilitate intentional communication
	Focus on social flourishing, classroom confidence and sense of agency
	Celebrate and emphasize all successes

(Continued)

Requirement	Description/Strategies
Affinity	Fun, playful, enjoyable activities built around shared interests and group goals
Inclusive	Environmental accommodations: supportive/adaptive seating, minimizing visual stimuli
	Individualized accommodations: noise reduction headphones, supporting praxis
	Cognitive support strategies: social stories, visual schedules
Nurturing	Developmentally appropriate, meeting the child where they are at
	Providing the "just right" success in multiple dimensions: sensory modulation/ sensorimotor/social emotional/ language/cognitive
	Transactional supports that respond to each child's needs/ interests
	Identify underlying contributors to challenges with participation
	Flexible expectations of performance
Therapeutic Use of Self	Attuned, connectedness, reading and respecting signs of overwhelm, identifying what works, active listening and waiting
	Intentional language use: less words, narration of what is happening, neutral language (nonjudgmental), validating
	Utilizing co-regulation strategies: constantly adjusting the pace to the group members, maintaining connection, comfortable with acknowledging emotions
Sensory Rich	Graded motor and sensory expectations, opportunities for whole body movements
	Considers all eight cross-modal, open sensory systems

School Based Services

The application of the STAR FoR in schools involves similarly tailored, client-centered support that integrates best evidence with professional judgement and expertise while considering client preferences (Miller et al., 2019b; Whiting, 2018). A continuum of therapy that aligns with the principles of the STAR FoR are offered within the multi-tiered systems of support (MTSS, formerly known as Response to Intervention) The clinician and team move to Tier 3 when Tier 1 and 2 supports are not enough and challenges with participation and function warrant specific skilled/individualized pull out intervention from an occupational therapist (OT) (Miller et al., 2019b). The evaluation process is identical to the process for an in-clinic evaluation with greater inclusion of the teacher alongside caregivers and other team members (see earlier).

Telehealth

When telehealth service provision is indicated, a few guiding principles are helpful to keep in mind. These are: parent empowerment, process based, and success-oriented whole-body therapeutic play. The environment and the tasks are different, but the core principles remain the same; telehealth sessions offer a unique and valuable opportunity to impact the level of therapeutic play occurring at home. These play sessions should always be SMART – Sensory Rich, Motor, Attuned, Relationship-rich, Time (Bialer & Miller, 2011; Miller et al., 2014). Telehealth remains true to the frame of reference, emphasizing the three domains of development but with an increased opportunity and responsibility for parent coaching. Exploration of the client's space with parental participation is a unique opportunity afforded by telehealth that supports lifestyle changes at home.

Parent empowerment during telehealth may involve preparation prior to the session so that the clinician and the parent feel they are on the same page. In keeping with clinic-based programs, separate parent education sessions to review how the telehealth process is going and protect space for parent coaching are included. The emphasis often needs to be on the importance of process over product in initial sessions and reminding families that treatment will continue to almost exclusively involve therapeutic play. By emphasizing fun and relationships we take the pressure off performing and are able to enter into all the therapeutic qualities of play. One strategy for being "in the moment" involves narrating the experiences of the session. Narration done in a playful and engaging way with deliberate use of affect. Can you describe what your client is experiencing; thinking about; how they are moving their bodies; the expressions on their face; the physical and sensory properties of the toys they are showing you or playing with; the furniture they are climbing; the food they are eating etc. Is there a way to join in the activities? Do you have the same toy, or can you do the same big silly whole-body movements in your own space?

Success oriented telehealth sessions support mastery, build confidence, and avoid introducing novel ideas too soon. Degrees of challenge are added incrementally and in keeping with the principles of the *just right success*. Sessions continue to be child-led and exploit therapeutic opportunities as they arise. If a child was seen in the clinic, telehealth provides an opportunity to coach the parents around how to apply the strategies that worked in the sensory gym within the home context.

Whole-body sensory-rich play can be achieved in the home through play outside, on the sofa, on beds and with cushions and mattresses. Children may often have gross motor play equipment that can be used during telehealth sessions. Consider asking the family to log-in on a mobile device so that as much movement as possible can be incorporated into the play. Keeping focused on SMART play and reinforcing how the session was therapeutically beneficial in follow up conversations empowers parents to continue play at home. Telehealth sessions can be the perfect vehicle for parent education and empowerment.

Research

The STAR FoR contributes to the body literature on interventions appropriate for and effective with children who have sensory integration and processing challenges. Years of application have contributed to the accumulation of clinically observed, and meaningful outcomes. Scientifically rigorous research demonstrating its effectiveness is emerging. Outcome/Effectiveness data exclusive to the STAR FoR is available from a retrospective chart review (Schoen et al., 2018) and several single subject studies (Carder et al., 2020; Schoen et al., 2019b). Data is also available from application of the STAR FoR in therapy groups (e.g., trampoline exercise group and bike riding training group). Current research is being conducted in school-based practice.

Relevant to this presentation of evidence is an examination of the individual elements of the STAR FoR. As described within this chapter, the theoretical framework/foundation of the STAR FoR attends to three cornerstones of human development: sensory integration/processing, relationship, and regulation. Thus, evidence for the effectiveness of this intervention is derived from Ayres Sensory Integration (ASI™) therapy and relationship-based interventions (based on DIR/Floortime). A key component of relationship-based interventions is the inclusion of parent education, parent collaboration, and parent coaching. This section concludes with a summary of the growing body of evidence specific to the STAR FoR.

The Sensory Integration/Processing Component

There is increasing support for the importance of addressing the sensory component of function and the impact the sensory component has on the health and wellness of children/adults. This evidence comes from studies of sensory integration intervention, based on the principles of Ayres (1972). Two systemic reviews highlighted in Chapter 2 showed the efficacy of the ASI™ therapy (Schaaf et al., 2018; Schoen et al., 2019a), and deemed it an evidence-based practice based on the standards of the Council for Exceptional Children (Schoen et al., 2019a). Further, the National Clearinghouse on Autism Treatment at the University of North Carolina also determined that sensory integration was an evidenced based intervention (Steinbrenner et al., 2020). This accumulating research provides important support for the STAR FoR, which emphasizes directing interventions to the unique sensory challenges of each individual relative to modulation, discrimination, posture, and praxis.

The Relationship Component

The relationship component is supported by an increased awareness/recognition that parents are central to and a necessity for a child's growth/development and learning (Ginsburg, 2007). This principle is supported by a review paper by Wallace and Rogers (2010), which purports that parent involvement in intervention is a critical component of effective interventions and needs to include coaching on responsivity and sensitivity to a child's cues. The effectiveness of relationship-focused interventions that capitalize on the parent-child relationship and an intentional focus on social engagement and social emotional development supports this component of the STAR FoR (Casenhiser et al., 2013; Liao et al., 2014; Pajareya & Nopmaneejumruslers, 2011; Reis et al., 2018; Solomon et al., 2014). Recent systematic reviews reinforce the strength of this evidence by showing the benefits of parental participation not only for children on the autism spectrum but also for children with idiopathic sensory processing challenges (Boshoff et al., 2020; Miller-Kuhaneck & Watling, 2018). The literature further suggests that significant gains are obtained when parent directed interventions are provided in conjunction with a therapist led intervention (Wilkes-Gillan et al., 2014).

The Regulation Component

The evidence for addressing the regulation component of the STAR FoR is supported by more than 50 studies, identified in a comprehensive literature review (Rosanbalm & Murray, 2017) indicating that parental warmth, responsiveness, and sensitivity, support the development of self-regulation. Physiological evidence suggests that arousal level changes across treatment and is modified by the sensory and relationship characteristics of the activities (Hedman et al., 2020). Including a continuous measure of arousal regulation will allow more specific identification of regulation/co-regulation procedures that are embedded within the STAR FoR. Additionally, current research suggests synchrony in electrodermal activity may be an important feature of attunement and social engagement. We suggest that behavioral and physiological synchrony is achieved when the therapist-child or parent-child dyads are fully immersed/engaged in attuned, playful interactions (Chaspari et al., 2014). Thus, it is likely this co-variation of physiological shifts supports regulation, engagement, and social interaction within the context of the STAR FoR therapy.

Putting it all together: STAR Frame of Reference

The evidence supporting the STAR FoR is emerging. The unique combination of research described earlier provides a foundation of support for its effectiveness. Additionally, research has been conducted specific to the application of the STAR FoR. A retrospective chart review of 179 children showed gains in adaptive behavior, emotional function, and sensory processing as reported by parents as well as motor improvements on standardized scales (Schoen et al., 2018). Gains in adaptive behaviors were reflected in functional communication, self-direction, self-care, home living, health and safety, leisure, and social skills. There was a reduction in problem behaviors related to externalizing, internalizing which included hyperactivity, aggression, anxiety depression, withdrawal, and inattention. Motor performance gains were reflected in fine motor, gross motor, and visual motor domains. Also noted was a decrease in sensory symptoms with less atypical sensory related behaviors reflective of over responsivity, under responsivity or craving. A nonconcurrent, multiple baseline, repeated measures research study of four boys showed gains in play level as well as an association between parent participation and associated changes (Schoen et al., 2019b). Another multiple baseline study of three toddlers showed a significant decrease in vestibular over-responsivity as reflected by decreased protests during diapering at home as well as an increase in time spent playing on a piece of suspended therapy equipment (Carder et al., 2020).

Research related to application of the STAR FoR to group interventions is supported by two studies, one using trampoline exercise and one using bike training. Both studies utilized a movement-based focus as the shared occupation of the participants. Results indicated improvement not only in motor performance/motor abilities, but additionally gains were reported in psychosocial and social emotional functioning (Schoen et al., 2020a, 2020b). Trampoline group participants showed improvement in social competency and social participation, while individuals in the bike group showed similar gains as well as improvements in self-confidence and self-esteem. Participation in daily routines and participation in community and extracurricular activities also improved.

Future Directions

The evidence base for this FoR is still emerging. Studies are in progress that examine the impact of the STAR FoR on expanded populations e.g., application with adolescents and adults, and related to different participation outcomes, e.g., outcomes related to school readiness and quality of life measures. Future studies should examine the impact of the frequency, duration, and intensity of "intensive" programs, as well as their lasting effects in order to better understand the benefits of this dosage. Inclusion of examiner administered tools and physiological measures would provide more objective measures of social interaction, engagement in activities and participation in childhood occupations. Importantly, measures of caregiver satisfaction and family empowerment should be included to substantiate the relative value of including parent collaboration, parent training and parent coaching.

References

Ayres, A. J. (1972). The art of therapy. In *Sensory integration and learning disorders* (pp. 256–265). Western Psychological Services.

Ayres, A. J., & Robbins, J. (2005). *Sensory integration and the child: Understanding hidden sensory challenges* (25th Anniversary ed.). Western Psychological Services.

Bialer, D. S., & Miller, L. J. (2011). *No longer A SECRET: Unique common sense strategies for children with sensory or motor challenges.* Sensory World.

Boshoff, K., Bowen, H., Paton, H., Cameron-Smith, S., Graetz, S., Young, A., & Lane, K. (2020). Child development outcomes of DIR/floor time TM-based programs: A systematic review. *Canadian Journal of Occupational Therapy, 87*(2), 153–164. https://doi.org/10.1177/0008417419899224

Burman, J. T., Green, C. D., & Shanker, S. G. (2015). On the meanings of self-regulation: Digital humanities in service of conceptual clarity. *Child Development, 86*(5), n/a-n/a. https://doi.org/10.1111/cdev.12395

Carder, D., Boucher, H., & Schoen, S. (2020). A preliminary study of treatment effectiveness for toddlers with vestibular over responsivity. *Manuscript Submitted for Publication.*

Casenhiser, D. M., Shanker, S. G., & Stieben, J. (2013). Learning through interaction in children with autism: Preliminary data from a social-communication-based intervention. *Autism: The International Journal of Research and Practice, 17*(2), 220–241. https://doi.org/10.1177/1362361311422052

Cermak, S. (2001, January). The effects of deprivation on processing, play, and praxis. *Understanding the Nature of Sensory Integration with Diverse Populations,* 385–408. www.researchgate.net/publication/230788536_The_Effects_of_Deprivation_on_Processing_Play_and_Praxis

Chaspari, T., Goodwin, M., Wilder-Smith, O., Gulsrud, A., Mucchetti, C. A., Kasari, C., & Narayanan, S. (2014). *A non-homogeneous poison process model of skin conductance responses integrated with observed regulatory behaviors for autism intervention.* 2014 IEEE International Conference on Acoustics, Speech and Signal Processing (ICASSP), pp. 1611–1615. https://doi.org/10.1109/ICASSP.2014.6853870

DeSantis, A., Coster, W., Bigsby, R., & Lester, B. (2004). Colic and fussing in infancy, and sensory processing at 3 to 8 years of age. *Infant Mental Health Journal, 25*(6), 522–539. https://doi.org/10.1002/imhj.20025

Ginsburg, K. R. (2007). The importance of play in promoting healthy child development and maintaining strong parent-child bonds. *PEDIATRICS, 119*(1), 182–191. https://doi.org/10.1542/peds.2006-2697

Greenspan, S. I., DeGangi, G., & Wieder, S. (2001). *The functional emotional assessment scale for infancy and early childhood: Clinical and research applications.* Interdisciplinary Council on Developmental and Learning Disorders.

Greenspan, S. I., & Wieder, S. (1998). *The child with special needs: Encouraging intellectual and emotional growth.* Perseus Books.

Greenspan, S. I., & Wieder, S. (2006a). *Engaging autism: Using the floor time approach help children, relate, communicate, and think.* De Capo Press/Lifelong Books.

Greenspan, S. I., & Wieder, S. (2006b). *Infant and early childhood mental health.* American Psychiatric Association.

Hedman, E., Schoen, S. A., Miller, L. J., & Picard, R. (2020, October). Wireless measurement of sympathetic arousal during in vivo occupational therapy sessions. *Frontiers in Integrative Neuroscience, 14,* 1–12. https://doi.org/10.3389/fnint.2020.539875

Kiresuk, T. J., Smith, A., & Cardillo, J. E. (2014). *Goal attainment scaling: Applications, theory, and measurement.* Psychology Press.

Lane, S. J., Bundy, A. C., & Gorman, M. (2019). Composing a theory: An historical perspective. In A. C. Bundy, S. J. Lane, & E. A. Murray (Eds.), *Sensory integration theory and practice* (3rd ed., pp. 40–54). F.A. Davis.

Liao, S. T., Hwang, Y. S., Chen, Y. J., Lee, P., Chen, S. J., & Lin, L. Y. (2014). Home-based DIR/Floortime™ intervention program for preschool children with autism spectrum disorders: Preliminary findings. *Physical and Occupational Therapy in Pediatrics, 34*(4), 356–367. https://doi.org/10.3109/01942638.2014.918074

Miller-Kuhaneck, H., & Watling, R. (2018). Parental or teacher education and coaching to support function and participation of children and youth with sensory processing and sensory integration challenges: A systematic review. *American Journal of Occupational Therapy, 72*(1). https://doi.org/10.5014/ajot.2018.029017

Miller, L. J., Fuller, D. A., & Roetenberg, J. (2014). *Sensational kids revised edition: Hope and help for children with sensory processing disorder (SPD).* Penguin.

Miller, L. J., Schoen, S. A., & Spielmann, V. (2019a). A frame of reference for sensory processing difficulties: Sensory therapies and research (STAR). In P. Kramer, J. Hinojosa, & T.-H. Howe (Eds.), *Frames of reference for pediatric occupational therapy* (4th ed., pp. 159–204). Wolters Kluwer.

Miller, L. J., Schoen, S. A., Whiting, C. C., & Ochsenbein, M. (2019b). *School-based intensive for occupational therapy practitioners [Webinar].* www.spdstar.org/basic/school-based-intensive-for-occupational-therapy-practitioners

Mueller, I., & Tronick, E. (2020). Sensory processing and meaning making in autism spectrum disorder. In *Autism 360°.* Elsevier Inc. https://doi.org/10.1016/b978-0-12-818466-0.00014-9

Pajareya, K., & Nopmaneejumruslers, K. (2011). A pilot randomized controlled trial of DIR/Floortime™ parent training intervention for pre-school children with autistic spectrum disorders. *Autism, 15*(5), 563–577. https://doi.org/10.1177/1362361310386502

Parham, L. D., Cohn, E. S., Spitzer, S. L., Koomar, J. A., Miller, L. J., Burke, J. P., Brett-Green, B., Mailloux, Z., May-Benson, T. A., Roley, S. S., Schaaf, R. C., Schoen, S. A., & Summers, C. A. (2007). Fidelity in sensory integration intervention fidelity in sensory integration intervention research. *Department of Occupational Therapy Faculty Papers, 25*(2), 216–227. https://doi.org/10.5014/ajot.61.2.216

Reis, H. I. S., Pereira, A. P. S., & Almeida, L. S. (2018). Intervention effects on communication skills and sensory regulation on children with ASD. *Journal of Occupational Therapy, Schools, and Early Intervention, 11*(3), 346–359. https://doi.org/10.1080/19411243.2018.1455552

Rosanbalm, K. D., & Murray, D. W. (2017). *Promoting self-regulation in early childhood: A practice brief* (OPRE Brief# 2017–79). Office of Planning, Research, and Evaluation, Administration for Children and Families, US. Department of Health and Human Services.

Schaaf, R. C., Dumont, R. L., Arbesman, M., & May-Benson, T. A. (2018). Efficacy of occupational therapy using Ayres Sensory Integration®: A systematic review. *American Journal of Occupational Therapy, 72*(1). https://doi.org/10.5014/ajot.2018.028431

Schoen, S. A., Ferrari, V., & Valdez, A. (2020a). It's not just about bicycle riding: Sensory motor, social and emotional benefits for children with developmental disabilities. *Unpublished manuscript.*

Schoen, S. A., Lane, S. J., Mailloux, Z., May-Benson, T., Parham, L. D., Smith Roley, S., & Schaaf, R. C. (2019a). A systematic review of Ayres sensory integration intervention for children with autism. *Autism Research, 12*(1), 6–19. https://doi.org/10.1002/aur.2046

Schoen, S. A., Miller, L. J., Camarata, S., & Valdez, A. (2019b). Use of the STAR PROCESS for children with sensory processing challenges. *The Open Journal of Occupational Therapy*, 7(4), 1–17. https://doi.org/10.15453/2168-6408.1596

Schoen, S. A., Miller, L. J., & Flanagan, J. (2018). A retrospective pre-post treatment study of occupational therapy intervention for children with sensory processing challenges. *The Open Journal of Occupational Therapy*, 6(1). https://doi.org/10.15453/2168-6408.1367

Schoen, S. A., Valdez, A., Ferrari, V., & Spielmann, V. (2020b). A trampoline exercise group: Feasibility, implementation, and outcomes. *American Journal of Occupational Therapy*, 74(4_Supplement_1), 7411520478p1. https://doi.org/10.5014/ajot.2020.74s1-po4113

Shanker, S. G. (2010). Self-regulation: Calm, alert and learning. *Education Canada*, 50(3), 4–7. https://doi.org/Volume 53 Issue 1

Solomon, R., Van Egeren, L. A., Mahoney, G., Quon Huber, M. S., & Zimmerman, P. (2014). PLAY project home consultation intervention program for young children with autism spectrum disorders. *Journal of Developmental & Behavioral Pediatrics*, 35(8), 475–485. https://doi.org/10.1097/DBP.0000000000000096

Spitzer, S. L., & Smith Roley, S. (2001). Sensory integration revisited. In S. Smith Roley, E. I. Blanche, & R. C. Schaaf (Eds.), *Understanding the nature of sensory integration with diverse populations* (pp. 3–27). Pro-ed.

Steinbrenner, J. R., Hume, K., Odom, S. L., Morin, K. L., Nowell, S. W., Tomaszewski, B., Szendrey, S., McIntyre, N. S., Yücesoy-Özkan, S., & Savage, M. N. (2020). *Evidence-based practices for children, youth, and young adults with autism.* The University of North Carolina at Chapel Hill, Frank Porter Graham Child Development Institute, National Clearinghouse on Autism Evidence and Practice Review Team.

Vygotsky, L. S. (1978). Mind in society: The development of higher psychological processes. In *Memory: Vol. Mind in So.* https://doi.org/(Original manuscripts [ca. 1930–1934])

Wallace, K. S., & Rogers, S. J. (2010). Intervening in infancy: Implications for autism spectrum disorders. *Journal of Child Psychology and Psychiatry*, 51(12), 1300–1320. https://doi.org/10.1111/j.1469-7610.2010.02308.x

Whitcomb, D. A., Carrasco, R. C., Neuman, A., & Kloos, H. (2015). Correlational research to examine the relation between attachment and sensory modulation in young children. *American Journal of Occupational Therapy*, 69(4). https://doi.org/10.5014/ajot.2015.015503

Whiting, C. C. (2018). Trauma and the role of the school-based occupational therapist. *Journal of Occupational Therapy, Schools, & Early Intervention*, 11(3), 291–301. https://doi.org/10.1080/19411243.2018.1438327

Wieder, S. (2017). The power of symbolic play in emotional development through the DIR lens. *Topics in Language Disorders*, 37(3), 259–281. https://doi.org/10.1097/TLD.0000000000000126

Wilkes-Gillan, S., Bundy, A., Cordier, R., & Lincoln, M. (2014). Evaluation of a pilot parent-delivered play-based intervention for children with attention deficit hyperactivity disorder. *American Journal of Occupational Therapy*, 68(6), 700–709. https://doi.org/10.5014/ajot.2014.012450

Yogman, M., Garner, A., Golinkoff, R. M., Hirsh-Pasek, K., & Hutchinson, J. (2018). The power of play: A pediatric role in enhancing development in young children. *Pediatrics*, 142(3), e20182058. https://doi.org/10.1542/peds.2018-2058

15 Community Programs

Program 1: Steppin' Up Transition Group Program for High School Students With Developmental Disabilities in High-Risk Areas

Bonnie Nakasuji

Type of program	Group Transition Program to prepare high school students for "life-after-high-school"
Population served	High school students with developmental disabilities in high-risk areas
Context	School-based
Frequency	One 1 hour, once per week
Program goals/objectives	To help high school students with intellectual disabilities develop the skills necessary to engage successfully in life skills as an adult.
Blended approaches	Group activities that encourage self-determination and mindfulness including sensory awareness, and which incorporate motor skill development, sensory strategies, appropriate social interactions, pre-vocational preparation and for some, leadership skills

Adolescence is naturally a challenging developmental period in life. Having a disability and/or growing up in an environment with limited available resources can exponentially reduce adult outcomes including independent living and employment (Blaskowitz et al., 2020; Human Services Research, 2012; Theobald et al., 2018).

Sensory processing difficulties (Crasta et al., 2020; Horder et al., 2014; Kinnealey et al., 2015) and decreased physical fitness (Hilton et al.,

DOI: 10.4324/9781003050810-18

2020; Sarris, 2018) are common, with physical fitness linked to executive functioning as well (Protic & Valkova, 2018; Savina et al., 2016). Both can result in reduced quality-of-life outcomes. Life skills related to self-determination (Ankeny & Lehmann, 2010), and social participation and vocation (Chiang et al., 2017; Griswold & Lange, 2015; Mazzotti et al., 2016; Theobald et al., 2018) are also commonly compromised for "at risk" individuals, potentially impacting ability to be integrated in educational and community contexts sufficiently.

The "Steppin' Up" group transition program was created to provide opportunities for "at-risk" adolescents to work on skills necessary for "life-after-high-school." These included providing them with more opportunities to formulate and express their own opinions, make relevant occupational choices, understand and develop healthier habits, and learn skills to live independently and productively.

Description of the Program

Intervention focus: This program design addressed four primary life skill areas, developed using a needs-assessment (interview with high-risk adults).

- Social skills:

  Communicating with others, including how communication can vary based on context (family, friends, work colleagues, boss/professors)
  Making and keeping friends
  Working with others, for example to solve problems.

- Mindfulness/Self-Determination

  Learning how to identify, interpret, respect, and communicate feelings (anxiety, sadness, etc.)
  Learning self-respect: forming and offering their opinions
  Understanding sensory processing and how it impacts one's emotion, behavior, motor skills and learning how to use sensory strategies for self-regulation
  Learning how to advocate for oneself (or for others)

- Physical fitness

  Engaging in physical activities
  Discovering which physical activities are enjoyable
  Promoting physical fitness habits

- Prevocational skills

  Developing motor skills (especially fine motor, bilateral motor coordination, tool use, etc.)

    Exploring job readiness (ability to focus, understanding and follow-
        ing directions, organization of work) through work experience
    Developing work habits (getting to work on time, being properly
        dressed, etc.)

The Steppin' Up program operates at high schools in lower socioeconomic and high-risk communities in Los Angeles County. Participating
students are part of the special education system, however, this program is
considered to be part of "curriculum enrichment" and is not driven by an
Individualized Educational Plan (IEP). Parents provide written consent
allowing their children to participate. The group meets once per week for
1 hour. Special education administrators select specific students or entire
self-contained classrooms to participate in the program. The students'
general level of intellectual abilities determine emphasis of the program
for each group. For example, the focus for students with moderate intellectual disabilities is in activities of daily living and instrumental activities
of daily living; and for higher functioning students is on preparing to
attend college, live independently and develop leadership skills. One regular topic of discussion for all groups is on sensory processing strategies to
help the students gain awareness of their comfort level, and learn to use
sensory strategies to self-regulate. Occupational therapists (OTs) also provide education to school personnel regarding the purpose of the activities
used in group for example activity analysis and the use of sensory processing and regulation strategies. The program has been implemented at two
to four high schools every semester since the summer 2014.

    The OT designed and supervised students in actual job experiences to
integrate skills learned in the Steppin' Up group program. High school
students are given an opportunity to identify career choices for the
future. Responses include "being a policeman," "opening up my own restaurant," "teaching Spanish" and "running a business." The OT guides
students to explore their choices, even if they are unrealistic, recruiting
school district employees who allow one or two students to work with
them for one period per week, accompanied by an OT as a "job-coach."
For example, one student who identified being a policeman as a career
choice assisted a campus security-guard to unlock classrooms in the
morning and check hall pass on fellow students walking around campus.
Other students interested in running their own businesses worked with
front office staff stamping envelopes, and sorting and distributing mail
into teachers' boxes. These work experiences furthered their training
in professional behaviors and work ethics. The students also uncovered
specific job skills that were lacking such as a student who could alphabetize the first letter in a name/word, but did not know how to alphabetize
the second letter in that name/word.

    Occupational therapy providers: Licensed occupational therapists
with experience in the use of sensory integration strategies, adolescent
mental health, school-based practice, and OT trainees.

Funding: By utilizing OT trainees, the cost to run the program is decreased.

Documentation: Completed by all staff and includes the following:

- Identifying information: name of student, date of session, session activity/activities with brief description of activity purpose.
- Brief description of the student's significant behavior during activity session (concerns or strengths)
- Hypotheses related to observed behavior(s)
- Description of strategies implemented during the session to promote success, and just-right-challenge
- Strategies for future use (directed to the student, school personnel and/or by OT professionals during subsequent sessions)

Finalized versions of the consultations are made available to the school district occupational therapist to be shared with school staff. Consultations include a summary form completed at the end of each semester for each student identifying significant changes, including improvements made in behaviors and performance. Summary reports annually presented to the district school board successfully justified continued funding.

Standardized measures used: Sensory Profile (Adolescent form), Children's Assessment of Participation and Enjoyment/Preferences of Activities in Children (CAPE/PAC) and/or an occupation-readiness scale (Double OT (DOT) currently being standardized (Haworth & Cyre, 2017; King et al., 2004). These assessments contribute to the student's self-awareness regarding their sensory processing profiles, interests, community resources, strengths, and areas to work on in the future; these are not designed to provide objective outcome measures resulting from participation in the Steppin' Up program.

Results: A retrospective review of 162 notes from six participating students (three male, three female, ages 13 to 20 years) from one high school was conducted. Results identified the students' primary challenges to be with social behaviors, communication skills with peers, adherence to group rules, sustained attention, sequencing steps in an activity, and motor skills. Documented improvements included attention-to-task, group participation, social behaviors, abilities to serve as a leader, participation in group discussion, adherence to group rules, motor skills and hand strength. Although this study identified several limitations, the results are encouraging and provide key points for making improvements in future programming (Merz et al., 2020).

References

Ankeny, E. M., & Lehmann, J. P. (2010). Journey toward self-determination: Voices of students with disabilities who participated in a secondary transition program on a community college campus. *Remedial and Special Education,* 20(10), 1–11. https://doi.org/10.1177/0741932510362215

Blaskowitz, M. G., Famularo, E., Lonergan, M., McGrady, E., Layer, L., Randall, L., & Zelenko, M. (2020). Developing inclusive higher-education (IHE) programs for youth with intellectual and developmental disabilities at the intersection of research and practice. *American Journal of Occupational Therapy,* 74(4). https://doi.org/10.5014/ajot.2020.74s1-po2209 volume 74 issue 4_Supplement_1 on page7411500014p1

Chiang, H., Ni, X., Lee, Y. (2017). Life skills training for middle and high school students with Autism. *Journal of Autism and Developmental Disorders,* 47(4), 1113–1121. https://doi.org/10.1007/s10803-017-3028-1

Crasta, J., Davies, P., & Gavin, W. (2020). Sensory processing mediates the relationship between attention and social responsiveness in young adults with and without autism spectrum disorder. *American Journal of Occupational Therapy,* 74(1), 164–183. https://doi.org/10.5014/ajot.2020.74s1-rp103a

Griswold, L. A., & Lange, J. (2015, July). Promoting social interaction skills to influence employment for older youth with autism spectrum disorders. *American Journal of Occupational Therapy,* 69, 6911515234p1. https://doi.org/10.5014/ajot.2015.69s1-po7083

Haworth, C., & Cyre, G. (2017, August 12). Supporting transitions to the workforce for at-risk youth: Development and using an occupation-based work skills assessment. *AOTA Occupational Therapy Practice,* 21–24.

Hilton, C., Ratcliff, K., Collins, D., & Jones, J. (2020). Physiological and cognitive effects of daily exercise on adolescents with autism spectrum disorder. *American Journal of Occupational Therapy 4* (Suppl. 1). https://doi.org/10.5014/ajot.2020.74s1-po2111 on page7411515358p1

Horder, J., Wilson, C. E., Mendez, A., & Murphy, D. G. (2014). Autistic traits and abnormal sensory experiences in adults. *Journal of Autism and Developmental Disorders,* 44, 1461–1469. https://doi.org/10.1007/s10803-013-2012-7

Human Services Research Institute. (2012). *Working in the community: The status and outcomes of people with intellectual and developmental disabilities in integrated employment,* National Core Indicators Data Brief. Human Services Research Institute.

King, G., Law, M., King, S., Hurley, P., Rosenbaum, P., Hanna, S., . . . Young, N. (2004). *Children's assessment of participation and enjoyment and preferences for activities of children.* Pearson.

Kinnealey, M., Riuli, V., & Smith, S. (2015). Case study of an adult with sensory modulation disorder. *AOTA Sensory Integration Special Interest Section Quarterly,* 38(1), 1–4.

Mazzotti, V. L., Rowe, D. A., Sinclair, J., Poppen, M., Woods, W. E., & Shearer, M. L. (2016). Predictors of post-school success: A systematic review of NLTS2 secondary analyses. *Career Development and Transition for Exceptional Individuals,* 39(4), 196–215. https://doi.org/10.1177/2165143415588047

Merz, J. A., Nakasuji, B., & Mollo, K. S. (2020). Occupational therapy group programming for adolescents with developmental and learning disabilities: A retrospective documentation review. *The open Journal of Occupational Therapy,* 8(3), 1–18. https://doi.org/10.15453/2168-6408.1675

Protic, M., & Valkova, H. (2018). The relationship between executive functions and physical activity in children with an intellectual disability. *Journal of Physical Education and Sport ® (JPES)*, *18*(2), 844–952.

Sarris, M. (2018, June 20). *The challenge of physical fitness for people with autism* (Rev.). Interactive Autism Network.

Savina, E., Garrity, K., Kenny, P., & Doerr, C. (2016). The benefits of movement for youth: A whole child approach. *Contemporary School Psychology, 20*(3), 282–292. https://doi.org/10.1007/s40688-016-0084-z

Theobald, R. J., Goldhaber, D. D., Gratz, T. M., & Holden, K. L. (2018). Career and technical education, inclusion, and postsecondary outcomes for students with learning disabilities. *Journal of Learning Disabilities.* https://doi.org/10.1177/0022219418775121

Program 2: Therapy West Integrated Specialized Play Program (TWISPP)

Sophia Magaña, Janet S. Gunter, and Erna Imperatore Blanche

Type of program	Early intervention (EI) evidenced based group program. Staffing ratio is three children to one adult staff minimum, with program capacity dependent on the facility size.
Population	Children ages 18 to 36 months. Designed to meet the needs of typically developing children, children at risk for developmental delays, and children identified with developmental disorders including genetic disorders, cerebral palsy, and autism spectrum disorder.
Context	Center-based, sensory enriched environment, caregiver training
Number of sessions	Three to five times per week, three hours a day
Program Goals/ Objectives	Developed to meet the child's individualized needs within a group setting.
Blended approaches	Coaching, Sensory Integration Theory and Treatment (SI), Biomechanical, Developmental, Cognitive, Behavioral, Oral Motor and Feeding, Neurodevelopmental Treatment (NDT), Motor Learning Theory, Activities of Daily Living training, Developmental Individualized-differences and Relationship Based (DIR)

Program Rationale

Early intervention (EI) programs for children under 3 years are delivered in many different ways. Some are individualized, others are in groups, some programs are delivered in the homes and others are delivered in community settings. Effective programs include critical and key components of active parent involvement and training, opportunities for learning and development through a play-based environment, and direct involvement of an interdisciplinary approach (Kingsley & Mailloux, 2013; Sullivan et al., 2014; Wallace & Rogers, 2010). In general, EI programs that have shown to be effective tend to include a large amount of parent involvement (Dawson et al., 2010; Prizant et al., 2003). Individuals with Disabilities Education Act, Part C (IDEA) also proposes recommendations for funding and guides the delivery of most EI programs in the United States; developmental skill based services focus on enhancing specific skills such as motor or cognitive development; and relationship based approaches focus on the importance of the parent-child interaction in the therapeutic process (Bailey et al., 2012; Bruder, 2010).

Program Description

TWISPP (Therapy West, Inc. 2020, 2010) is a manualized, evidence based, preventative enrichment and intervention program provided in a playful, sensory enriched environment that specifically incorporates principles of sensory integration (SI) theory (Ayres, 2005; Barton & Lissman, 2015; Blanche et al., 2016; Case-Smith, 2013; Frolek Clark & Schlabach, 2013) in conjunction with other intervention approaches identified on Table 15.2. The core elements include the following: sensory rich environment; multi-modal delivery; context of play and child directed; just right challenge/individualized group; context of social interactions; interdisciplinary team and blended approaches (see Table 15.1).

TWISPP was created with a strong foundation of therapeutic collaboration to ensure children's needs are being supported and met. Occupational therapists (OT), physical therapists (PT), and speech-language pathologists (SLP) created center times and activities based on goals related to typical development. The curriculum is focused on communication, social, cognitive, motor, and adaptive behaviors, and activities of daily living (ADLs) skill development. During program delivery, therapists collaborate with caregivers to create individualized goals for children who are identified with developmental needs. Goals for each child may include sensorimotor development, play, language and communication, socialization, ADLs, and caregiver goals. A variety of frames of reference and intervention approaches are used to support and guide intervention for the individual needs of each child and the needs of the group as well as to continually support overall development in activity centers (see Table 15.2). Table 15.2 presents the program centers, goals, and commonly used approaches specific to each center. The approaches are often delivered in a blended format in order to maximize client outcomes.

Table 15.1 TWISPP Core Elements

Sensory rich environment	Developed based on the theory of SI to support the development of motor, language, emotional regulation, and social skills. Sensory rich play activities and environment are presented within the routine to support sensory organization and nourishment. Sensory strategies are also embedded.
Multi-modal delivery	Caregiver training on self-identified topics of interest. Caregivers actively participate in the program, home visits, community fieldtrips, caregiver conferences and consultations. Inclusion of typically developing peers provides natural social environment and modelling.
Context of play and child directed	Developed based on the concept that play is one of the main occupations of a child. Play is utilized to facilitate self-awareness, autonomy, exploration, mastery of motor, language and communication, social interaction, socio-emotional, self-help, and cognitive skills and competence in natural environments. Capitalizes on the child's intrinsic motivation to master the environment.
Just right challenge /Individualized group	Developed to meet the individual child's needs within a group setting. Therapists collaborate and prepare activities to challenge the child's development. Children are supported to have purposeful and meaningful interactions with others and their environment.
Context of social interactions	Opportunities for social interactions are supported throughout routines such as taking turns, greeting peers, sharing materials, etc.
Use of outcome measures	Bayley-III administered upon entering the program and at approximately 4-month intervals throughout attendance or until exit at age 3 years. Currently Bayley-IV being used.
Interdisciplinary team and blended approaches	Specialists in the fields of OT, SLP, PT, and mental health support children through a variety of approaches specific to their scope of practices as well as in collaboration with one another and the family for an interdisciplinary and blended approach to best meet the needs of the children.

TWISPP has also been delivered in a telehealth format with groups of 3 to 4 children with one therapist. Children are seen in one and a half hour increments with a caregiver supporting them to participate in the program activities. Caregivers are sent a list of materials and activities the week prior to sessions to allow adequate time for preparation. Therapist guides the children and caregivers through shortened centers.

Table 15.2 TWISPP Activity Center Goals and Approaches Utilized

Center Time	Overall Goals	Approaches									
		ADL Training	Behavioral	Biomechanical	Cognitive	Developmental	DIR	Motor Learning	NDT	Oral Motor and Feeding	SI
Exploratory Play	Attention and purposeful play based on theme and concepts of month										
	Executive functioning skills										
	Organize arousal level and self-regulation	X		X	X	X	X	X			X
	Social interactions and turn taking										
	Functional language										
Circle Time (Open and Closing)	Functional language										
	Executive functioning skills		X	X	X	X	X		X		X
	Independent sitting										
	Imitation and motor planning										
	Identification of self and peers										
	Social interactions										
	Sensory play										
	Regulation of arousal level as needed										
	Safety awareness in play										
	Executive functioning skills										
	Social interactions										

Activity	Skill					
Toileting and Handwashing	ADLs					
	Executive functioning skills	X			X	
	Social interactions for turn taking					
	Functional language					
Snack	ADLs					
	Executive functioning skills	X			X	
	Social interactions		X			X
	Functional language		X			X X
	Oral motor/feeding skills					
Movement and Music Time/ Sensory Organization	Functional language		X			
	Sensory organization					
	Imitation and motor planning skills					
	Executive functioning skills	X	X		X	X
Creative Expression	Creative art					
	Functional language	X	X	X	X	X
	Social interactions			X		
	Sensory play					
	Fine and visual motor performance					
	Executive functioning skills					
	Imitation and sequencing					
	Independent sitting					

Centers are shortened to accommodate and support the children's ability to engage through virtual platforms. This format has been used when children have not been able to access in-person services due to Covid-19 pandemic as well as caregiver preference.

Measured Results/Outcomes

Children who attend this program are administered the Bayley Scales of Infant and Toddler Development, Third Edition (Bayley-III, 2006) upon entering the program and at approximately 4-month intervals or until they exit. A retrospective study conducted by Blanche et al. (2016) on the effectiveness of the TWISPP program, reported results which included statistically significant improvements in the areas of fine motor, gross motor, receptive language, expressive language and cognition of children who attended the program. Children identified as having sensory processing difficulties (as identified by the Sensory Profile, Dunn, 2002) were found to have made significant improvements in more developmental areas than children without sensory processing difficulties. Outcomes were measured based on data analysis from the Bayley-III administered to 71 children who participated in this group program. Currently the Bayley-IV is being used. Caregiver goals are documented at entry and approximately 6-month intervals until exiting the program. Parenting Stress Index (Abidin, 2012) is completed at entry and exit. Blanche (2019), in an additional retrospective study to analyze the effects of dosage of intervention (defined as number of intervention sessions within a set time frame), identified that children in TWISPP maintained gains over time per results of the Bayley-III and that progress and rate of progress were found to vary based on dosage of the intervention. For example, although children made significant changes in all five areas between the first and second measurement, they only made significant changes in language skills and gross motor areas between the second and third time measurement (Blanche, 2019).

References

Abidin, R. R. (2012). *Parenting stress index, fourth edition: Professional manual.* Psychological Assessment Resources, Inc. https://doi.org/10.1037/t02445-000

Ayres, A. J. (2005). *Sensory integration and the child* (25th Anniversary ed.). Western Psychological Service.

Bailey, D. B., Raspa, M., & Fox, L. C. (2012). What is the future of family outcomes and family centered services, *Topics in Special Early Childhood Special Education, 31*, 216–223. https://doi.org/10.1177/0271121411427077

Barton, E. E., & Lissman, D. C. (2015). Group parent training combined with follow-up coaching for parents of children with developmental delays. *Infants & Young Children, 29*(3), 220–236. https://doi.org/10.1097/iyc.0000000000000036

Bayley, N. (2006). *Bayley scales of infant and toddler development,* third edition. San Antonio: Harcourt Assessment.

Blanche, E. I. (2019, June 21). *How often should I treat? Dosage in early intervention* [Conference presentation]. European Congress of Sensory Integration 2019, Thessaloniki, Greece.

Blanche, E. I., Chang, M. C., Gutiérrez, J., & Gunter, J. (2016). Effectiveness of a sensory-enriched early intervention group program for children with developmental disabilities. *The American Journal of Occupational Therapy, 70*(5), 7005220010p1–7005220010p8. https://doi.org/10.5014/ajot.2016.018481

Bruder, M. B. (2010). Early childhood intervention: A promise to children and families for their future. *Exceptional Children, 76,* 339–355. https://doi.org/10.1177/001440291007600306

Case-Smith, J. (2013). Systematic review of interventions to promote socio-emotional development in young children with or at risk for disability. *The American Journal of Occupational Therapy, 67,* 395–404. https://doi.org/10.5014/ajot.2013.004713

Dawson, G., et al. (2010). Randomized, controlled trial of an intervention for toddlers with autism: The early start denver model. *Pediatrics, 125,* e17–e23. http://dx.doi.org/10.1542/peds.2009-0958

Dunn, W. (2002). *Infant/toddler sensory profile manual.* Psychological Corporation.

Frolek Clark, G. J., & Schlabach, T. L. (2013). Systematic review of occupational therapy interventions to improve cognitive development in children ages birth–5 Years. *The American Journal of Occupational Therapy, 67,* 425–430. https://doi.org/10.5014/ajot.2013.006163

Kingsley, K., & Mailloux, Z. (2013). Evidence for the effectiveness of different service delivery models in early intervention services. *The American Journal of Occupational Therapy, 67,* 431–436. http://dx.doi.org/10.5014/ajot.2013.006171

Prizant, B. M., Wetherby, A. M., Rubin, E., & Laurent, A. (2003). The SCERTS model: A transactional, family centered approach to enhancing communication and socioemotional abilities of children with autism spectrum disorder. *Infants and Young Children, 16,* 296–316. https://doi.org/10.1097/00001163-200310000-00004

Sullivan, K., Stone, W. L., & Dawson, G. (2014). Potential neural mechanisms underlying the effectiveness of early intervention for children with autism spectrum disorder. *Research in Developmental Disabilities, 35*(11), 2921–2932. https://doi.org/10.1016/j.ridd.2014.07.027

Therapy West, Inc. (2020, 2010). *Revised therapy west infant specialized play program manual.* Unpublished manuscript.

Wallace, K. S., & Rogers, S. J. (2010). Intervening in infancy: Implications for autism spectrum disorders. *Journal of Child Psychology and Psychiatry, 51*(12), 1300–1320. https://doi.org/10.1111/j.1469-7610.2010.02308.x

Program 3: The Moving to Make Friends © Program

Karrie L. Kingsley

Type of program	Activity-based, group social intervention
Population served	School-aged children with social interaction needs, for example, diagnoses and eligibilities of Attention Deficient Hyperactivity Disorder, Autism Spectrum Disorder, Sensory Processing Disorder, Developmental Coordination Disorder, and Specific Learning Disability
Context	School setting
Number of sessions per week	1 hour per week for 8–10 weeks
Number of sessions	Three to five times per week, three hours a day
Program goals/ objectives	To facilitate social interaction, promote friendships, and facilitate generalization of social performance within the natural setting
Type of interventions utilized	Group activities that encourage self-determination and social participation

The focus of school is the meaningful participation and engagement in classroom and social activities, with the goal of students progressing in their abilities in both realms. Social competence is the ability to utilize one's social skills across various contexts and social partners (Kauffman & Kinnealey, 2015). Several studies have found children with disabilities, independent of eligibility category or diagnosis, demonstrate lower participation in social activities and lower social competence with peers and adults than their typically developing peers (Eriksson et al., 2007; Kauffman & Kinnealey, 2015).

Social skills and competence will have a direct impact on a child's abilities to make friends, participate in play occupations, and access community-based leisure activities. Gresham (2015) found that social competence and resulting positive behaviors were enablers for academic achievement. A literature review by *What Works Clearinghouse* (2013) identifies research evidence on the positive impact of social skills training on cognition and social emotional development and behavior. Furthermore, Segrin and Flora (2000) report that individuals with poor social skills are vulnerable to increased depressive symptoms, loneliness, and social anxiety and that strong social skills act as a protective factor from depression during stressful life events. Therefore, social skills and competency are highly important for both academic and psychosocial outcomes. This program illustrates how principle of sensory integration theory can be combined with other theories and approaches within the context of a school setting in order to promote social participation.

The Moving to Make Friends © program (MTMF) is one example of an activity-based group social intervention, based on key occupational science and occupational therapy principles including creating a social context using occupations, tapping on intrinsic motivation, and applying principles of Sensory Integration theory. The MTMF program utilizes movement-based play activities facilitated by an occupational therapy practitioner (OTP). Depending on the setting, students are referred by teachers through a multi-tiered system of support. The actual implementation of the program is intended to be dynamic, student-centered, and integrated within the school setting through consistent feedback with teachers, parents, and other professionals to maximize carry-over. The goals of the MTMF program are to facilitate generalization of social participation within the natural settings and promote friendships.

Program Description and Key Concepts

The creation of a social context depends on the concepts of occupational intactness and context. Occupational intactness refers to the extent to which therapeutic use of occupation occurs in the natural context (Pierce, 2001). By allowing the participants to co-construct their social context during the sessions they are able to practice skills in more intact occupational conditions leading to greater likelihood of skill generalization across settings (Humphry, 2005; Lawlor, 2003).

This program uses concepts from occupational science and ideas about co-occupations. Humphry (2005) describes co-occupational engagement "where doing and experiencing meaning go beyond the individual and take place in an interpersonal space" (p. 40). Lawlor (2003) adds that children as what she terms as "socially occupied being" co-create their play with others in a variety of natural environments. These concepts led to the inclusion of a cooperative element in every session. This inherent cooperation, a key concept for the purposes of the MTMF program, promotes peer interactions versus child and adult interactions. The cooperative element creates a social context within which the participants can practice social interactions in an environment that represents their natural play settings.

Intrinsic motivation is evident when children engage in an activity for the value of participating in the activity (Rom á n-Oyola et al., 2018). MTMF's use of sensory-based and cooperative activities resembles the developmental play level of elementary school-age children. Play at this age includes daring physical play involving strength and skill, engagement in games with rules, and cooperative play (Parham & Fazio, 2008).

Research has examined the relationship between sensory processing disorders (SPD) and social participation. One group of authors suggested children with SPD experience adverse impact on their social competence due to a variety of factors, including self-regulation, and recommend that interventions must target access to social interaction with peers (Cosby et al., 2010). In another study with children diagnosed with autism and developmental delay, Watson et al. (2011) found children identified as hyporesponsive to sensory information and those who engaged in high levels of sensory seeking behaviors were found to have greater severity of social communication symptoms whereas children identified as hyperresponsive had no significant differences in their severity of social communication symptoms.

MTMF focuses on providing occupation-based treatment within the naturally occurring setting of schools. Students are grouped depending on age and identified areas of focus in dyads, triads, and foursomes. In order to successfully implement the MTMF Program, observations of the students should be conducted prior to and after the program. Occupational therapists can utilize interviews and design questionnaires to gain valuable information regarding the child's performance both in and outside of the classroom. This data will be valuable when establishing effectiveness of the MTMF implementation as well as assessing whether or not generalization of skills demonstrated during the MTMF sessions occurs.

Programmatic length depends on the group and each student's goals, but ranges from 8–10 weeks (one session per week). This allows for students to then demonstrate and generalize skill acquisition independently. The program can then be re-established for any student depending on any ongoing or new needs. Every MTMF session includes a sensory-motor based play activity, an inherently cooperative element, and a foil. A foil is when the therapist purposely creates a problem that needs to be solved. The role of the adult is to plan the sessions and supervise for child safety (see Table 15.3). If the session is well planned, and/or as social interaction abilities progress, the adult child interaction

Table 15.3 Activity Planning Template: Boxcar Racing

Brief description of sensory-motor activity:

Students must take turns pushing each other in a boxcar constructed from a cardboard box and a scooter board. They can set up different tracks to race on.

Describe foils built into the activity:

1. Oversized box for scooter board – leads to problem-solving when the box falls off the scooter.
2. Allowing students to change the track – provides opportunities for interaction and agreement.

Describe Inherent Cooperative Element:

To propel the boxcar, one of the members has to push, and the other cannot propel from within the box. The boxcar does not remain on the scooter if it is pushed without someone in it.

should decrease. The session creates a social context where children interact and adults only facilitate when a natural learning opportunity arises, using shaping and reinforcement techniques. Typically, the reinforcement comes from the successful problem solving and intrinsically motivated, cooperative play with a peer.

Case Example

Eli and Danny were both fourth grade students enrolled in general education classrooms with special education support. Danny qualified for special education services under the eligibility of emotional disturbance; Eli under specific learning disability. Both Danny and Eli had previously received and been exited from occupational therapy services. They were receiving counseling from the school psychologist. Eli was taking medication for Attention Deficit Hyperactivity Disorder (ADHD) throughout his participation in this program.

Danny and Eli both reported that their favorite activities involved a "racing" component, so activities were geared toward this to maximize engagement. Additionally, quantitative data supported that these activities yielded more interactions, and the activity that resulted in the most spontaneous interactions was one in which the activity required constant dialogue to successfully achieve the goal, as one child was wearing a blindfold and relied on his partner to assist the dyad with navigating a scooter-board through space.

The previous example highlights one specific activity as part of the curriculum for Danny and Eli. While activities can be adapted and modified for use with different students, it is important to stress that activities are tailored for each dyad or group. The first session within the curriculum focuses on establishing one's current state and ways to attain optimal self-regulation. As previously noted, each activity has a therapist-driven foil to create opportunities for problem-solving and social participation.

Conclusion

The MTMF program utilizes a blended approach to address social interaction in elementary school-age children. It is informed by concepts from occupational science, principles of Sensory Integration, play, and social learning theories. Elements from these theories drive the MTMF program at both the conceptual and session level. Cognitive-behavioral approaches to self-regulation facilitate optimal arousal states for play in the natural context, while the interaction of these other concepts facilitates children co-constructing the social and play contexts in order to interact with one another.

To explicate the impact of the guiding concepts we see that Eli and Danny preferred to race and compete during their sessions. Their self-reports of levels of enjoyment being higher during sessions with preferred elements reinforces the importance of intrinsic motivation from play theories, leading to better performance during sessions. Additionally, self-regulation is addressed with principles of sensory integration theory.

References

Cosby, J., Johnston, S. S., & Dunn, M. L. (2010). Sensory processing disorders and social participation. *American Journal of Occupational Therapy, 64*, 462–473.

Eriksson, L., Welander, J., & Granlund, M. (2007). Participation in everyday school activities for children with and without disabilities. *Journal of Developmental and Physical Disabilities, 19*(5), 485–502.

Gresham, F. (2015). Evidence-based social skills interventions for students at risk for EBD. *Remedial and Special Education, 36*(2), 100–104.

Humphry, R. (2005). Model of processes transforming occupations: Exploring societal and social influences. *Journal of Occupational Science, 12*(1), 36–44.

Kauffman, N. A., & Kinnealey, M. (2015). Comprehensive social skills taxonomy: Development and application. *American Journal of Occupational Therapy, 69*(2), 6902220030p1–6902220030p10.

Lawlor, M. (2003). The significance of being occupied: The social construction of childhood occupations. *American Journal of Occupational Therapy, 57*, 424–434.

Parham, L. D., & Fazio, L. S. (Eds.). (2008). *Play in occupational therapy for children*. Mosby.

Pierce, D. (2001). Occupation by design: Dimensions, therapeutic power, and creative process. *American Journal of Occupational Therapy, 55*(3), 249–259.

Román-Oyola, R., Figueroa-Feliciano, V., Torres-Martínez, Y., Torres-Vélez, J., Encarnación-Pizarro, K., Fragoso-Pagán, S., & Torres-Colón, L. (2018). Play, playfulness, and self-efficacy: Parental experiences with children on the autism spectrum. *Occupational Therapy International, 2018.*

Segrin, C., & Flora, J. (2000). Poor social skills are a vulnerability factor in the development of psychosocial problems. *Human Communication Research, 26*(3), 489–514.

Watson, L. R., Patten, E., Baranek, G. T., Poe, M., Boyd, B. A., Freuler, A., & Lorenzi, J. (2011). Differential associations between sensory response patterns and language, social, and communication measures in children with autism or other developmental disabilities. *Journal of Speech Language and Hearing Research, 54*(6), 1562–1576. doi:10.1044/1092-4388(2011/10-0029)

What Works Clearinghouse. (2013). *Procedures and standards handbook* (Version 3.0). http://ies.ed.gov/ncee/wwc/documentsum.aspx?sid=19

Program 4: The Kid Power Program: A Clinical Program to Enhance Spontaneous Bimanual Use and Achieve Functional Goals

M. Angelica Barraza and Takako Shiratori

Type of program	Interdisciplinary, home, and clinic-based program
Population served	Children with hemiplegia
Ages	3 to 15 years
Diagnoses or functional issues	Cerebral palsy and any other neurologic trauma resulting in hemiplegia and presenting with functional limitations in activities of daily living (ADL)
Context	Individual home program followed by individualized intensive in a group clinical program
Number of sessions/hours	60 to 100 hours of home programming followed by a three-week clinical program (three hours per day/five days per week
Program Objectives	Increase spontaneous bimanual use to meet functional goals
Blended Approaches	Forced Use, bimanual intensive therapy, parent education, and sensory integration (SI)

Program Rationale

Hemiplegia is the most common form of cerebral palsy, accounting for 30 percent of these children (Motta et al., 2010). Although many children with hemiplegia can utilize their affected hand in functional activities, they tend to favor their non-affected upper extremity (UE) and use a unimanual approach during bimanual tasks. This phenomenon is termed "developmental non-use" (Aarts et al., 2011). Even if the skill of the affected hand itself is relatively good, this does not necessarily translate to spontaneous bimanual use. This disparity between unimanual skill and functional bimanual use has been termed "developmental disregard" (Aarts et al., 2011). Therapeutic interventions for children with hemiplegia include intense delivery of repeated movement

practice to improve individual-specific goals and spontaneous bimanual use (i.e., Constraint-Induced Movement Therapy [CIMT], Hand
Arm Bimanual Intensive Training, and forced use). See Chapter 5 for
details on CIMT.

Program Description

The Kid Power Program is an evidence-based program that is a result of
11 years of multidisciplinary collaboration between outpatient occupational therapists (OTs), physical therapists (PTs), and researchers. Our
clinical program uses two phases, home-based forced-use followed by
clinical intensive bimanual therapy (IBT). Forced-use is a method utilized to increase the skill of the affected UE by constraining the unaf-
fected UE without the shaping and guided mass practice that is usually
delivered with CIMT models (Motta et al., 2010; Psychouli et al., 2010).
Then, IBT is delivered without a constraint, promoting bimanual hand
use with play and functional tasks in a structured, repetitive, adaptive
manner, in an engaging environment (Klepper et al., 2017). Sensory
integration theory is applied in both phases to help promote self-regulation and skill acquisition.

The validity of the Kid Power Program was established over 3 years of
data collection and program evaluation using the Assisting Hand Assessment (AHA) and the Canadian Occupational Performance Measure
(COPM). Data collected on five children showed that all participants
improved in bimanual hand function and individual goal areas from
both forced use and IBT camp phase and maintained gains 6 months
post-camp (Barraza et al., 2015). This pilot was crucial in establishing the
current program described herein.

Phase One: Forced-Use at Home

Clients ages 3 to 15 years old referred to the camp receive a one- to two-
hour OT/PT assessment to establish baseline functioning. The following
evaluation tools are used depending on the areas of need:

1. Select gross motor and fine motor elements of the Peabody Development Motor Scale, 2nd edition or the Bruininks-Oseretsky Test of
   Motor Proficiency – 2
2. Timed Up and Go
3. 30 Second Sit to Stand
4. COPM
5. Sensory Processing Measure (SPM)

During the initial evaluation, the appropriateness of camp and functional goals are discussed with families. There are no motor exclusion

criteria, but participants may be excluded secondary to the inability to follow one-step directions or significant self-regulation issues. If sensory processing issues are reported or suspected secondary to the participant's history or therapist observations, parents complete the SPM, and the child's sensory needs are accommodated during treatment planning.

After families select either a removable or non-removable constraint, this constraint is worn for 100 hours during this phase. Children with the removable thermoplastic constraint wear the constraint for a minimum of 3.5 hours a day for 4 weeks. Those with the non-removable constraint wear the constraint for 20 consecutive days, equating a day to a minimum of 5 hours per day of affected UE activity. Parents are educated on when the removable constraint should be worn, taking into account activity demands, child abilities, sensory profile, and emotional state of the child. Application of sensory strategies based on sensory integration (SI) theory to be used in the home setting is reviewed to help parents adjust activities and decrease frustration. Family support is available on a needs basis. Constraint wearing schedule may be modified to accommodate individual family and client needs. Concurrently, parents submit a request on topics for the parent education series that will occur during the IBT phase.

Forced use is intended to increase the capacity in the affected UE preparing it for mass bimanual practice in the subsequent IBT phase. The implementation of forced-use at home and not in the clinic allows the program to be more cost-effective while also achieving the intensity of practice reported in the literature. The evidence supports goal-directed home occupational therapy program is effective in promoting UE function (Novak et al., 2009; Sakzewski et al., 2014).

Phase Two: Camp Kid Power (IBT)

Evidence supports that one-handed training followed by bimanual training enhances UE capacity (Aarts et al., 2011; Barraza et al., 2015). Camp Kid Power uses bimanual training to build upon the unimanual skills acquired with forced use in phase one. Camp Kid Power is a three-week (15 days) three hours per day program delivering bimanual training in an intensive group therapy format that is informed by SI theory.

The camp uses foundational elements of SI to guide task selection and environmental modification to increase the client's intrinsic motivation and internal control (Bundy & Lane, 2020). Emphasis is placed on promoting friendship and peer support in a playful and motivating environment. Campers collaborate on activity choices as they are engaged in daily decisions of projects and themes (i.e., dance party, tie-dye, crazy hair day) to help keep camp novel and exciting (Parham et al., 2011). Throughout the camp, therapists facilitate improved hand function by paying close attention to individual needs and respond with grading of tasks, environmental modification, and/or sensory-motor based activities. Activities are modified to provide the "just right challenge" and ensure success when needed (Parham et al., 2011). Campers are also encouraged to motivate each other and share individual successes in the daily wrap-up sessions and/or posting them on a "win wall."

At the beginning of camp, all campers are videotaped performing their functional goals. The camp is staffed with one therapist for two children and one camp counselor for every child to help co-regulate campers and organize activities. The camp day is divided into various sections that address impairments and promote spontaneous bimanual use. Each day includes active lengthening, postural activation, bi-manual coordination (gross and fine), goal simulation, ADLs, i.e., dressing, meal preparation, and elements of SI to address self-regulation as needed. To continue to build on the child's internal drive and foster a therapeutic alliance between staff and client, the order of activities and time spent on activities is individually adjusted and often determined by the child with support from a therapist (Bundy & Lane, 2020; Parham et al., 2011).

Caregiver education is a significant component of Camp Kid Power and is intended to empower families and promote the carryover to the home environment. Family training occurs weekly on topics selected by the families (alignment, childhood nutrition, review of current research, and community resources) and is conducted by staff, guest lecturers, and when appropriate, led by a caregiver. Parents have reported positive benefits from family training, as one parent said, "It has been invaluable sharing thoughts and ideas with parents going through this. I know I am not alone but it's so nice to be reminded." Many of the campers are repeat participants, allowing older children and parents to share information and take a mentorship role with younger campers and their families. Repeat camper participation also allows the therapist to monitor long-term changes and progress.

During the last day, individual outcome measures are collected for assessment purposes. Children in the program make significant gains in goal areas, hand function, coordination, and fitness. Return campers are maintaining skills from the previous year(s), with exception of campers that have experienced new neurological insults or significant mental health issues.

Telehealth Feasibility

In the current health care environment, the telehealth feasibility of The Kid Power Program must be explored. Training parents to administer the testing has already been utilized in a home-based bimanual program (Ferre et al., 2016) and could be done in our program. Few adaptations would be needed in the first phase of the program as it is already delivered in the home setting. Current evidence supports the plausibility of transferring the IBT camp to a telehealth model. A systematic review of home-based programs for children with cerebral palsy (Beckers et al., 2017) found moderate to high parent compliance. Also, a home-based bi-manual program with a therapist supervising parents and child via webcam one hour a week for nine weeks produced meaningful bimanual functional change for the family (Ferre et al., 2016).

With the help of video conferencing platforms, Camp Kid Power could be adapted to fit a telehealth model by:

1. Educating caregivers to deliver Camp in a 3 hours program divided into synchronous group time and asynchronous time.
2. Using video telehealth technology during synchronous group time to deliver a virtual group supervised by therapists, promoting the benefits of positive peer interaction.
3. Implementing off-camera asynchronous time, supervised by a caregiver, as an opportunity to complete therapist-assigned activities and practice goals.
4. Having therapists available to answer questions, provide daily guidance and problem solve issues during asynchronous time.

Summary

The Kid Power Program is a culmination of knowledge from research and clinical foundations blending forced use, intensive bimanual training, and SI principles to improve UE bimanual function for children with hemiplegia. The program continues to evolve with annual evaluation and modification using feedback from therapists, clients, and their families, outcome results, updated research evidence, and adjusting to circumstances such as those experienced during the pandemic. In the future, we look forward to adapting this intensive model to other diagnoses and welcome collaboration with other clinics in adopting and implementing the Kid Power Program.

References

Aarts, P. B., Jongerius, P. H., Geerdink, Y. A., van Limbeek, J., & Geurts, A. C. (2011). Modified constraint induced movement therapy combined with bimanual training (mCIMT-BiT) in children with unilateral spastic cerebral palsy: How are improvements in arm-hand use established? *Research in Developmental Disabilities, 32*, 271–279. https://doi.org/10.1016/j.ridd.2010.10.008

Barraza, M. A., Jensen, J., & Shiratori, T. (2015, May). SuperKids: A clinical program to enhance bimanual skills for children with hemiplegia. *OT Practice, 11*(8), 11–16.

Beckers, L., Schnackers, M., Janssen-Potten, Y., Kleijnen, J., & Steenbergen, B. (2017). Feasibility and effect of home-based therapy programmes for children with cerebral palsy: A protocol for a systematic review. *BMJ Open, 7*(2), e013687. https://doi.org/10.1136/bmjopen-2016-013687

Bundy, A. C., & Lane, S. (2020). *Sensory integration: Theory and practice* (3rd ed., pp. 286–298). F. A. Davis.

Ferre, C., Brandão, M., Surana, B., Dew, A., Moreau, N., & Gordon, A. (2016). Caregiver directed home-based intensive bimanual training in young children with unilateral spastic cerebral palsy: A randomized trial. *Developmental Medicine & Child Neurology, 59*(5), 497–504. https://doi.org/10.1111/dmcn.13330

Klepper, S., Clayton Krasinski, D., Gilb, M., & Khalil, N. (2017). Comparing unimanual and bimanual training in upper extremity function in children with unilateral cerebral palsy. *Pediatric Physical Therapy, 29*(4), 288–306. https://doi.org/10.1097/pep.0000000000000438

Motta, F., Antonello, C. E., & Stignani, C. (2010). Forced-use, without therapy, in children with hemiplegia: Preliminary study of a new approach for the upper limb. *Journal of Pediatric Orthopaedics, 30,* 582–587. https://doi.org/10.1097/bpo.0b013e3181e88ee4

Novak, I., Cusick, A., & Lannin, N. (2009). Occupational therapy home programs for cerebral palsy: Double-blind, randomized, controlled trial. *Pediatrics, 124,* e606–e614. https://doi.org/10.1542/peds.2009-0288

Parham, L. D., Roley, S. S., May-Benson, T., Koomar, J., Brett-Green, B., Burke, J. P., & Schaaf, R. C. (2011). Development of a fidelity measure for research on ayres sensory integration. *American Journal of Occupational Therapy, 65,* 133–142. https://doi.org/10.5014/ajot.2011.000745

Psychouli, P., Burridge, J., & Kennedy, C. (2010). Forced use as a home-based intervention in children with congenital hemiplegic cerebral palsy: Choosing the appropriate constraint. *Disability & Rehabilitation: Assistive Technology, 5,* 25–33. https://doi.org/10.3109/17483100903121489

Sakzewski, L., Gordon, A. M., & Eliasson, A. C. (2014). The state of the evidence for intensive upper limb therapy approaches for children with unilateral cerebral palsy. *Journal of Child Neurology, 29,* 1077–1090. https://doi.org/10.1177/0883073814533150

Program 5: Blue Bird Day Program

Alexa Greif, Laura Mraz, Leah Dunleavy, Sarah Hirschman, and Erin Harvey

Type of Program	Interdisciplinary, early childhood program
Population served	Children with autism, sensory processing challenges, Down syndrome, cerebral palsy, developmental delays, and complex medical conditions
Context	Intensive program in a clinical setting
Number of sessions	Six hours daily, four to five days per week
Program goals	Implementation of intensive, inter-professional, coordinated programming that is family-centered and evidence-based to enhance participation outcomes
Types of interventions	Sensory Integration, Intentional Relationship Communicative Model (IRM), Model of Human Occupation, Developmental, Applied Behavioral Analysis

Participation in daily activities, considered the ultimate health and educational outcome, is an indicator of children's well-being and linked to developmental outcomes (WHO, 2010; Gorter et al., 2011). A focus on participation is central to occupational therapy (OT), defined as the "therapeutic use of everyday life occupations with persons, groups, or populations for the purpose of enhancing or enabling participation" (AOTA, 2020). Participation centered outcomes, as well as ongoing shifts in health care towards evidence-based practice and cost-effectiveness are opportunities for occupational therapists to demonstrate the unique value of OT while advancing its contribution to the realm of health care.

A systematic review on effectiveness of interventions aimed to improve participation outcomes for children with disabilities supports individually tailored programs. The, evidence suggests that interventions which use multiple approaches for improving participation are effective, highlighting the idea of increased participation being achieved via many pathways (Adair et al., 2015). By promoting client experiences directed towards positive health outcomes, along with blending multi-disciplinary interventions to enhance participation, the following program, Blue Bird Day (BBD), was developed.

BBD an intensive, interdisciplinary program demonstrates an approach focused on participation and the blending of different measures and interventions impacting outcomes at the body structure/function and activity – participation levels of the ICF-CY model. The program's name BBD highlights a shared vision of an optimal "blue bird day" or a clear blue-sky perfect day, the ultimate goal for all families enrolled in the program.

Program Description

BBD serves children ages 2 to 7 years old and their families, with a primary focus on children with autism, sensory processing challenges, Down syndrome, cerebral palsy, developmental delays, and complex medical conditions. BBD clients seek services due to participation restrictions and display performance deficits across meaningful areas of occupation and environments.

BBD provides daily occupational therapy, speech therapy, physical therapy, developmental therapy, applied behavioral analysis, medical nutrition therapy and social work services within clinic and home contexts. Clients receive daily intensive services tailored to the unique needs of clients utilizing a blend of approaches through BBD's small group Therapy Rotations © and individual therapies.

BBD's therapy spaces include a combination of sensorimotor gyms, sensory retreat rooms, small treatment rooms, classroom like spaces, and lunchrooms. All contexts are arranged to support the child's safe and active participation in meaningful sensory based therapeutic play activities that are of interest to the child.

BBD was developed with a focus on family-centered, evidence-based, sensory, and relationships-focused, programming resulting in enhanced participation outcomes for clients and families. BBD services occur in a peer-oriented environment, designed to promote the client's successful transition to an academic setting. Clients receive daily services simulating a preschool or kindergarten day. Each client is assigned to a "classroom" team of therapists and peers with a SW providing the role of "teacher" Classrooms are split into bird groups, based on developmental level, and move through discipline specific rotations with assigned peer group and receive individual therapy outside of rotations.

BBD is primarily informed by sensory integration treatment (SIT), the model of human occupation (MOHO) along with therapist's use of the intentional relationship model (IRM) to support the development of the therapeutic alliance between the child, the family, and the therapist. Applied behavioral analysis is incorporated as an adjunctive therapy used for skill building with children referred as part of their enrollment.

IRM, a theoretical model integrating interpersonal approaches, provides tools for effective therapeutic relationships, and demonstrates how to employ interpersonal strategies while using occupation as the central mechanism of change. According to IRM, the therapist is responsible for bringing an interpersonal skill base, therapeutic modes and capacity for interpersonal reasoning to the therapist-client interaction (Taylor, 2020). IRM defines six modes of relating to a client including empathizing, collaborating, instructing, advocating, problem solving and encouraging (Taylor, 2020). IRM is meant to complement other therapeutic models instead of being a stand-alone approach and elaborates upon therapeutic use of self, a core component of sensory integration treatment. All therapists involved with BBD programming are trained in using the IRM approach.

In IRM terms, therapeutic use of self may be viewed as the extent to which one possesses a knowledge base and interpersonal skills applied thoughtfully to common interpersonal events in practice (Taylor, 2020). It explains the relationship that naturally exists between client and therapist, consisting of four central elements: the client, interpersonal events occurring in therapy, the therapist and occupation (Taylor, 2020). Along with a focus on the power of relationships, effective communication and self-reflection, the treatment approaches used at BBD are informed by a child centered SI approach with all disciplines trained in SIT and oriented to the process and structural elements comprising sensory integration treatment (Bundy & Lane, 2020).

Objectives

The goal of BBD is for clients to develop foundational skills across developmental domains in order to participate in meaningful daily life activities, specifically supporting the transition to the least restrictive academic environment. Disciplines collaborate in teams to meet the unique needs of clientele through BBD's Therapeutic Rotations ©. For example, the physical therapy rotation focuses on gross motor skills, while the OT rotation targets sensory integration treatment, however, both aim to promote independence in daily life activities. BBD Therapy Rotations© seamlessly complement each other to address all developmental skills necessary for meaningful participation in everyday life. It also provides a clear framework for therapists and support staff to understand their role within the interdisciplinary team.

It is recognized in the literature that conceptual clarity is required to fully understand participation as an outcome. Therefore, BBD processes of evaluation, intervention and outcome measurement are modeled after the Family of Participation-Related Constructs (fPRC), an evidence-based, contemporary framework designed to model participation and its related concepts within pediatric practice (Imms et al., 2017). The fPRC notes participation is objectively measured by physical attendance and captured as frequency and/or diversity of activities, whereas subjective components refer to the experience of participation, such as volition (Imms et al., 2017). Finally, participation-related concepts include those that are person and environmentally focused, including activity competence and sense of self. BBD recognizes this complexity and aims to capture all elements of fPRC through a comprehensive approach (Figure 15.1).

Outcomes

Enrollment in BBD begins with a comprehensive evaluation in which caregivers complete the Young Children's Participation and Environment Measure (YC-PEM; Khetani et al., 2013) or the Participation and Environment Measure-Children and Youth (PEM-CY; Coster et al., 2010).

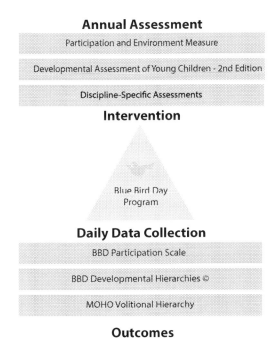

Annual Assessment

Participation and Environment Measure

Developmental Assessment of Young Children - 2nd Edition

Discipline-Specific Assessments

Intervention

Blue Bird Day Program

Daily Data Collection

BBD Participation Scale

BBD Developmental Hierarchies ©

MOHO Volitional Hierarchy

Outcomes

Developmental

Functional

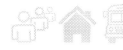
Participation

Figure 15.1

These tools evaluate participation in the home, school, and community, and collect information on the contextual factors influencing engagement within each setting. These measures are unique as they allow the team to understand more about the child's baseline levels of participation while initiating conversations surrounding a caregiver's current strategies to better support their child's engagement in daily life. The results of this measure are used to develop family-centered goals, which provides a strong foundation for family engagement upon entering BBD. Family-centered care is an essential component of this program as caregiver involvement is supported in the evidence as studies have found that parents' perceptions of their self-efficacy were both a predictor of children engaging in diversity in activities and a facilitator for increased participation (Soref et al., 2012).

Following the PEM, clients are evaluated by an interdisciplinary team, with each discipline focusing on a different developmental domain. This is completed holistically with a single global development tool, the Developmental Assessment of Young Children-2nd Edition (DAYC-2). This assessment provides baseline information regarding a child's development across domains of cognition, communication, social-emotional development, physical development and adaptive behavior. It is implemented yearly to capture changes in percent developmental delay. Depending on the client, additional discipline-specific assessments are implemented to measure potential areas impacting development. For example, the OT may utilize a version of the Sensory Profile-2 in order to understand how the child's sensory differences impact participation and functional performance.

Once a client begins services, data towards client goals are collected daily, utilizing BBD's Developmental Hierarchies ©, which encompass all areas of development deemed necessary to promote progress towards

Table 15.4 Measures Across ICF-CY Levels

Measure	Collection Frequency	Data Source	ICF Level
PEM	Annually	Caregiver	P & E
DAYC-2	Annually	Interdisciplinary team	BSF & A
Discipline-specific assessments	Annually	Caregiver/therapist	BSF & A & E
Developmental Hierarchies©	Daily in each rotation	Interdisciplinary team	BSF, A & P
BBD Participation Scale	Daily in each rotation	Interdisciplinary team	A & P
Volitional Hierarchy	Daily in each rotation	Interdisciplinary team	Person

BSF=Body Structure and Function, A=Activity, E= Environment, P= Participation

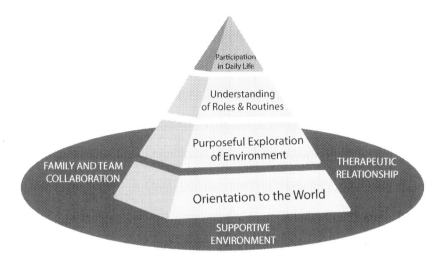

Figure 15.2 Blue Bird Day Pyramid

the outcome of participation. Hierarchies of skills are designated per discipline and are tracked upwards through four levels of the BBD Approach to Learning© Pyramid (Figure 15.2). The primary focus of the Developmental Hierarchies© is capturing changes in factors thought to influence participation through interventions provided at these levels. In addition to collecting data on developmental skills, data on the child's participation within each therapeutic rotation is collected on a 5-point scale, modeled after the Assistance to Participate Scale (Bourke-Taylor et al., 2013). Finally, data is collected on the development of each child's volition, or the motivation to act. This is done utilizing a volitional hierarchy, modeled after the MOHO-based Pediatric Volitional Questionnaire (Basu et al., 2008).

With increased participation in BBD rotations over time, progress towards long-term, family-centered outcomes can be correlated with mastery of hierarchy targets. This data is utilized to demonstrate how interventions are effective to promote development of foundational skills, improved functional performance and thus enhance participation in meaningful areas of life. The initial program level outcomes data emerges from the annual PEM measures, depicting the total number of caregivers reporting a decrease in their desired change regarding their child's participation across the home, community and/or school environments (Table 15.5). Recent data indicates that more than 50 percent of 56 caretakers participating in completing outcome data on their child's participation in the program reported a decrease in desired change in the home, daycare/ school, and the community (see Table 15.5).

Table 15.5 Outcomes Data

Caregiver reported decrease in desired change in home	Caregiver reported decrease in desired change in community	Caregiver reported decrease in desired change in daycare or school
n=33	n=35	n=29*

Total n=56 *Missing data on PEM reports
Change over one year in program

References

Adair, B., Ullenhag, A., Keen, D., Granlund, M., & Imms, C. (2015). The effect of interventions aimed at improving participation outcomes for children with disabilities: A systematic review. *Developmental Medicine & Child Neurology*, 57(12), 1093–1104. doi:10.1111/dmcn.12809

American Occupational Therapy Association. (2020). Occupational therapy practice framework: Domain and process Fourth edition. *American Journal of Occupational Therapy*, 74 (Suppl. 2), 1–87. https://doi.org/10.5014/ajot.2020.74S2001

Basu, S., Kafkes, A., Schatz, R., Kiraly, A., & Kielhofner, G. (2008). *A user's manual for the pediatric volitional questionnaire* (21st ed.). Model of Human Occupation Clearinghouse, Department of Occupational Therapy, University of Illinois at Chicago.

Bourke-Taylor, H. M., Law, M., Howie, L., & Pallant, J. F. (2013). *Assistance to participate scale for children with disabilities participation in play and leisure information booklet*. https://canchild.ca

Bundy, A., & Hacker, C. (2020). The art of therapy. In A. Bundy & S. Lane (Eds.), *Sensory integration: Theory and practice* (pp. 286–299). F. A. Davis.

Coster, W., Law, M., & Bedell, G. (2010). *Participation & environment measure-children & youth [assessment tool]*. https://doi.org/10.1037/t34829-000

Gorter, J. W., Stewart, D., & Woodbury-Smith, M. (2011). Youth in transition: Care, health and development. *Child Care and Health Development*, 37, 757–763. doi:10.1111/j.1365-2214.2011.01336.x

Khetani, M., Coster, W., Law, M., & Bedell, G. (2013). *Young children's participation & environment measure [assessment tool]*. doi:10.1080/01942638.2017

Imms, C., Granlund, M., Wilson, P. H., Steenbergen, B., Rosenbaum, P. L., & Gordon, A. M. (2017). Participation, both a means and an end: A conceptual analysis of processes and outcomes in childhood disability. *Developmental Medicine & Child Neurology*, 59(1), 16–25. https://doi.org/10.1111/dmcn.13237

Soref, B., Ratzon, N. Z., Rosenberg, L., Leitner, Y., Jarus, T., & Bart, O. (2012). Personal and environmental pathways to participation in young children with and without mild motor disabilities. *Child: Care, Health & Development*, 38(4), 561–571. doi:10.1111/j.1365-2214.2011.01295.x

Taylor, R. R. (2020). *The intentional relationship: Occupational therapy and use of self* (2nd ed.). F. A. Davis Company.

World Health Organization. (2010). *International classification of functioning, disability and health: Children and youth version (ICF-CY)*. World Health Organization. doi:10.3109/09638288.2010.516787

Appendix A
Assessment Table

Resources of Recommended Standardized Assessments in Pediatrics

Assessment	Research Comments
ACTIVLIM-CP: Bleyenheuft et al., 2017 Criterion based parent questionnaire; measures ADL performance in CP. 2–18 yrs. Available free online at www.rehab-scales	Measures changes in performance after motor training intervention and medical intervention i.e., lower extremity Botox-A injection in children with CP (Paradis et al., 2018) Discriminates differences in activities limitations in children with CP compared to typical age expected activity performance manual and gross motor function abilities II-V (Paradis et al., 2020)
Ages and Stages Questionnaire (ASQ-3, ASQ:SE-2): Bricker et al., 1999 Developmental questionnaire 0–5 yrs., 6 mos.	Recommended to screen for ASD (CDC, 2020) Identified 87% of children who screened positive on M-CHAT-R with follow-up and 95% of those diagnosed with ASD (Hardy et al., 2015)
Alberta Infant Motor Scale (AIMS): Piper et al., 1992 Observational, norm-referenced measure of gross motor development in various positions. Birth-18 mos.	Capacity to predict abnormal motor development varies by age. Provides superior specificity and sensitivity at eight months (Spittle et al., 2008) Based on systematic review, AIMS is used to identify atypical motor development in children born premature (Fuentefria et al., 2017)
Assisting Hand Assessment (AHA) 5.0: Krumlinde-Sundholm et al., 2014	Excellent reliability for adolescent AHA and valid for use with adolescents (Louwers et al., 2016, 2017)

(*Continued*)

Assessment	Research Comments
Criterion-referenced observational instrument for unilateral disability i.e., hemiplegia cerebral palsy, obstetric brachial plexus palsy; assesses bimanual hand use. Assesses how effectively the more affected upper extremity (UE) is used with the less affected UE during bimanual tasks. School Kids AHA and Adolescent AHA handling of objects occurs within the context of board games (Krumlinde-Sundholm & Wagner, 2019; Louwers et al., 2017) Standardized for children from 18 months - 18 years: Small Kids AHA: 18 mos.–5 yrs. School Kids AHA: 6–12 yrs. Adolescent AHA: 13–18 yrs.	Effective in showing change from intervention, tracks changes longitudinally; used in research and clinical practice (Krumlinde-Sundholm & Wagner, 2019) Used as an outcome measurement in intervention studies with children with CP (Geerdink et al., 2013; Klingels et al., 2013)
Autism Diagnostic Interview-Revised (ADI-R): Le Couteur et al., 2003 Diagnostic test; interview for caregivers of children and adults. Mental ages 18 mos. and above	Individuals with more severe forms or high rate of autism Identify clinical needs using subgroups & categories
Autism Diagnostic Observation Schedule-2 (ADOS-2): Lord et al., 2012 Diagnostic test; observation and coding of behaviors. 12 mos. - adulthood	Considered a gold standard in children Early childhood screening, treatment planning, and program evaluation
Bayley-IV: Bayley & Aylward, 2019 Structured assessment and parent questionnaire for development across: cognitive, language, motor development, social-emotional and adaptive behaviors. 16 days–42 mos.	Bayley-III can substitute for PDMS-2 for children 8–24 mos. (Connolly et al., 2012) Bayley-III has motor outcome predictive validity at age 2 (Griffiths et al., 2018)
Beery-Buktenica Developmental Test of Visual Motor Integration (Beery VMI): **Beery & Beery, 2010** Measures visual and motor skills; copying geometric forms arranged in increasing difficulty. Two supplemental tests, Visual Perception and Motor Coordination for screening. 2 yrs.–adult (short form for ages 2–7 yrs.)	Although often used to measure change, does not correlate with functional improvement in children (Ohl et al., 2020)

(*Continued*)

Assessment	*Research Comments*
Both Hands Assessment (BoHA): Elvrum et al., 2017 Criterion-referenced test measures bimanual upper extremity (UE) activity and unilateral performance in children with CP MACS Level I-III. 22 mos.–13 yrs.	Appropriate observational measure for CP with bilateral UE (Burgess et al., 2020)
Bruininks-Oseretsky Test of Motor Proficiency, 2nd Edition (BOT-2): Bruininks & Bruininks, 2005 Performance-based, norm-referenced, eight subtests of fine and gross motor skills: fine motor precision; fine motor integration; manual dexterity; bilateral coordination; balance; running speed and agility; upper limb coordination and strength. 4–21 yrs.	BOT2-SF suggested as valid tool to evaluate upper limb activities for children with CP as significant correlation demonstrated with MACS (Selves et al., 2019) BOT-2 assesses motor skills in children with ASD. Poor scores in the BOT-2 may be associated with poor social skills (Liu et al., 2019) Recommendations (Griffiths et al., 2018): • distinguishes between non-clinical and specific clinical groups (DCD, high-functioning ASD, mild to moderate, intellectual disabilities). • test-retest reliability is highest in BOT-2, MABC-2, PDMS-2 and TGMD-2, when compared to other motor assessments (Bayley-3, McCarron Assessment of Neuromuscular Development (MAND), Neurological Sensory Motor Developmental Assessment (NSMDA) Recommendations (Blank et al., 2019) for DCD: • use with adolescents and adults • use as secondary measure to assess motor problems if there is insufficient evidence of DCD in children being evaluated using the MABC-2 • adapted culturally, German version very good sensitivity • cut-off score for determining diagnosis of DCD using the BOT-2 is 2 SD or more below the mean based on total score

(*Continued*)

Assessment	*Research Comments*
Canadian Occupational Therapy Performance Measure (COPM): Law et al., 2019 Instrument measuring problems in daily life and aids in goal setting. Covers three domains in semi-structured interview; self-management, productive, and leisure activities. Parents/child rates importance, performance and satisfaction of daily tasks in three domains. All ages	Responsive measure to aid in setting and evaluating treatment goals in DCD population and used as evaluative instrument in multiple DCD treatment studies (Heus et al., 2020) Several studies (Dunford, 2011; Miller et al., 2001; Thornton et al., 2016) found that children treated for DCD improved over time on both performance and satisfaction scale.
CARE Index: Crittenden, 2010 Assesses quality of caregiver – infant interaction; measures overall sensitivity of adult within context of caregiver-child dyad. Observes caregiver facial expression, verbal expression, position and body contact, affection, turn-taking contingencies, control and choice of activity. Birth-4 yrs.	Research shows significant relationship between maternal sensitivity and attachment security of the child (Crittenden et al., 2005) Effectively identifies two opposite forms of insensitivity: over- and under-engagement with the infant (Künster et al., 2010). Used to measure maternal sensitivity with premature infants (Fuertes et al., 2006) From Farnfield et al. (2010): • Adult sensitivity to infant state (2–3 mos. age) • Dyadic turn-taking and shared joint pleasure for 3–9 mos. • Shared joint play with patterned sequences around 9–15 mos. • Object based play and non-verbal negotiation of differences at 15–24 mos. • Linguistic mediation of play, reciprocal communication
Cassidy Marvin Preschool Attachment Coding System (MAC): Cassidy et al., 1992 Classification based on their attachment behaviors into secure category, insecure/organized categories (insecure-avoidant and insecure-ambivalent), or one of three insecure-disorganized categories for children with disrupted caregiver attachment 3–5 yrs.	Identifies children at risk, but not sensitive enough to identify nuances of insecurity in the normative population. (Crittenden et al., 2007) Added category of Disorganized Attachment to previously identified secure and insecure patterns Research conducted on children experiencing maltreatment, maternal anxiety disorders, drug use and institutionalization (Crittenden et al., 2007)

(*Continued*)

Assessment	*Research Comments*
Childhood Autism Rating Scale, Second Edition (CARS-2): Schopler et al., 2010 Two rating scales completed by a clinician and one form for caregivers 2 yrs. and up	Identification and severity of ASD; discrimination between ASD and cognitive impairments Adequate evidence supporting the CARS-2 as a tool for making a differential diagnosis for individuals with autism and high-functioning autism (McLellan, 2014)
Crittenden's Preschool Attachment Assessment (PAA): Crittenden, 2006 Preschool Assessment of Attachment (PAA) is an instrument for assessing patterns of attachment. 18 mos.–5 yrs.	Excellent identification of children at risk for maltreatment (Farnfield et al., 2010) PAA is developmentally and clinically fine-tuned to tap the attachment behavior of endangered children (Farnfield et al., 2010) PAA differentiates between typical anxious patterns (Type A1–2, Type c 1–2), where actual danger is likely to be low, and higher patterns where an intervention may be needed (Teti & Gelfand, 1997; Vondra et al., 1999)
DCD DAILY: Van der Linde et al., 2013 Standardized, clinical test measures quality and speed of performing tasks; covers domains of self-care (feeding and dressing), school (writing, crafts, coloring, cutting) and play (hopping). 5–8 yrs.	Evaluative instrument used in multiple DCD treatment studies Recommended in Dutch DCD guidelines to use for evaluation of treatment outcomes Differentiate between children with and without DCD Reliable and valid instrument for use in clinical practice
DCDDaily-Q: Moraal- van der Linde et al., 2014 Parent questionnaire, 23 items, includes self-care-maintenance, productivity, schoolwork, leisure and play items. Examines how children perform ADL, whether they have taken longer to learn ADL compared to peers, and how often they perform ADL. 5–8 yrs.	DCDDaily-Q better predicted DCD than currently used questionnaires such as MABC-2 Checklist and DCDQ. Designed to identify children at risk for DCD
The Developmental Coordination Disorder Questionnaire Revised (DCDQ-R)'07: Wilson & Crawford, 2007	Recommended as preferred screening tool for clinical population but sensitivity too low to be used in general population to screen for DCD (Blank et al., 2019).

(Continued)

Assessment	*Research Comments*
(Wilson & Crawford, 2012) Parent questionnaire and screening tool to identify DCD and motor, coordination problems in three domains: postural control during movement, fine motor/handwriting and general coordination. 5–15 yrs. http:www.dcdq.ca	Most studied and evaluated DCD questionnaire (Asunta et al., 2019) even more than MABC-2 Checklist (Blank et al., 2019) DCDQ-R extended to ages 3 and 4 years as the Little DCDQ (Blank et al., 2019) Cross culturally adapted in many countries (Blank et al., 2019); Brazil MABC correlates with DCDQ-BR
The Functional Emotional Assessment Scale (FEAS): Greenspan et al., 2001 Criterion-referenced; assesses functional, emotional, developmental level 7 mos. - 4 yrs.	Systematic assessment of child/caregiver's functional emotional capacities. Evaluates caregiver capacity to support child's development in all assessed areas (Greenspan & DeGangi, 2001) Based upon the sensitivity calculations, FEAS appears to be well suited for children with regulatory disorders, particularly between 7 and 24 mos. (Greenspan et al., 2001)
Gilliam Autism Rating Scale – Second Edition (GARS-3): Gilliam, 2014 Rating scale designed to help clinicians diagnose autism and its severity 3–22 yrs.	Psychometric properties of the GARS-3 have been replicated in international samples (Gorji et al., 2020; Minaei & Nazeri, 2018) GARS-3 includes items to reflect ASD diagnostic criteria based on the DSM-V-
Gross Motor Function Measure 2nd Ed. (GMFM-66 & GMFM-88): Russell et al., 2013 **GMFM-88** Five level classification consistent with ICF to describe gross motor function and change for children with CP. Focuses on self-initiated movements during mobility, sitting and transfers. **GMFM-66** Subtest of original GMFM-88 used to assess change within a child with Cerebral Palsy over time or to compare patterns of change among children. 5 mos. - 16 yrs.	Internationally accepted, universal standard is a valid and reliable tool for research and clinical purposes and available in multiple languages. Useful in setting realistic goals and determining within child change over time and patterns of change. From www.cpnet.canchild.ca/en/resources/44-gross-motor-function-measure-gmfm: • **GMFM 88** for young children or more complex motor disabilities such as those functioning in GMFCS level V • **GMFM 88** used for children using ambulatory aids and/or orthoses or shoes • **GMFM-66** test performed barefoot • **GMFM-66** takes less time than GMFM-88 and items are ordered by difficulty • All versions of GMFM demonstrate strongest evidence for responsiveness and validity for children with CP (Ferre-Fernandez et al., 2020)

(*Continued*)

Assessment	Research Comments
Hammersmith Infant Neurological Examination (HINE): Haataja et al., 1999 Detects motor impairment for risk of CP; items assessing posture, movements, tone, reflexes and responses, motor milestones and behavior 2–24 mos. http://hammersmith-neuro-exam.com	High sensitivity and predictability (90%) for infants/toddlers at risk for CP (Novak et al., 2017) Good sensitivity and specificity to identify risk of cognitive delays in preterm infants after 3 mos. with and without CP (Romeo et al., 2020) Used on preterm and term infants at risk for developing CP and provides information on type and severity of CP (Romeo et al., 2015
Hand Assessment for Infants (HAI): Krumlinde-Sundholm et al., 2017 Norm referenced and criterion referenced; assess unilateral and bilateral hand use in infants and to identify any upper extremity (UE) asymmetries identifying those at risk for unilateral CP 3–12 mos.	Used to evaluate development and deviations in UE development (Krumlinde-Sundholm & Wagner, 2019) Can measure atypical hand use in infants to detect early UE asymmetries during functional use (Ek et al., 2019)
Little Developmental Coordination Disorder Questionnaire (Little DCDQ-CA): Wilson & Creighton, 2015 Parent report screens for coordination difficulties in gross/fine motor skills at home and preschool during play 3–5 yrs. www.dcdq.ca	Not used for diagnosis of DCD, in reporting, describe results as "suspect for" or "probable DCD" Little DCDQ-CA evolved from DCDQ'07 to identify younger children suspect for motor problems with sensitivity higher than specificity.
The Melbourne Assessment of Unilateral Upper Limb Function (MA2): Randall et al., 2012 MA2: Adapted from MUU: Criterion-Referenced assessment measures upper extremity function in unilateral or bimanual CP. Consists of 14 items evaluating quality of upper limb movement including: range of movement at each joint; accuracy of reach and placement; dexterity of grasp, release and manipulation; and fluency of movement (Krumlinde-Sundholm & Wagner, 2019; Randall et al., 2012) 2–15 yrs.	Used as outcome measurement in intervention studies with CP (Geerdink et al., 2013; Klingels et al., 2013) Valid tool for research and clinical use (Wang et al., 2017)

(*Continued*)

Assessment	*Research Comments*
Miller Function and Participation Scales (M-FUN): Miller, 2006 Standardized developmental assessment for fine/gross motor, visual motor, and participation. Each domain assesses aspects of postural abilities; hand function; executive function and participation; and non-motor visual perception 2 yrs., 6 mos. - 7 yrs., 11 mos.	Scores on the M-FUN (visual motor subscale) had a high correlation with the DTVP-2 (Diemand & Case-Smith , 2013) Designed to identify children who exhibit moderate pre-academic problems.
Mini Assisting Hand Assessment (AHA): Greaves et al., 2013 Measures use of affected upper extremity during bimanual play for unilateral CP. 8–18 mos.	Useful to evaluate functional hand use and the effects of intervention in an age group when potential for change is high (Greaves et al., 2013)
The Modified Checklist for Autism in Toddlers, Revised with Follow-Up (M-CHAT-R/F): Robins et al., 2009 Free caregiver questionnaire focusing on assessing risk and identification of ASD 16–30 mos. https://mchatscreen.com/	Children in the validation study were diagnosed 2 years younger than the national median age of diagnosis (Robins et al., 2014)
Motor Observation Questionnaire for Teachers-(MOQ-T): Shoemaker, 2003 Teacher questionnaire, 18 items, identifies children with clumsiness or DCD; fine and gross motor items divided into general motor functions (dressing, playing ball) and handwriting 5–11 yrs.	Developed by van Dellon et al. (1990) and first called Groninger Motor Observation Scale. Original version revised by Shoemaker (Cancer et al., 2020) From Asunta et al., 2019: • Good cross-cultural validity • Discriminative validity between MOQ-T and DCDQ • Concurrent validity of MOQ-T with MABC and DCDQ • Easy to complete and described well therefore highly usable tool for teachers
Movement Assessment Battery for Children-2 (MABC-2 Test): Henderson et al., 2007 Norm referenced movement assessment, identifies motor function impairments and DCD. Includes eight tasks assessing manual dexterity (3), aiming and catching (2), and balance across three separate age groups. 3–16 yrs.	From Blank et al., 2019: • Fair to good construct and concurrent validity with BOT-2 • MABC and MABC-2 are most used and best studied standardized motor tests for individuals with DCD and are moderate to good in informing diagnosis of DCD. • Lack of research on discriminant validity • Culturally adapted, 10 countries and languages

(*Continued*)

Assessment	*Research Comments*
Movement Assessment Battery for Children Checklist – Second Edition (MABC-2-C): Henderson et al., 2007 Checklist for parent or teacher to make qualitative judgment about movements in natural contexts. Developed as a complement to MABC-2. Focuses on individual's activity level and has items for self-care, classroom skills, and physical recreational skills. Screens for needing further testing with MABC-2. 5–12 yrs.	From Blank et al., 2019: • Significant correlation (concurrent) between Checklist/Test and DCDQ'07 • Designed for broad population with motor impairments and predicts motor impairment better than the DCDQ'07. • Less examined than DCDQ-R • Translated into many countries (Asunta et al., 2019)
Mullen Scales of Early Learning (MSEL): Mullen, 1995 Developmental standardized assessment measuring gross motor, fine motor, visual reception, receptive and expressive language Birth-68 mos.	Children with ASD are assessed quickly with the MSEL, but they display significantly more off tasks behaviors (Akshoomoff, 2006) MSEL was administered to children with ASD, CP and EPI; they demonstrated significant differences when compared with typical children (Burns et al., 2013)
Peabody Developmental Motor Scales, 2nd Edition (PDMS-2): Folio & Fewell, 2000 Performance based assessment of Reflexes, Stationary, Locomotion, Object Manipulation, Grasping, Visual-Motor Integration. Birth - 5 yrs., 11 mos.	Moderate concurrent validity with MABC-2 and BOT-2 (Blank et al., 2019) Evaluative motor measure for children with CP aged 2 to 5 years (Wang et al., 2006). Reliable and valid for assessing motor function of low birth weight pre-term infants (Tavasoli et al., 2014). PDMS-FM-2 may not be sensitive enough for children with fine motor problems (van Hartingsveldt et al., 2005) PDMS-2 determined differences in fine and gross motor skills in infants with perinatal risk factors i.e., prematurity, hypoxia compared to typical infants (Karimi et al., 2016) PDMS has been used to document motor skill competency in children with ASD and association with other domains of function (Holloway et al., 2018)

(*Continued*)

Assessment	*Research Comments*
The Pediatric Balance Scale (PBS): Franjoine et al., 2003 Modified from Berg Balance Scale, PBS measures balance in children With mild to moderate motor impairment i.e., CP 5–15 yrs.	Scores correlate with gross motor function on GMFM (88 & 66) in children with CP and can assess balance related to standing and walking (Yi et. al., 2012) Used to quantify balance in children with CP (Sharma & Thapar, 2018)
Pediatric Evaluation of Disability Inventory (PEDI)-CAT Q-Global: Haley et al., 2020 Computer adaptive test (CAT) of original PEDI developed in 1992 based upon real-time responses, limits items reducing respondent burden. Estimates abilities within functional domains: Daily Activities, Mobility and Social/Cognitive with assistance required and modifications needed. Responsibility domain measures extent caregiver or child take responsibility for managing life tasks. Two versions, speedy and content-balanced.	PEDI-CAT (ASD) is a module of the assessment for children with ASD with additional items for daily activities, social/cognitive, and responsibility (Kramer et al., 2016) PEDI-CAT differentiates children with a diagnosis of ASD from those who are typically developing (Kao et al., 2012) Clinicians and parents report that PEDI-CAT items represent relevant domains for children with ASD (Kramer et al., 2012) Useful for measuring functional and participation changes over time and program evaluation (Dumas et al., 2012)
PEDI-CAT (ASD) for Autism: Haley et al., 2020 Module of PEDI-CAT validated for ASD. Includes instructions to help parents select appropriate ratings and items added to Daily Activities, Social/Cognitive and Responsibility domains based on unique patterns of ASD. Birth - 20 yrs.	PEDI-CAT used to assess the same child; there is no minimum time requirement for re-assessment (Kramer et al., 2016)
Prechtl's Qualitative Assessment of General Movement (GMA): Einspieler et al., 2004 Gross motor spontaneous movements are videotaped. Identifies absent or abnormal general movements. Preterm-20 weeks (corrected age)	Requires standardized training (Spittle et al., 2008) When given during fidgety general movements (10–20 weeks corrected age) has strongest sensitivity, specificity and predictive validity for CP (Kwong et al., 2018) Predictive tool with 98% sensitivity of identifying cerebral palsy in infants under 5 months adjusted age (Novak et al., 2017)

(*Continued*)

Assessment	*Research Comments*
Screening Tool for Autism in Toddlers and Young Children (STAT™): Stone et al., 2000, 2008 12 interactive, play-based items that can be administered in 20 minutes to screen for autism 2–3 yrs. https://stat.vucinnovations.com/	Differentiates ASD from other developmental disorders (Stone et al., 2000) STAT can be administered by community service providers Different play activities assess communicative behaviors, play, imitation, directing attention and requesting Sample of children who have an older brother with autism or that were referred because of autism concerns was investigated with the STAT. False positives were highest for the 12–13 mo. old group and decreased for 14 mo. or older (Stone et al., 2008)
Sensory Processing Measure (SPM): Parham et al., 2007 Parent and teacher questionnaires examining sensory domains (vision, hearing, touch, body awareness, balance, and motion) planning and ideation, & social participation in different activities & contexts. Total score includes all areas including taste and smell but not social participation **SPM Home Form (SPM-Home): Parham & Ecker, 2007** **SPM Main Classroom Form: Miller-Kuhaneck, Henry, & Glennon, 2007** **SPM School Environments Form: Miller-Kuhaneck, Henry, Glennon, & Mu, 2007** 5–12 yrs. **SPM-Preschool (SPM-P): Miller-Kuhaneck et al., 2010** 2 yrs.–5 yrs.	Adequate face, content and construct, good ability to distinguish between clinical and typical samples (Glennon et al., 2011) Useful for team collaboration on assessing and implementing interventions for sensory processing issues across contexts Useful for typical and at-risk children for demonstrating sensory processing issues (Premature, ASD, Regulatory Disorders). Increasingly used in studies with children identified as DCD and having sensory processing problems. (Allen & Casey, 2017)
Sensory Profile 2: Dunn, 2014 Assessments – Infant Sensory Profile 2, Toddler Sensory Profile 2, Child Sensory Profile 2, Short Sensory Profile 2 (research version), and School Companion Sensory Profile 2	Yields three group of scores: sensory pattern, sensory system and behavioral pattern, interpreted together. Moderate correlation between the Sensory Over-Responsivity Inventory and the Adolescent/ Adult Sensory Profile (Kanda et al., 2017)

(*Continued*)

Assessment	Research Comments
Judgement based questionnaires; provides a standard method to document child's sensory processing patterns in context of everyday life Birth - 14 yrs., 11 mos.	Children with CP demonstrated differences in sensory processing in 16 out of 23 items on the SP when compared to children with typical development (Pavão & Rocha, 2017) Identifies difficulties in sensory processing in infants at high risk for developing sensory processing disorder (Flanagan et al., 2019) Useful for typical and at-risk children for demonstrating sensory processing issues (premature, ASD, DCD, ADHD) Increasingly used in studies with children identified as DCD and having sensory processing problems. (Allen & Casey, 2017) Small to moderate correlations with SOSI-M, observational measure, suggest observational tools need to be used when assessing motor performance (Blanche et al., 2021)
Social Responsiveness Scale (SRS-2): Constantino & Gruber, 2012 Rating scale completed by caregivers or teachers (e.g., social awareness & communication) Identifies and describes social difficulties and severity. Includes total score and scores on different subscales including social awareness, social cognition, social communication, social motivation and, restricted and repetitive behavior. 2.6 years – adulthood	SRS-2 assesses social deficits from different perspectives. The instrument has school age, preschool, adult (relative) and adult self-report formats (Constantino & Gruber, 2012). SRS-s has shown adequate concurrent and predictive validity in a sample of adults with a diagnosis of autism (Chan et al., 2017). Distinguishes individuals with autism from controls and also from other clinical groups (Constantino & Gruber, 2012). Caution should be used when using SRS to differentiate between ASD and related conditions (Zwaigenbaum & Penner, 2018).
Structured Observations of Sensory Integration-Motor (SOSI-M) and Comprehensive Observations of Proprioception (COP-R): Blanche et al., 2021 Observational tool measuring sensory-motor skills and their relationship to proprioception and vestibular functions 5–14 yrs.	From Blanche, Bodison, Chang, & Reinoso, 2012; Blanche, Reinoso, Chang, & Bodison, 2012: • SOSI-M and COP-R are assessments of motor performance linked to sensory processing observations. • SOSI-M and COP-R evaluate proprioceptive, vestibular, motor planning, and postural control skills. • SOSI-M and COP-R are based on nationally representative US sample:

(Continued)

Assessment	Research Comments
	pilot testing in several international clinical sites.
	• SOSI-M national sample yielded adequate psychometric properties for clinical applications and research.
	• Standardization included Spanish speaking children and Spanish instructions (Imperatore Blanche et al., 2016)
The Systematic Detection of Writing Problems (SOS-2-NL): Smits-Engelsmen et al., 2014 Normative measure to detect writing problems (quality and speed), child copies standard text 7–12 yrs.	Recommended by international DCD guidelines to detect writing problems, culturally adapted (Blank et al., 2019)
Test of Infant Motor Performance (TIMP): Campbell et al., 2012 Observed, elicited postural and selective motor control for functional skills assessment 34 weeks (gestational)-4 mos. (corrected)	TIMP most predictive under four mos. (Spittle et al., 2008) Identifies atypical motor development in high risk infants under 5 mos. corrected age in conjunction with general movement assessment (GMA) (Novak et al., 2017) Strongest predictive validity for neurodevelopmental outcome along with the GMA for premature infants (Craciunoiu & Holsti, 2016)
Test of Sensory Functions in Infants (TSFI): Degangi & Greenspan, 1989 Performance-based measure for infants or children who are at risk for or demonstrating sensory processing issues (premature, ASD, Regulatory Disorder). Five domains of sensory reactivity and processing (touch pressure and vestibular reactivity, visual and tactile integration, ocular-motor control, and adaptive motor functions) 4–18 mos.	Measures sensory processing in infants but recommended to be used with a sensory parent questionnaire to identify sensory processing problems (Eelles et al., 2012).

Note: Reliability and validity rating of excellent, good etc. are as described in the research article referenced

Value of screen is to accurately identify those with a condition (sensitivity) as compared to accuracy of incorrectly identifying those without a condition (specificity)

Contributions by Lisa R. Reyes, MSCS, MS, OTR/L

References

Akshoomoff, N. (2006). Use of the Mullen scales of early learning for the assessment of young children with autism spectrum disorders. *Child Neuropsychology: A Journal on Normal and Abnormal Development in Childhood and Adolescence, 12*(4–5), 269–277. https://doi.org/10.1080/09297040500473714

Allen, S., & Casey, J. (2017). Developmental coordination disorders and sensory processing and integration: Incidence, associations and co-morbidities. *British Journal of Occupational Therapy, 80*(9), 549–557. https://doi.org/10.1177/0308022617709183

Asunta, P., Viholainen, T., Ahonen, T., & Rintala, P. (2019). Psychometric properties of observational tools for identifying motor difficulties. *BMC Pediatrics, 19,* 322. https://doi.org/10.1186/s12887-019-1657-6

Bayley, N., & Aylward, G. P. (2019). *Bayley scales of infant and toddler development screening test* (4th ed.). Technical Manual Pearson.

Beery, K. E., & Beery, N. A. (2010). *Beery VMI administration, scoring, and teaching manual. 6th.* NCS Pearson Inc.

Blanche, E. I., Bodison, S., Chang, M., & Reinoso, G. (2012). Development of the comprehensive observations of proprioception (COP): Validity, reliability and factor analysis. *American Journal of Occupational Therapy, 66*(6), 691–698.

Blanche, E. I., Reinoso, G., Chang, M., & Bodison, S. (2012). Evaluation of the comprehensive observations of proprioception scale (COP) on children with autism spectrum disorders and developmental disabilities. *American Journal of Occupational Therapy, 66*(5), 621–624.

Blanche, E. I., Reinoso, G., & Blanche Kiefer, D. (2021). *Structured observations of sensory integration-motor (SOSI-M) & comprehensive observations of proprioception (COP-R).* Administration Manual. Academic Therapy Publications (ATP).

Blank, R., Barnett, A. L., Cairney, J., Green, D., Kirby, A., Polatajko, H., . . . Vincon, S. (2019). International clinical practice recommendations on the definition, diagnosis, assessment, intervention, and psychosocial aspects of developmental coordination disorder. *Developmental Medicine & Child Neurology, 61,* 242–285. https://doi.org/10.1111/dmcn.14132

Bleyenheuft, Y., Paradis, J., Renders, A., Thonnard, J. L. & Arnould, C. (2017). ACTIVLIM-CP a new Rasch-built measure of global activity performance for children with cerebral palsy. *Research in Developmental Disabilities, 60,* 285–294, https://doi.org/10.1016/j.ridd.2016.10.005

Bricker, D., Squires, J., Mounts, L., Potter, L., Nickel, R., Twombly, E., & Farrell, J. (1999). *Ages and stages questionnaire.* Paul H. Brookes.

Bruininks, R., & Bruininks, B. (2005). *Bruininks-Oseretsky test of motor proficiency – 2nd edition (BOT-2): Manual.* AGS Publishing.

Burgess, A., Boyd, R., Ziviani, J., & Sakzewski, L. (2020). A systematic review of upper limb activity measures for 5- to 18-year-old children with bilateral cerebral palsy. *Australian Occupational Therapy Journal, 66,* 552–567. https://doi.org/10.1111/1440-1630.12600

Burns, T. G., King, T. Z., & Spencer, K. S. (2013). Mullen scales of early learning: The utility in assessing children diagnosed with autism spectrum disorders, cerebral palsy, and epilepsy. *Applied Neuropsychology: Child, 2*(1), 33–42. https://doi.org/10.1080/21622965.2012.682852

Campbell, S., Girolomi, G., Kolobe, T. H. A., Osten, E. T., & Lenke, M. C. (2004, 2012). *Test user's manual for the test of infant motor performance V.3 for the TIMP version 5*. S. K. Campbell. www.thetimp.com

Cancer, A., Minoliti, R., Crepaldi, M., & Antonietti, A. (2020). Identifying developmental motor difficulties: A review of tests to assess motor coordination in children. *Journal of Functional Morphology and Kinesiology*, 5(16). https://doi:10.3390/jfmk50100016

Cassidy, J., Marvin, R. S., & The MacArthur Working Group. (1992). *Attachment organization in preschool children: Procedures and coding manual*. Unpublished manuscript, University of Virginia, 125–131.

Centers for Disease Control and Prevention. (2020, February 11). *National center on birth defects and developmental disabilities*. www.cdc.gov/ncbddd/autism/hcp-screening.html

Chan, W., Smith, L. E., Hong, J., Greenberg, J. S., & Mailick, M. R. (2017). Validating the social responsiveness scale for adults with autism. *Autism Research: Official Journal of the International Society for Autism Research*, 10(10), 1663–1671. https://doi.org/10.1002/aur.1813

Connolly, B. H., McClune, N. O., & Gatlin, R. (2012). Concurrent validity of the Bayley-III and the Peabody developmental motor scale – 2. *Pediatric Physical Therapy*, 24(4), 345–352. https://doi.org/10.1097/pep.0b013e318267c5cf

Constantino, J. N., & Gruber, C. P. (2012). *Social responsiveness scale-second edition (SRS-2)*. Western Psychological Services.

Craciunoiu, O., & Holsti, L. (2016). A systematic review of the predictive validity of neurobehavioral assessments during the preterm period. *Physical & Occupational Therapy in Pediatrics*, 37(3), 292–307. https://doi.org/10.1080/01942638.2016.1185501

Crittenden, P. M. (2006). A dynamic-maturational model of attachment. *Australian and New Zealand Journal of Family Therapy*, 27(2), 105–115. https://doi.org/10.1002/j.1467-8438.2006.tb00704.x

Crittenden, P. M. (2010). *CARE-index. Infants. Coding manual*. Family Relations Institute.

Crittenden, P. M., Claussen, A., & Kozlowska, K. (2007). Choosing a valid assessment of attachment for clinical use: A comparative study. *Australian and New Zealand Journal of Family Therapy*, 28(2). https://doi.org/10.1375/anft.28.2.78

Crittenden, P. M., Der, C. A. R. E., & Früherkennung, I. (2005). *Using the CARE-index for screening, intervention, and research*. Online verfügbar unter www. patcrittenden. com/images/CARE-Index. pdf, zuletzt aktualisiert am, 3, 2009.

DeGangi, G. A., & Greenspan, S. I. (1989). *Test of sensory functions in infants*. Western Psychological Services.

Diemand, S., & Case-Smith, J. (2013). Validity of the Mi ller function and participation scales. *Journal of Occupational Therapy, Schools, & Early Intervention*, 6(3), 203–212 https://doi.org/10.1080/19411243.2013.850937

Dumas, H. M., & Fragala-Pinkham, M. A. (2012). Concurrent validity and reliability of the pediatric evaluation of disability inventory-computer adaptive test mobility domain. *Pediatric Physical Therapy: The Official Publication of the Section on Pediatrics of the American Physical Therapy Association*, 24(2), 171–176. https://doi.org/10.1097/PEP.0b013e31824c94ca

Dunford, C. (2011). Goal oriented group intervention for children with developmental coordination disorder. *Physical and Occupational Therapy in Pediatrics*, 31(3), 288–300. https://doi.org/10.3109/01942638.2011.565864

Dunn, W. (2014). *Sensory profile™2*. Pearson.

Eelles, A., Spittle, A., Anderson, P., Brown, N., Lee, K., Boyd, R., & Doyle, L. (2012). Assessments of sensory processing in infants: A systematic review. *Developmental Medicine & Child Neurology*, 55(4), 314–326. https://doi.org/10.1111/j.1469-8749.2012.04434.x

Einspieler, C., Prechtl, H. F., Bos, A. F., Ferrari, F., & Cioni, G. (2004). Prechtl's method on the qualitative assessment of general movements in preterm, term and young infants. In *Clinics in developmental medicine* (p. 167). Mac Keith Press.

Ek, L., Eliasson, A., Sicola, E., Sjöstrand, L., Guzzetta, A., Sgandurra, G., et al. (2019). Hand assessment for infants: Normative reference values. *Developmental Medicine & Child Neurology*, 61(9), 1087–1092. https://doi.org/10.1111/dmcn.14163

Elvrum, A.-K. G., Zethræus, B.-M., & Krumlinde-Sundholm, L. (2017). *Both hands assessment administration and scoring manual*. Bversion 1.1 English. Handfast. https://doi.org/10.1080/01942638.2017.1318431

Farnfield, S., Hautamäki, A., Nørbech, P., & Sahhar, N. (2010, July). DMM assessments of attachment and adaptation: Procedures, validity and utility. *Clinical Child Psychology and Psychiatry*, 5(3), 313–328. https://doi.org/10.1177/1359104510364315

Ferre-Fernández, M., Murcia-González, M. A., Espinosa, M. D. B., & Ríos-Díaz, J. (2020). Measures of motor and functional skills for children with cerebral palsy: A systematic review. *Pediatric Physical Therapy*, 32(1), 12–25

Flanagan, J., Schoen, S., & Miller, L. (2019). Early identification of sensory processing difficulties in high-risk infants. *American Journal of Occupational Therapy*, 73(2), 7302205130p1. https://doi.org/10.5014/ajot.2018.028449

Folio, M. R., & Fewell, R. R. (2000). *Peabody developmental motor scales. Examiners manual*. Pro-ED.

Franjoine, M., Gunther, J., & Taylor, M. (2003). Pediatric balance scale: A modified version of the berg balance scale for the school-age child with mild to moderate motor impairment. *Pediatric Physical Therapy*, 15(2), 114–128. https://doi.org/10.1097/01.pep.0000068117.48023.18

Fuentefria, R., Silveira, R., & Procianoy, R. (2017). Motor development of preterm infants assessed by the Alberta infant motor scale: Systematic review article. *Jornal De Pediatria*, 93(4), 328–342. https://doi.org/10.1016/j.jped.2017.03.003

Fuertes, M., Santos, P. L. D., Beeghly, M., & Tronick, E. (2006). More than maternal sensitivity shapes attachment: Infant coping and temperament. https://doi.org/10.1196/annals.1376.037

Geerdink, Y., Aarts, P., & Geurts, A. (2013). Motor learning curve and long-term effectiveness of modified constraint-induced movement therapy in children with unilateral cerebral palsy: A randomized controlled trial. *Research in Developmental Disabilities*, 34(3), 923–931. https://doi.org/10.1016/j.ridd.2012.11.011

Gilliam, J. E. (2014). *Gilliam autism rating scale – third edition (GARS-3)*. ProEd.

Glennon, T. J., Miller Kuhaneck, H., & Herzberg, D. (2011). The sensory processing measure – preschool (SPM-P) – Part one: Description of the tool and its use in the preschool environment. *Journal of Occupational Therapy, Schools, & Early Intervention*, 4(1), 42–52.

Gorji, R., Hassanzadeh, S., Ghasemzadeh, S., & Qolamali Lavasani, M. (2020). Sensitivity and specificity Gilliam autism rating scale (GARS) in diagnosis autism spectrum disorders: Systematic review. *Shefaye Khatam*, 8(4), 80–89. http://shefayekhatam.ir/article-1-2157-en.html

Greaves, S., Imms, C., Dodd, K., & Krumlinde-Sundholm, L. (2013). Development of the mini-assisting hand assessment: Evidence for content and internal scale validity. *Developmental Medicine & Child Neurology, 55*(11), 1030–1037. https://doi.org/10.1111/dmcn.12212

Greenspan, S. I., DeGangi, G., & Wieder, S. (2001a). *The functional emotional assessment scale (FEAS): For infancy & early childhood.* Interdisciplinary Council on Development & Learning Disorders.

Greenspan, S. I., DeGangi, G., & Wieder, S. (2001b). Research on the FEAS: Test development, reliability, and validity studies. In *The functional emotional assessment scale (FEAS) for infancy and early childhood. Clinical and research applications* (pp. 167–247). ICDL.

Griffiths, A., Toovey, R., Morgan, P. E., & Spittle, A. J. (2018). Psychometric properties of gross motor assessment tools for children: A systematic review. *BMJ Open, 8*(10), e021734. http://dx.doi.org/10.1136/bmjopen-2018-021734

Haataja, L., Mercuri, E., Regev, R., Cowan, F., Rutherford, M., Dubowitz, V., Dubowitz, L. (1999). Optimality score for the neurologic examination of the infant at 12 and 18 months of age. *Journal of Pediatrics, 135*(2 Pt 1), 153–161. https://doi.org/10.1016/s0022-3476(99)70016-8

Haley, S. M., Coster, W. J., Dumas, H. M., Fragala-Pinkham, M. A., & Moed, R. (2020). *Pediatric evaluation of disability inventory computer adaptive test – PEDI CAT: Administration manual.* Pearson.

Hardy, S., Haisley, L., Manning, C., & Fein, D. (2015). Can screening with the ages and stages questionnaire detect autism? *Journal of Developmental and Behavioral Pediatrics: JDBP, 36*(7), 536–543. https://doi.org/10.1097/DBP.0000000000000201

Henderson, S. E., Sugden, D. A., & Barnett, A. L. (2007). *Movement assessment battery for children-2: Movement ABC-2: Examiner's manual.* Pearson.

Heus, I., Weezenberg, D., Severijnen, S., Vlieland, T. V., & van der Holst, M. (2020). Measuring treatment outcomes in children with developmental coordination disorder; Responsiveness of six outcome measures. *Disability and Rehabilitation,* 1–12. https://doi.org/10.1080/09638288.2020.1785022

Holloway, J. M., Long, T. M., & Biasini, F. (2018). Relationships between gross motor skills and social function in young boys with autism spectrum disorder. *Pediatric Physical Therapy: The Official Publication of the Section on Pediatrics of the American Physical Therapy Association, 30*(3), 184–190. https://doi.org/10.1097/PEP.0000000000000505

Imperatore Blanche, E., Reinoso, G., Blanche-Kiefer, D., & Barros, A. (2016). Desempeño de niños típicos entre 5 y 7.11 años de edad en una selección de observaciones clínicas: Datos preliminares y propiedades psicométricas en una muestra Chilena. *Revista Chilena de Terapia Ocupacional* (1), 17–26.

Kanda, M., Ruzzano, L., Cohen, E., & Cermak, S. (2017). The association between two sensory processing measures: The sensory over-responsivity inventory and the adolescent/adult sensory profile. *American Journal of Occupational Therapy, 71*(4_Supplement_1), 7111500033p1–7111500033p1. https://doi.org/10.5014/ajot.2017.71s1-po3035

Kao, Y. C., Kramer, J. M., Liljenquist, K., Tian, F., & Coster, W. J. (2012). Comparing the functional performance of children and youths with autism, developmental disabilities, and no disability using the revised pediatric evaluation of disability inventory item banks. *The American Journal of Occupational Therapy:*

Official Publication of the American Occupational Therapy Association, 66(5), 607–616. https://doi.org/10.5014/ajot.2012.004218

Karimi, H., Aliabadi, F., Hosseini-Jam, M. & Afsharkhas, L. (2016). Evaluation of motor skills in high risk infants based on Peabody developmental motor scales (PDMS-2). *International Journal of Children and Adolescents, 2*(1), 4–7.

Klingels, K., Feys, H., Molenaers, G., Verbeke, G., Van Daele, S., & Hoskens, J., . . . De Cock, P. (2013). Randomized trial of modified constraint-induced movement therapy with and without an intensive therapy program in children with unilateral cerebral palsy. *Neurorehabilitation and Neural Repair, 27*(9), 799–807. https://doi.org/10.1177/1545968313496322

Kramer, J. M., Coster, W. J., Kao, Y. C., Snow, A., & Orsmond, G. I. (2012). A new approach to the measurement of adaptive behavior: Development of the PEDI-CAT for children and youth with autism spectrum disorders. *Physical & Occupational Therapy in Pediatrics, 32*(1), 34–47. https://doi.org/10.3109/019 42638.2011.606260

Kramer, J. M., Liljenquist, K., & Coster, W. J. (2016). Validity, reliability, and usability of the pediatric evaluation of disability inventory-computer adaptive test for autism spectrum disorders. *Developmental Medicine and Child Neurology, 58*(3), 255–261. https://doi.org/10.1111/dmcn.12837

Krumlinde-Sundholm, L., Ek, L., Sicola, E., Sjöstrand, L., Guzzetta, A., Sgandurra, G., . . . Eliasson, A.- C. (2017). Development of the hand assessment for infants: Evidence of internal scale validity. *Developmental Medicine & Child Neurology, 59*(12), 1276–1283. https://doi.org/10.1111/dmcn.13585

Krumlinde-Sundholm, L., Holmefur, M., & Eliasson, A. (2014). *Manual: Assisting hand assessment – kids, 18 months to 12 years, β-version 5.0, English.* Karolinska Institutet.

Krumlande-Sundholm, L., & Wagner, L. V. (2019). Upper extremity assessment and outcome evaluation in cerebral palsy. In F. Miller, S. Bachrach, N. Lennon, & M. O'Neil (Eds.), *Cerebral Palsy.* Springer. https://doi.org/10.1007/978-3-319-74558-9_108

Künster, A. K., Fegert, J. M., & Ziegenhain, U. (2010). Assessing parent – child interaction in the preschool years: A pilot study on the psychometric properties of the toddler CARE-Index. *Clinical Child Psychology and Psychiatry, 15*(3), 379–389. https://doi.org/10.1177/1359104510367585

Kwong, A., Fitzgerald, T., Doyle, L., Cheong, J., & Spittle, A. (2018). Predictive validity of spontaneous early infant movement for later cerebral palsy: A systematic review. *Developmental Medicine & Child Neurology, 60*(5), 480–489. https://doi.org/10.1111/dmcn.13697

Law, M., Baptiste, S., Carswell, A., McColl, M. A., Polatajko, H., & Pollock, N. (2019). *Canadian occupational performance measure* (5th ed.). COPM.

Le Couteur, A., Lord, C., & Rutter, M. (2003). *The autism diagnostic interview – revised (ADI-R).* Western Psychological Services.

Liu, T., Vineela, K., Litchke, L. G. (2019). Motor competence and social function in children with autism spectrum disorder. *The Journal of Neuroscience, 3,* 007. https://doi.org/10.3390/medicina55050135

Lord, C., Rutter, M., DiLavore, P., Risi, S., Gotham, K., & Bishop, S. L. (2012). *ADOS-2, autism diagnostic observation schedule, Part 1: Modules 1–4* (2nd ed.). Western Psychological Services.

Louwers, A., Beelen, A., Holmefur, M., & Krumlinde-Sundholm, L. (2016). Development of the assisting hand assessment for adolescents (Ad- AHA) and validation of the AHA from 18 months to 18 years. *Developmental Medicine & Child Neurology, 58*(12), 1303–1309. https://doi.org/10.1111/dmcn.13168

Louwers, A., Krumlinde-Sundholm, L., Boeschoten, K., & Beelen, A. (2017). Reliability of the assisting hand assessment in adolescents. *Developmental Medicine & Child Neurology, 59*(9), 926–932. https://doi.org/10.1111/dmcn.13465

McLellan, M. J. (2014). Test review of childhood autism rating scale, second edition. In J. F. Carlson, K. F. Geisinger, & L. Jonson (Eds.), *The nineteenth mental measurements yearbook*. http://marketplace.unl.edu/buros/

Miller, L. J. (2006). *Miller function and participation scales: Examiners manual*. PsychCorp Harcout Assessment.

Miller, L. T., Polatajko, H. J., Missiuna, C., Mandich, A. D., & Macnab, J. J. (2001). A pilot trial of a cognitive treatment for children with developmental coordination disorder. *Human Movement Science, 20*(1–2), 183–210. https://doi.org/10.1016/s0167-9457(01)00034-3

Miller-Kuhaneck, H., Ecker, C. E., Parham, L. D., Henry, D. A., & Glennon, T. J. (2010). *Sensory processing measure-preschool (SPM-P): Manual*. Western Psychological Services.

Miller-Kuhaneck, H., Henry, D. A., & Glennon, T. J. (2007). *Sensory processing measure (SPM) school environments form*. Western Psychological Services.

Miller-Kuhaneck, H., Henry, D. A., Glennon, T. J., & Mu, K. (2007). Development of the sensory processing measure – School: Initial studies of reliability and validity. *American Journal of Occupational Therapy, 61*(2), 170–175.

Minaei, A., & Nazeri, S. (2018). Psychometric properties of the Gilliam autism rating scale – third edition (GARS-3) in individuals with autism: A pilot study. *JOEC, 18*(2), 113–122. http://joec.ir/article-1-847-en.html

Mullen, E. M. (1995). *Mullen scales of early learning: Administration manual*. Pearson.

Novak, I., Morgan, C., Adde, L., Blackman, J., Boyd, R. N., Brunstrom-Hernandez, J., & De Vries, L. S. (2017). Early, accurate diagnosis and early intervention in cerebral palsy: Advances in diagnosis and treatment. *JAMA Pediatrics, 171*(9), 897–907. https://doi.org/10.1001/jamapediatrics.2017.1689

Ohl, A., Schelly, D., & Sharpe, S. (2020). Establishing the minimal clinically important difference of the beery-Buktenica developmental test of visual-motor integration (VMI). *American Journal of Occupational Therapy, 74*(4_Supplement_1), 7411500011p1–7411500011p1. https://doi.org/10.5014/ajot.2020.74s1-po2112

Paradis, J., Arnould, C., & Bleyenheuft, Y. (2020). Normative values and discriminative ability across functional levels of ACTIVLIM-CP, a measure of global activity performance for children with cerebral palsy. *Disability and Rehabilitation, 42*(19), 2790–2796.

Paradis, J., Arnould, C., Thonnard, J., Houx, L., Pons-Becmeur, C., Renders, A., . . . Bleyenheuft, Y. (2018). Responsiveness of the ACTIVLIM-CP questionnaire: Measuring global activity performance in children with cerebral palsy. *Developmental Medicine & Child Neurology, 60*(11), 1178–1185. https://doi.org/10.1111/dmcn.13927

Parham, L. D., & Ecker, C. (2007). *Sensory processing measure: Home form (SPM – Home)*. Western Psychological Services.

Parham, L. D., Kuhaneck, H., Ecker, C., Henry, D. A., & Glennon, T. J. (2007). *SPM sensory processing measure*. Western Psychological Services.

Pavão, S. L., & Rocha, N. A. C. F. (2017). Sensory processing disorders in children with cerebral palsy. *Infant Behavior and Development, 46,* 1–6. https://doi.org/10.1016/j.infbeh.2016.10.007

Piper, M. C., Pinell, L. E., Darrah, J., Maguire, T., & Byrne, P. J. (1992). Construction and validation of the Alberta infant motor scale (AIMS). *Canadian Journal of Public Health = Revue Canadienne De Sante Publique, 83* (Suppl 2), S46–S50.

Randall, M., Johnson, L., & Reddihough, D. (2012). *The Melbourne assessment 2: A test of unilateral upper limb function.* www.rch.org.au/melbourneassessment

Robins, D. L., Casagrande, K., Barton, M., Chen, C. M. A., Dumont-Mathieu, T., & Fein, D. (2014). Validation of the modified checklist for autism in toddlers, revised with follow-up (M-CHAT-R/F). *Pediatrics, 133*(1), 37–45.

Robins, D. L., Fein, D., & Barton, M. (2009). The modified checklist for autism in toddlers, revised with follow-up (M-CHAT-R/F). *Pediatrics, 133,* 37–45.

Romeo, D., Cowan, F., Haataja, L., Ricci, D., Pede, E., & Gallini, F., . . . Mercri, E. (2020). Hammersmith infant neurological examination for infants born preterm: Predicting outcomes other than cerebral palsy. *Developmental Medicine & Child Neurology.* https://doi.org/10.1111/dmcn.14768

Romeo, D., Ricci, D., Brogna, C., & Mercuri, E. (2015). Use of the hammersmith infant neurological examination in infants with cerebral palsy: A critical review of the literature. *Developmental Medicine & Child Neurology, 58*(3), 240–245. https://doi.org/10.1111/dmcn.12876

Russell, D. J., Rosenbaum, P., Wright, M., & Avery, L. M. (2013). *Gross motor function measure (GMFM-66 & GMFM-88) user's manual* (2nd ed.). MacKeith Press.

Schopler, E., Reichler, R. J., & Renner, B. R. (2010). *The childhood autism rating scale (CARS).* Western Psychological Services.

Selves, C., Stoquart, G., Renders, A., Detrembleur, C., Lejeune, T., &., & Gilliaux, M. (2019). Reliability and concurrent validity of the Bruininks-Oseretsky test in children with cerebral palsy. *Biomedical Journal of Scientific and Technical Research, 18*(5), 13961–13967.

Sharma, P., & Thapar, S. (2018). Balance assessment in cerebral palsy children using pediatric reach test and pediatric balance scale. *Indian Journal of Public Health Research & Development, 9*(5), 1. https://doi.org/10.5958/0976-5506.2018.00403.5

Shoemaker, M. (2003). Manual of the motor observation questionnaire for teachers. In *Groniongen: Center for human movement sciences.* Dutch Internal Publication.

Smits-Engelsmen, B. C. M., van Bommel-Rutgers, I., & van Waelvelde, H. (2014). *Systemattische opsporing schriffproblemen: SOS-2-NL.* Technische Handleiding.

Stone, W. L., Coonrod, E. E., & Ousley, O. Y. (2000). Brief report: Screening tool for autism in two-year-olds (STAT): Development and preliminary data. *Journal of Autism and Developmental Disorders, 30*(6), 607.

Stone, W. L., McMahon, C. R., & Henderson, L. M. (2008). Use of the screening tool for autism in two-year-olds (STAT) for children under 24 months: An exploratory study. *Autism, 12*(5), 557–573. https://doi.org/10.1177/1362361308096403

Spittle, A. J., Doyle, L. W., & Boyd, R. N. (2008). A systematic review of the clinimetric properties of neuromotor assessments for preterm infants during the first year of life. *Developmental Medicine & Child Neurology*, *50*(4), 254–266. https://doi.org/10.1111/j.1469-8749.2008.02025.x

Tavasoli, A., Azimi, P., & Montazari, A. (2014). Reliability and validity of the Peabody developmental motor scales-second edition for assessing motor development of low birth weight preterm infants. *Pediatric Neurology*, *51*(4), 522–526. https://doi.org/10.1016/j.pediatrneurol.2014.06.010

Teti, D. M., & Gelfand, D. M. (1997). The preschool assessment of attachment: Construct validity in a sample of depressed and nondepressed families. *Development and Psychopathology*, *9*(3), 517–536. https://doi.org/10.1017/s0954579497001284

Thornton, A., Licari, M., Reid, S., et al. (2016). Cognitive orientation to (daily) occupational performance intervention leads to improvements in impairments, activity and participation in children with developmental coordination disorder. *Disability in Rehabilitation*, *38*(10), 979–986. https://doi.org/10.3109/09638288.2015.1070298

Van Dellon, T., Vaessen, W., & Schoemaker, M. M. (1990). Clumsiness: Definition and selection of subjects. In A. F. Kalverboer (Ed.), *Developmental biopsychology, experimental and observational studies in children at risk* (pp. 135–152). University of Michigan Press.

van der Linde, B. W., van Netten, J. J., Otten, B., Postema, K., Geuze, R. H., & Schoemaker, M. M. (2013). Development and psychometric properties of the DCDDaily: A new test for clinical assessment of capacity in activities of daily living in children with developmental coordination disorder. *Clinical Rehabilitation*, *27*(9), 834–844. doi:10.1177/0269215513481227

van der Linde, B. W., van Netten, J. J., Otten, B., Postema, K., Geuze, R. H., & Schoemaker, M. M. (2014). Psychometric properties of the DCDDaily-Q: A new parental questionnaire on children's performance in activities of daily living. *Research in Developmental Disabilities*, *35*(7), 1711–1719. http://dx.doi.org/10.1016/j.ridd.2014.03.008

van Hartingsveldt, M. J., Cup, E. H., & Oostendorp, R. A. (2005). Reliability and validity of the fine motor scale of the Peabody developmental motor scales – 2. *Occupational Therapy International*, *12*(1), 1–13. https://doi.org/10.1002/oti.11

Vondra, J. I., Hommerding, K. D., & Shaw, D. S. (1999). Stability and change in infant attachment in a low-income sample. *Monographs of the Society for Research in Child Development*, 119–144. https://doi.org/10.1111/1540-5834.00036

Wang, H. H., Liao, H. F., & Hsieh, C. L. (2006). Reliability, sensitivity to change, and responsiveness of the Peabody developmental motor scales – second edition for children with cerebral palsy. *Physical Therapy*, *86*(10), 1351–1359. https://doi.org/10.2522/ptj.20050259

Wang, T., Liang, K., Liu, Y., Shieh, J., & Chen, H. (2017). Psychometric and clinimetric properties of the Melbourne assessment 2 in children with cerebral palsy. *Archives of Physical Medicine and Rehabilitation*, *98*(9), 1836–1841. https://doi.org/10.1016/j.apmr.2017.01.024

Wilson, B. N., & Crawford, S. G. (2007). *The developmental coordination disorder questionnaire 2007(DCDQ'07). Administration manual for the DCDQ'07 with psychometric properties.* www.dcdq.ca

Wilson, B. N., & Crawford, S. G. (2012). *The developmental coordination disorder questionnaire 2007 (DCDQ'07). Administration manual for the DCDQ'07 with psychometric properties.* www.dcdq.ca

Wilson, B. N., & Creighton, D. (2015). *The little developmental coordination disorder questionnaire – Canadian (Little DCDQ-CA)*. www.dcdq.ca

Yi, S., Hwang, J., Kim, S., & Kwon, J. (2012). Validity of pediatric balance scales in children with spastic cerebral palsy. *Neuropediatrics, 43*(6), 307–313. https://doi.org/10.1055/s-0032-1327774

Zwaigenbaum, L., & Penner, M. (2018). Autism spectrum disorder: Advances in diagnosis and evaluation. *BMJ*, 361. https://doi.org/10.1136/bmj.k1674

Appendix B
Approaches Table

After the therapist has identified problem areas, sensory integration may be combined with multiple approaches as part of the intervention process.

	Problem Areas	Intervention Approaches	
If the child. . .	. . . has impaired movement characteristics impacting postural control and functional movement. . .	. . . consider combining principles of **SENSORY INTEGRATION** with. . .	. . . a **NEURO-DEVELOPMENTAL TREATMENT** approach
	. . . has difficulty performing functional tasks. . .		. . . a **MOTOR TASK TRAINING** approach
	. . . has physical limitations, such as range of motion, strength, endurance, edema affecting function. . .		. . . a **BIOMECHANICAL** approach
	. . . has disruptive or avoidant behaviors that impact participation or performance of activities. . .		. . . a **BEHAVIORAL** approach based on behaviorism
	. . . has motor coordination and motor planning problems. . .		. . . the **COGNITIVE ORIENTATION TO DAILY OCCUPATIONAL PERFORMANCE** approach

(Continued)

Problem Areas	*Intervention Approaches*	
. . . has difficulties with social-emotional engagement and communication. . .		. . . a **DEVELOPMENTAL, INDIVIDUAL DIFFERENCE, RELATIONSHIP-BASED (DIR)/ FLOORTIME** approach
. . . has difficulty with child-caregiver attachment and/ or has experienced life trauma. . .		. . . a **HEALING CENTERED ENGAGEMENT** or **MODIFIED INTERACTIONAL GUIDANCE** approach
. . . and caregiver can benefit from directed support for sustained functional progress. . .		. . . a caregiver **COACHING** approach

Approach	*Informed By*	*Key Concepts & Goals of Intervention*
SENSORY INTEGRATION Ayres, 1972, 1979, 1985, 1989; Bundy & Lane, 2020)	Neurosciences, Behavioral Sciences, Occupational Science	Use of child-directed sensory activity to increase sensory processing, self regulation, and adaptive motor skills. Basic elements of Sensory Integration Treatment are sensory experiences, challenge and adaptive responses, in the context of play, therapeutic alliance and an enriched environment.
NEURO-DEVELOPMENTAL TREATMENT (Bierman et al., 2016; Bobath, 1948; Kalisperis et al., 2019)	Neurosciences, Motor Control, Motor Learning	Use of therapeutic handling based on movement analysis to address optimal sensorimotor processing, task performance and acquisition of functional motor skills. Improve functional movement performance by addressing impairments impacting posture and movement using therapeutic handling to: guide active, goal-directed movement; redirect ineffective movement and assist in learning more efficient movements to increase activities and participation.

(*Continued*)

Approach	Informed By	Key Concepts & Goals of Intervention
TASK TRAINING (Shumway-Cook & Woollacott, 2017)	Neurosciences, Motor Learning, Psychology	Acquisition of skills through practice and experience that are task-specific, and contextually based. Practicing parts of the task can be done but should be practiced within the context of the whole task and variability of the task, in many contexts and environments, so that it can be generalized into new situations. Improved functional abilities through facilitated practice of movement in contextualized environments.
BIOMECHANICAL (Colangelo & Shea, 2018)	Kinesiology, Physiology, Anatomy	Promotes independent participation through external supports or development of functional strength, joint alignment, range of motion in order to enhance function.
BEHAVIORAL (Howe et al., 2018; Martin & Pear, 2015)	Psychology	Behavior can be observed, measured and shaped through skill training, chaining, modeling, reinforcement, and practice.
COGNITIVE ORIENTATION TO DAILY OCCUPATIONAL PERFORMANCE (Missiuna et al., 2001; Polatajko, Mandich, Miller et al., 2001; Polatajko, Mandich, Missiuna et al., 2001)	Psychology, Education	Utilizes a cognitive approach to problem-solve occupational performance challenges through a child-centered, solution-oriented approach. Foster skill acquisition and carry over for occupational performance in variety contexts and environment.
DEVELOPMENTAL, INDIVIDUAL DIFFERENCE, RELATIONSHIP-BASED (DIR)/ FLOORTIME (Greenspan & Wieder, 2008)	Human Development, Psychology	Use of play as intervention to facilitate parent responsiveness to increase the child's cognitive, emotional and communication functions. Create foundations for social, emotional, and intellectual capacities.

(Continued)

Approach	Informed By	Key Concepts & Goals of Intervention
HEALING CENTERED ENGAGEMENT (Ginwright, 2018) **MODIFIED INTERACTIONAL GUIDANCE** (Benoit, 2001; Madigan et al., 2006; Tooten et al., 2012).	Psychology	Addresses cultural, spiritual, and civic elements to support the collective healing process. Guides parents to increase the sensitivity of their attunement skills in a play context through videotape analysis and modeling. Improve dyadic co-regulation and safety to facilitate the child's social/emotional development and self-regulatory skills.
CAREGIVER COACHING (Graham et al., 2009; Graham, 2020; Kraversky, 2019; Rush & Sheldon, 2011)	Social Sciences	Guides parents to identify and implement social and physical environmental changes that support successful occupational performance. Process may include identifying barriers and challenges, discussing potential solutions, and following up.

References

Ayres, A. J. (1972). *Sensory integration and learning disorders.* Western Psychological Services. https://doi.org/10.1177/002221947200500605

Ayres, A. J. (1979). *Sensory integration and the child.* Western Psychological Services.

Ayres, A. J. (1985). *Developmental dyspraxia and adult onset apraxia.* Sensory Integration International.

Ayres, A. J. (1989). *Sensory integration and praxis test – SIPT manual.* Western Psychological Services.

Benoit, D. (2001–2002, Winter). Modified Interaction Guidance. *Newsletter of the Infant Mental Health Promotion Project, 32,* 61–65.

Bierman, J., Franjoine, M., Howle, J., Hazzard, C., & Stamer, M. (2016). *Neurodevelopmental treatment: A guide to NDT clinical practice.* Thieme Medical Publishers Incorporated.

Bobath, B. (1948). A new treatment of lesions of the upper motor neurone. *British Journal of Physical Medicine, 11*(1), 26–30.

Bundy, A. C., & Lane, S. J. (Eds.). (2020). *Sensory Integration: Theory and Practice* (3rd ed.). F. A. Davis Company.

Colangelo, C. A., & Shea, M. (2018). A biomechanical frame of reference to position children for function. In P. Kramer (Ed.), *Frames of reference for pediatric occupational therapy.* Lippincott, Williams & Wilkins.

Ginwright, S. (2018). The future of healing: Shifting from trauma informed care to healing centered engagement. *Occasional Paper, 25.*

Graham, F. (2020). *Occupational performance coaching (OPC) logic model.* University of Otago. https://otago.ac.nz/opc.

Graham, F., Rodger, S., & Ziviani, J. (2009). Coaching parents to enable children's participation: An approach for working with parents and their children. *Australian Occupational Therapy Journal, 56*(1), 16–23.

Greenspan, S., & Wieder, S. (2008). *DIR®/Floortime™ model.* The International Council on Developmental and Learning Disorders. https://www.stanley-greenspan.com

Howe, H. T., Kramer, P., & Hinojosa, J. (2018). Developmental perspective: Fundamentals of developmental theory. In P. Kramer (Ed.), *Frames of reference for pediatric occupational therapy.* Lippincot, Williams & Wilkins.

Kalisperis, F. R., Shanline, J. M., & Styer-Acevedo, J. (2019). Neurodevelopmental treatment clinical practice model's role in the management of children with cerebral palsy. In F. Miller, S. Bachrach, N. Lennon, & M. O'Neil (Eds.), *Cerebral palsy.* Springer.

Kraversky, D. G. (2019). *Occupational performance coaching as an ultimate facilitator.* American Occupational Therapy Association. www.aota.org/~/media/Corporate/Files/Publication/CE-Articles/CE_Article_November_2019.pdf

Madigan, S., Hawkins, E., Goldberg, S., & Benoit, D. (2006). Reduction of disrupted caregiver behavior using modified interaction guidance. *Infant Mental Health Journal: Official Publication of The World Association for Infant Mental Health, 27*(5), 509–527. https://doi.org/10.1002/imhj.20102

Martin, G., & Pear, J. J. (2015). *Behavior modification: What it is and how to do it.* Psychology Press.

Missiuna, C., Mandich, A. D., Polatajko, H. J., & Malloy-Miller, T. (2001). Cognitive orientation to daily occupational performance (CO-OP) part I-theoretical foundations. *Physical & Occupational Therapy in Pediatrics, 20*(2–3), 69–81.

Polatajko, H. J., Mandich, A. D., Miller, L. T., & Macnab, J. J. (2001a). Cognitive orientation to daily occupational performance (CO-OP) part II the evidence. *Physical & Occupational Therapy in Pediatrics, 20*(2–3), 83–106.

Polatajko, H. J., Mandich, A. D., Missiuna, C., Miller, L. T., Macnab, J. J., Malloy-Miller, T., & Kinsella, E. A. (2001b). Cognitive orientation to daily occupational performance (CO-OP) part III-the protocol in brief. *Physical & Occupational Therapy in Pediatrics, 20*(2–3), 107–123.

Rush, D. D., & Sheldon, M. L. (2011). *The early childhood coaching handbook.* Paul H. Brookes.

Shumway-Cook, A., & Woollacott, M. H. (2017). *Motor control: Translating research into clinical practice* (5th ed.). Lippincott Williams & Wilkins.

Tooten, A., Hoffenkamp, H. N., Hall, R. A., Winkel, F. W., Eliëns, M., Vingerhoets, A. J., & van Bakel, H. J. (2012). The effectiveness of video interaction guidance in parents of premature infants: A multicenter randomised controlled trial. *BMC Pediatrics, 12*(1), 1–9.

Appendix C
Reproducible Working Documents

C1 – Hypotheses Generation Form With Conclusion

First Phase: Data *(Issues in participation, observations, other available information)*	Second Phase: *Hypotheses Generation/ Interpretations*	Third Phase: *Counting Data points and Conclusion.*
Reason for referral:		
Reason for referral:		
Sensory questionnaire and interview		
Sensory questionnaire and interview		
Observations in the classroom or community	⌂	
Observations in the classroom or community		
Observation in the specialized setting		
Observation in the specialized setting		
Structured observations in specialized setting:		
Structured observations in specialized setting:		
Standardized testing:		
Standardized testing:		
Standardized testing:		

Source: © Imperatore Blanche, 2021; can be copied for clinical use

Appendix C2 Incorporating SIT Elements With Other Intervention Approaches

SI PRINCIPLES	*USED IN MY SIT INTERVENTION*	*OTHER COMPREMENTARY INTERVENTIONS*
SENSORY SYSTEMS		
ADAPTIVE RESPONSE/ CHALLENGE		
CONTEXT OF PLAY/ CHILD CENTERED		
THERAPEUTIC ALLIANCE		
ENRICHED PHYSICAL ENVIRONMENT		

Source: © Imperatore Blanche, 2021 – Can be copied for clinical use

Index

[Note: numbers in *italics* indicate a figure. Numbers in **bold** indicate a table.]

Printed in the United States
by Baker & Taylor Publisher Services